COURAGE TO CARE

COURAGE to CARE

Responding
to the Crisis of
Children with AIDS

EDITED BY

Gary R. Anderson

Child Welfare League of America, Inc.
Washington, DC

CHILD WELFARE LEAGUE OF AMERICA, INC.
440 First Street, NW, Suite 310, Washington, DC 20001-2085

CURRENT PRINTING (last digit)
10 9 8 7 6 5 4 3 2 1

Cover design by Deborah Daly
Text design by Rose Jacobowitz

Printed in the United States of America

Library of Congress Cataloging-in-Publication Data

Courage to care : responding to the crisis of children with AIDS /
   edited by Gary R. Anderson.
        p.   cm.
   Includes bibliographical references (p.   ).
   ISBN 0-87868-384-4 : $24.95 — ISBN 0-87868-401-8 (pbk.) : $15.95
   1. AIDS (Disease) in children—Social aspects.   2. AIDS (Disease)
in children—Patients—Family relationships.   3. AIDS (Disease) in
children—Patients—Services for.   4. Health education.
I. Anderson, Gary R., 1952–   .   II. Child Welfare League of
America.
RJ387.A25C68   1990
362.1'98929792—dc20   90-2085
                                                                                    CIP

ISBN # 0-87868-384-4
ISBN # 0-87868-401-8 (pbk.)

Contents

APPENDICES

Acknowledgments

CREATING THIS BOOK REQUIRED THE COOPERATION OF MANY TALENTED and busy professionals. The contributors, pioneers in work with children and families with HIV infection, are in active service to families, and adding writing responsibilities to their other duties called for extraordinary commitment and courage. Many other contributors, noted throughout the book, provided information and insights.

It is also important to acknowledge the contributions of staff members of the Child Welfare League of America: Carl Schoenberg, whose editorial skills are evidenced throughout the book, Susan Brite, Jean Emery, and Eve Malakoff-Klein.

I would also like to thank the many persons who supported and encouraged this project, including Dean Harold Lewis and Professor George Getzel, of the Hunter College School of Social Work; William Guarinello, Rob Miss, and Mia Higgins, of the Catholic Guardian Society of Brooklyn; Paul Gitelson, of the Jewish Child Care Association, New York; members of the Child Welfare League of America Group Care Task Force; Cecelia Sudia and Jerry Silverman, of the U.S. Administration for Children, Youth and Families, Department of Health and Human Services; Joan Altman; Dorianne Perrucci, of Covenant House, New York; Phyllis Gurdin; Virginia Anderson; Richard and Carol Anderson; Lawrence and Jean Glesnes; Marilyn Hines; and Lauren Marie Anderson.

I would like to give special recognition to my wife, Valerie A. Glesnes-Anderson, of Newark Beth Israel Hospital, New Jersey, whose interest in, and concern about, AIDS in 1982 were the stimulus for my investigations, and whose loving support was vital to the creation and completion of this volume.

It is my hope that this book will be immediately helpful to families and those assisting families, and that AIDS prevention and medical interventions will be increasingly, and finally, so effective that they will replace the need for the assistance this volume describes.

Preface

IN THE EARLY 1980S, A NEW AND TERRIBLE ILLNESS WAS REPORTED IN LOS Angeles and New York City. Originally labeled a homosexual disease, this illness, soon called acquired immune deficiency syndrome (AIDS), was also found among intravenous drug users and some individuals, such as hemophiliacs, who had received blood products through transfusions.

It took several years before the findings of physicians, such as James Oleske in Newark and Arye Rubinstein in New York City, received attention. These physicians determined that chidren were also contracting AIDS. The number of children diagnosed with AIDS is now well over two thousand; over half have died. Thousands more are infected by the virus that eventually leads to AIDS, and these children live in every state throughout our nation.

We have learned about HIV-infected children in a disturbing manner. On television, we have seen homes firebombed, schools picketed, and the children and their families ostracized. There have been accounts of children who have been forced to move and, in some cases, to hide. One little girl was allowed to attend school only as long as she agreed to stay in a glass-walled bubble. Some of these youngsters have been abandoned by their caregivers and their parents; still others have been orphaned when their parents died of AIDS. We have seen children in confined and isolated hospital wards, long beyond any medical necessity for hospitalization, simply awaiting a home.

Yet, at the same time, there have been inspiring accounts of caring people who have opened their hearts and their homes to these children. We know of family members who have cared for these youngsters and fought for their right to a quality life—no matter how short the life span. And, in many instances, when family members have been unable to continue to provide care, others have cared for and given HIV-infected children a home. Many of these caregivers have done so quietly, unnoticed and without recognition, out of concern for the children's privacy and because of the stigma and misunderstanding surrounding AIDS.

The purpose of this book is to recognize some of the people and organizations that have responded responsibly and compassionately in the AIDS crisis. Through a range of services, these pioneers have provided a loving example for others to follow. This volume features only a few of these groups; they are representative of the many individuals and organizations that have reached out to children in need. This book is intended to inform, guide, and encourage others to provide the support and services that children and their families require when facing illness.

AIDS is not a disease of individuals alone; it is a disease of families and of communities. And the battle to overcome AIDS will be long and hard-fought. This is a fight that we can hope to win in only one way—together. It is my hope that this book will help.

DIONNE WARWICK
Ambassador of Health
The Warwick Foundation
Washington, D.C.

Introduction

THE WORLD HEALTH ORGANIZATION ESTIMATES THAT THE CUMULATIVE total of individuals with AIDS as of 1989 was over 500,000, and that five to ten million individuals are presently HIV-infected worldwide. The pandemic scope of AIDS has become reasonably well defined, and unprecedented progress has been made in a short time in understanding the structure of the AIDS virus and its mechanisms of spread. The consequences of HIV infection and the disease spectrum are also being unraveled expeditiously. The war on AIDS has been fought with passionate commitment, ingenuity, and courage by health care professionals and by scientists—all pioneers in the field. The range of the social and economic meaning of the AIDS pandemic on a local and global level has, however, not yet been fully perceived and appreciated.

The most challenging recent changes in the AIDS pandemic are the shift from homosexual to heterosexual transmission, from infected men to women of child-bearing age, and to children. In the last decade, a drastic increase in mortality among women 25 to 44 years old was noted in New York City, mostly related to HIV infection. In selected areas of New York City, the prevalence of HIV infection in pregnant women rose to eight percent. The effect of HIV infection on women and children has not yet been fully conveyed. Confronting AIDS demands of us the courage to extend our knowledge and actions beyond the mere limits of medical expertise to the psychosocial plights of our societies, to issues of poverty, of human rights and discrimination.

A number of these issues are captured in this comprehensive and timely book, *Courage to Care.* This volume is a fundamental source for those seeking a comprehensive review of the implications of AIDS on individuals, families, and society. Its diverse topics address better care for the sick, the young, and the disabled; better education for a range of concerned audiences; and preservation of human rights. It illuminates the social meaning of AIDS, without which no effective preventive measures can be taken to stem this epidemic even when the best scientists and clinicians are at hand. It is a must for those who treat, and offer care to, HIV-infected women, children, and families, and who are truly concerned about their fate.

ARYE RUBINSTEIN, M.D.
Professor of Pediatrics, Microbiology, and Immunology
Albert Einstein College of Medicine
Bronx, New York

1

Children and AIDS: Crisis for Caregivers

GARY R. ANDERSON

PROFESSIONALS AND FAMILIES CARING FOR CHILDREN, PARTICULARLY those from vulnerable or distressed families, are confronting a new and fearsome reality—acquired immune deficiency syndrome (AIDS). Selectively infecting immune system cells and incapacitating the system intended to guard against that type of invasion, this progressive and irreversible immune defect provides an opportunity for infections and other agents to afflict infected persons [Fauci 1988]. In less than a decade, AIDS has moved from an unknown term to a primary diagnosis for more than 100,000 Americans, over 50,000 of whom have died; the number of Americans with the human immunodeficiency virus (HIV) is estimated at over one million individuals [Institute of Medicine 1986]. The Public Health Service has predicted that by 1991 there will have been 270,000 cumulative cases of AIDS meeting the Centers for Disease Control (CDC) case definition, and 3,000 cases of pediatric AIDS.[1]

Originally called gay-related immune deficiency syndrome, AIDS was first identified among homosexual men in California and New York City [CDC 1981]. Later, identifying high-risk groups changed to an emphasis on high-risk behaviors. In early December 1982, the Centers for Disease Control reported three cases of children with AIDS: a

[1]The Congressional General Accounting Office has estimated there will be 300,000 to 400,000 Americans with AIDS by the end of 1991 [Thomas 1989].

1

20-month-old San Francisco boy who had received a blood transfusion, and two school-age children with hemophilia. Later that month, the CDC reported four infants with "unexplained cellular immunodeficiency and opportunistic infections" [CDC 1982]. It was increasingly reported that children were becoming ill, displaying characteristics similar to adults—weakened or almost nonexistent immune systems, persistent symptoms, and opportunistic infections, particularly a deadly pneumonia [Oleske et al. 1983; Rubinstein et al. 1983]. After brief consideration, a category of pediatric AIDS was accepted by the CDC [Falloon 1989]. Reviewing this period, Surgeon General Koop observed:

> By 1984 the numbers of children with AIDS had begun to escalate, especially in New York City, Newark, and Miami. The Division of Maternal and Child Health first held an ad hoc meeting to try to delineate the nature of the problem in New York City where infants were occupying acute hospital beds unnecessarily because no alternate living arrangements were available . . . Attendees at this meeting agreed that AIDS *did* occur in children, that the number of children involved was undercounted in the CDC surveillance system, and that infected infants and children and their families were subject to discrimination and sometimes barred from basic services [Koop 1987].

The fearsome reality for children and their families included social and psychological consequences in addition to medical complications and led to the need for assistance from a range of societal institutions and agencies.

Before HIV: Child Welfare's Steady State

After more than a decade of debate and study, the concept of permanency planning—preventing placement, reuniting families, or providing a permanent home for a child—was clinically accepted, legally sanctioned in 1980 by Public Law 96-272, and implemented under regulations. An optimistic outlook included the closing or limiting of institutions, the proliferation of family support and child abuse prevention strategies, a shrinking number of children in foster care, and those in care either rapidly returning home, placed with relatives, or preparing for an adoptive placement [Select Committee 1989]. At worst, responding to child abuse and neglect and providing child welfare services would remain difficult and uneven but within an identifiable range of circumstances to be countered with increasingly familiar interventions.

A Vulnerable State

A series of societal events in the 1980s began to undermine seriously the ability of families, communities, and social agencies to provide for children's best interests [Allen 1989]. To note several:

1. *The growth of poverty among children:* This number has increased by three million since 1979, and the number of single adolescent parent households has proliferated, with three out of four households headed by a mother under the age of 25 being poor. Although economics and family structure do not automatically determine risk for children, the needs of families and extended families caring for young children may often tax if not eclipse attainable resources: "Family dissolution and isolation, adolescent parenthood, and the feminizing of poverty may militate for increased child mortality and morbidity and for developmental attrition" [Newberger et al. 1986].

2. *The increase in the number of homeless families:* Although substandard and overcrowded housing and homelessness are not new phenomena, the past decade has found thousands of parents with children searching for housing and finding few alternatives to short-term, makeshift accommodations or shelters.

3. *The proliferation of drug use:* With the advent of "crack," a cocaine derivative that is initially inexpensive, easily obtained, and highly addictive, illegal drug use has spread to a larger population, with devastating social and physical effects.

4. *The dramatic rise in the number of child abuse and neglect reports:* The American Humane Association noted that the number of reports between 1981 and 1985 rose 55 percent. Others noted even greater increases. Included in these reports was a rise in concern about the sexual abuse of children.

The struggle to obtain the basic necessities of life engulfed families and children as the search for food, clothes, and shelter reduced the ability of parents to consider the needs of vulnerable children. For some parents, the search for drugs competed with basic needs and preempted personal and financial resources needed by the child and family. These issues—poverty, teen pregnancy, homelessness, drug abuse, and child abuse—have been generally beyond the curative powers of individual psychotherapy or the organizational strategies of individual agencies. The demand for substitute care began to rise. An ecological perspective might capably assess the demands and deficiencies of the environment, but the resources and capabilities to respond effectively to greater needs with new complications have been limited, at best.

A Crisis-Precipitating Event: AIDS

A stressor can be defined as a situation for which the individual, family, agency, or community has had little or no preparation, therefore posing a formidable problem with crisis potential [Hill 1958]. AIDS has proven to be such a stressor. For a reportable diagnosis of pediatric AIDS, the CDC initially required documentation of an opportunistic infection, such as pneumocystis carinii pneumonia, or an AIDS-associated malignancy, such as Kaposi's sarcoma, and the ruling out of alternate congenital disorders and infectious-agent explanations for immunological defects. In 1985, this definition was expanded to include children with lymphocytic interstitial pneumonia, and expanded again in 1987 to include one of a list of AIDS indicator diseases [CDC 1987; Falloon 1989]. Children's lives, however, have been medically threatened and psychosocially affected by falling anywhere on an HIV spectrum that ranges from being HIV-infected but evidencing no symptoms, to having HIV-related symptoms, to having a CDC case definition of AIDS.

Primarily through acquiring HIV from mothers with HIV/AIDS, by August 1989 the number of children with AIDS had surpassed 1,660 cases, spread through almost every state.[2] The number of children with HIV infection, not meeting CDC surveillance definitions, may be three to four times as many. HIV has posed a range of stressors in addition to the challenge of an unfamiliar and eventually fatal medical condition.

Various meanings are attached to stressful events, for in addition to medical definitions of HIV/AIDS there are also cultural definitions as framed by communities and subjective definitions composed by individuals [Hill 1958]. The meaning of HIV/AIDS may involve the following confrontations:

[2]There have been some cases of transmission from sexual abuse by HIV-infected men. States with no reported pediatric AIDS case are Montana, North and South Dakota, and Wyoming [CDC 1989].

1. Illness, suffering, and the deaths of infants, children, adolescents, and young adults, many of whose lives can be threatened by the severe symptoms of HIV infection without even progressing to a clinical diagnosis of AIDS
2. Sexuality, including homosexuality, adolescent sexuality, and, in some cases, sexual abuse
3. Drug addiction among adolescents, pregnant mothers, and parents
4. Ethical quandaries such as confidentiality and issues related to birth control and abortion

These issues raise the specter of one's own mortality, previous life losses, personal comfort about sexuality, homophobia, the ability to communicate about sexuality, prejudice, and personal values and religious beliefs. The different effects of the stress and the range of meanings attached to HIV infection guarantee that AIDS affects professionals and agencies in a variety of individualized ways.

For a child welfare agency, the effects may also include assessing social stigma, financial commitments, and legal complications. It is one more demand for resources from a vulnerable system already stretched or depleted by simultaneous stressors. Multiple definitions of children with HIV—reflecting value systems and previous experience in meeting crises—transform the stressful event into a potential crisis [Hill 1958].

Heading Off a Crisis: Employing Traditional Coping Mechanisms

When facing a threat, valuable lessons may be learned from past experiences, and a contemporary response can be formulated to contain threats to life and well-being. In public health, AIDS has prompted historical study to guide a present-day perspective even while public health officials have departed from some traditional responses to threats to public health [Brandt 1988; Cutler and Arnold 1988; Yankauer 1988]. Throughout American history, public health crises have resulted in ill families, dying children, and social stigma, but the pandemics of smallpox, typhoid fever, yellow fever, diphtheria, cholera, bubonic plague, even tuberculosis and polio may appear like ancient history to agencies that seem to have greater familiarity with psychotherapeutic rather than medical considerations.

Maintaining HIV-infected children with their parents, a primary goal of permanency planning, was difficult to achieve when parents were HIV-infected; dying; immersed in, or devastated by, a drug culture; isolated and stigmatized; or at times simply not to be found. Against tremendous odds, many parents continued to care for their children at home. They needed a range of support services that they found to be nonexistent or inaccessible. Potentially helpful people were frightened. When parental care was no longer possible, relatives were often sought for child placement; however, even relatives were hesitant to face what seemed to be a mystery illness, demanding resources that few families could provide. Even when fear could be overcome, the grief and stigma were heavy burdens for families mourning the HIV infection of their children and grandchildren. Similarly, foster parents were often afraid, unprepared, or lacking support services to meet the medical, developmental, and psychosocial challenges of caring for HIV-infected children.

Generalizing from adult AIDS to pediatric AIDS presented some complications as a number of differences emerged. Some opportunistic infections were less often noted, such as Kaposi's sarcoma; others, such as lymphoid interstitial pneumonitis, were much more common in children [Oleske 1987]. With children's less mature immune systems, a more rapid tempo of symptomatology and severe effect on a number of developing functions was noted [Katz and Wilfert 1989]. Complicating the ability to diagnose HIV was the presence of the mother's antibodies in her newborn child, requiring a 15- to 18-month period of diagnostic uncertainty for many newborns [Blanche et al. 1989].

A Crisis State

The drug culture provided no community, as the homosexual community had done, to mobilize care for its members and advocate for treatment and resources [Koop 1987]. Other mothers, having acquired HIV from heterosexual transmission rather than their own drug use, made the often shocking discovery of their infection after their child's HIV test or illness. Children whose HIV infection was due to blood transfusions or blood products (predominantly prior to the 1985 HIV screening tests) may have had the benefit of families with less vulnerability to disorganization, but even these faced social stigma and discrimination, in addition to coping with the child's illness and the family's sorrow.

By the end of February 1987, over 300 boarder babies in New York hospitals were awaiting homes because they were ready for discharge and could not return home. Some children with HIV infection spent most or all of their lives in a hospital room. Dr. John Hutchings, assistant director of the Division of Maternal and Child Health, DHHS, noted:

> The babies who are left in the hospital should be placed in homes . . . no matter how concerned and loving the hospital staff is, a home environment is still recognized as the best place for a child. There is a more stable environment in the home, and not such a crowd of people hovering over the baby. Also, socialization with other children, if it is possible or appropriate, is very important for the child [Gentry 1986].

Four years after the identification of pediatric AIDS, children were being raised in hospitals, few foster homes were available, many professionals were uncomfortable with serving HIV-infected persons, and many continued to believe that this was primarily a homosexual disease and restricted to coastal cities. Children with HIV were denied access to schools or confronted with unusual accommodations—such as isolated quarters or bubble-like environments. In some cases, families were forced to leave their communities; however, agency and individual attempts to reorganize, through trial and error as often as thoughtful planning, began to establish routines for responding to children and their families.

The Crisis for Black and Hispanic Children

A high number and disproportionate percentage of pediatric AIDS cases reported to the CDC are black and Hispanic children. Of 1,736 cases reported in August 1989, 918 were black children (52.9 percent of the total), 409 were Hispanic children (23.6 percent), and 392 were white children (22.6 percent); there were nine Asian/Pacific Islander children and four American Indian/Alaskan natives [CDC 1989]. A higher percentage of black and Hispanic children has been constant for many years, and the percentage in urban areas is even higher.[3] These alarming

---

[3]In the adult/adolescent AIDS population (100,885 August 1989), 57 percent of the cases were white (57,848), 27 percent were black (26,749), and 15 percent were Hispanic. In June 1987, the percentage of white adults was 61 percent, black 24 percent and Hispanic 14 percent. There appears to be a gradual shift in the adult AIDS racial composition. For cumulative incidence of AIDS, there were 58.2 Hispanic cases per 100,000 population, 65.9 black cases, and 21.5 white cases [COSSMHO 1989].

numbers have prompted special concern for preventing HIV transmission and for providing services for black and Hispanic families. Further concern has been expressed that stigmatization resulting from AIDS—heightened by high incidence rates in Africa, speculation that AIDS began in Africa, and the initial identification of Haitians as a high-risk group—would compound discrimination against people of color.

High incidence rates and the need for services have spurred calls for culturally sensitive responses to the AIDS crisis. This sensitivity has been described in the following ways:

1. An awareness of the high number of black and Hispanic children with AIDS and HIV infection so that community groups are encouraged to provide AIDS education and begin prevention initiatives, and funding groups are encouraged to provide resources for agencies and community organizations that effectively serve black and Hispanic families

2. An attentiveness to access to services so that good-quality medical, psychosocial, and concrete assistance programs, first, exist and, second, are located in accessible locations, preferably community clinics with experience in serving black and Hispanic families, with no obstacles to utilization

3. The creation of culturally and racially appropriate written materials, including the use of wording and language (e.g., bilingualism) that are understandable and effective; using pictures and images that reflect racial diversity, distributed through sites that are readily available to a large and potentially at-risk population

4. Similarly, the provision of services in the first language of the client, for example, HIV pre-test and post-test counseling, and no exclusion of Spanish-speaking clients from receiving services or participating in research [see, for example, Kegeles et al. 1989]

5. The identification of possible cultural characteristics that might influence prevention of AIDS transmission and response to the illness: some writers have noted the influence of men's and women's roles, fatalism, religious beliefs, views of illness, and the stigma of bisexuality and homosexuality in the black and Hispanic community [Medina 1987; Flaskerud and Rush 1989; Schilling et al. 1989]. These attempts to list and describe cultural/racial or ethnic traits, however, have met with some

concern about negative stereotyping, the failure to individualize persons served, and an ignoring of social and political changes to benefit black and Hispanic families [De La Cancela 1989]

6. The recognition of strengths of black and Hispanic families because a significant number of the caregivers for children with HIV/AIDS are black and Hispanic; because extended families provide a resource for ill family members and potentially orphaned children, and close families and community organizations can combat HIV transmission and the use of intravenous drugs—which is the primary means of HIV transmission for black and Hispanic pediatric cases [Schilling et al. 1989]

7. The inclusion of black and Hispanic patients in medical and social science clinical trials and research with potential benefits for participants

The need for outreach is all the more acute in light of the finding in recent surveys that black and Hispanic adolescents are at increased risk of HIV infection due to lack of knowledge and greater acceptance of misconceptions about the cause, transmission, and prevention of AIDS [DiClemente et al. 1988], as well as the tendency not to use accurate knowledge to alter their behaviors [Goodman and Cohall 1989]. Local and national organizations—such as Blacks Educating Blacks About Sexual Health Issues (BEBASHI) of Philadelphia, the Kupona Network of Chicago, the Health Education and Resource Organization of Baltimore, the Minority AIDS Project of Los Angeles, the National Coalition of Hispanic Health and Human Service Organizations (COSSMHO), and the National Minority AIDS Council—have mobilized to advance strategies and agendas and facilitate networking for better service provision [Deresiewicz 1988].

The Present and Future Crisis: Adolescents with HIV

Awareness is growing of a crisis within a crisis—concern for adolescents and the spread of HIV [Remafedi 1988; Hein 1989]. In 1987, Surgeon General Koop noted:

We are grateful that you have emphasized our ignorance about AIDS in adolescents. The CDC definition of pediatric AIDS ends at age 13; perhaps we have not given enough attention to this vulnerable group. I did say that adolescents may not know if they are homosexual or will be drug abusers and therefore might not heed or understand messages others might find pertinent. These youngsters must be reached and taught about risk behaviors that expose them to infection with the AIDS virus. We need to know how this virus affects youth during this second period of rapid growth [Koop 1987].

The ignorance of adolescents and their failure to change their risky behaviors even when informed and knowledgeable about HIV infection poses a challenge for educators and service providers and a fearful potential for the near future [DiClemente et al. 1988; Rickert et al. 1989].

A Response to the Crisis

The response to HIV has varied in relation to geographic location, and, in addition to innovative programs, solutions from the 1800s have been resurrected.

Geographic Location

Within the United States,[4] several areas have had particularly high numbers of children with AIDS and HIV infection: "Since 1982, the highest density of pediatric AIDS has been in New York City, Newark, New Jersey, and Miami" [Nicholas et al. 1989]. In addition to New York, New Jersey, and Florida, high-incidence states have included California, Texas, Pennsylvania, Connecticut, and Illinois. Within these states the experience of HIV infection has not been uniform. For example, one study indicated that women of child-bearing age in San Francisco have low seropositive rates [Darney et al. 1989]; another found relatively high rates of infection in Caribbean nations that may both reflect, and contribute to, the number of HIV-infected children in Florida or the New York City metropolitan area [Quinn et al. 1989; Thomas 1989]. As mentioned earlier, an examination of the spread of AIDS noted the disproportion-

[4]In comparison with the 1,346 pediatric AIDS cases in the United States at the close of 1988, Canada was reporting 38 cases.

ately high number of blacks and Hispanics reflecting the "high relative risk of HIV infection and AIDS among the members of these minority groups, who reside primarily in inner city populations of the Northeast section of the United States" [Quinn et al. 1989]. So the urgency of responding has varied.

Historical Responses

Some programs have taken on characteristics of historical responses to dependent children. One has proposed moving HIV-positive children from high-incidence cities to foster homes in a midwestern city. This proposal may be subject to many of the criticisms of the 1800s' practice of transporting children to midwestern and western farm families. It raises questions about the role of the extended family and attentiveness to race and culture, since the HIV-positive children are predominantly black and Hispanic, and the potential foster parents are predominantly white. It also seems to assume that other cities' programs have not been created or are not capable of serving high numbers of children and their families.

Prompted by the increase in the number of HIV-positive children, the projected high numbers of orphans, and the difficulty of finding a sufficient number of extended families and foster families, another response has been to open institutions for young children [Lambert 1989]. The creation of institutions, however, also raises historic and well-justified concerns about the quality of child care and the developmental appropriateness of congregate institutional care for very young children. In addition, the expense involved in maintaining a congregate residence is a cause for concern. A number of institutions are noted in this volume, but they have roles primarily as transitional residences, short-term respite care for foster families, and as a setting for children too ill or with too many complications to be in foster care but able to benefit from a more home-like environment than a hospital.

Necessary Qualities for a Successful Response

A crisis has the potential of strengthening or demoralizing individuals, families, agencies, and communities. Child welfare agencies that may be best able to respond positively to the AIDS crisis may possess the same qualities that assist families when encountering a crisis: *(1)* adaptability; *(2)* ability to work together in an integrated manner; *(3)* positive feelings for each other and for those served; *(4)* flexible, democratic decision making; and *(5)* adequate health and wealth [Hill 1958].

Innovations in Child Welfare Services

At the Attention to AIDS [1987] conference sponsored by the Child Welfare League of America, Dr. Virginia Anderson stated, "To really share your experiences and to learn from one another is an exemplary way to approach a crisis." Correspondingly, this volume has several purposes: *(1)* the description of a number of programs that have served HIV-positive children and their families to provide examples, guidance, and encouragement to programs that will be created or reorganized to serve such children; *(2)* the discussion of educational initiatives to give some suggestions for the implementation of directives to provide educational programs; and *(3)* the identification of resources that can be used by individuals, programs, and agencies to be better informed, to carry out initiatives, and to network with each other. This exchange of information will reduce the likelihood that wheels will be reinvented or that recommendations to begin educational programs will be delayed by a lack of information.

Programs

The programs described (in discrete chapters, by references and examples, or in Appendix C) were selected because of their pioneering work with HIV-positive children; many were the first programs of their type in the country. This volume is not an evaluation of their effectiveness, although some successes will be noted, as well as continuing struggles. Some have and will serve as models; some may have limited futures due to precarious funding. Many of the programs are those of voluntary, not-for-profit agencies, but many of these could not operate effectively without substantial support from public child welfare agencies, which also provide services to many families. Moreover, these are not the only programs serving HIV-positive children; there are many other fine programs, as well as dedicated individuals and families and child-care organizations across the country.

Program descriptions in this volume highlight common approaches to common problems, as well as variations in structure and design based on client needs, agency traditions, geographic location, and funding. There are many tasks to be done, and this work has attracted a number of compassionate and dedicated persons; the AIDS crisis has often united people within agencies and among agencies, professions, and territories. It is to be hoped that the examples of programs and of people who have had a vision for caring for HIV-positive children and their families will stimulate further compassion, creativity, and development.

Educational Initiatives and Resources

This section of the volume offers guidance for the content and presentation of HIV/AIDS educational programs for a variety of audiences. Its content concerning staff member education, responding to drug-using clients, foster parent education and support groups, prevention,[5] HIV testing and counseling, and grief education is of particular pertinence to child welfare agencies but has broader applicability as well. These initiatives are further informed by appendices, which comprise a glossary, case studies, bibliography, resource guide, and reprints from the American Academy of Pediatrics.

Conclusion

Without denying the terrible personal and family tragedies and obstacles to serving sick and stigmatized clients, a sense of optimism and hopefulness is sustained in this volume by the initial mobilization of services to HIV-positive children, the growing concern and knowledge about HIV and children, and the experiences of the programs that are described. Although this book focuses on services to children and their families, it is this author's hope that child welfare agencies will accept a growing responsibility to join in efforts at prevention of HIV infection and that resources for finding a cure will be ever more broadly marshalled and successful. Then perhaps the compassion, commitment, and resources that are being generated for the AIDS crisis can be reallocated to the continuing crises of children who are vulnerable to multiple societal ills.

REFERENCES

Allen, Mary Lee (Children's Defense Fund). Statement to the House Select Committee. Select Committee on Children, Youth and Families. U.S. House of Representatives,

---

[5]Prevention among adolescents, particularly teens involved in homosexual or bisexual behavior, is targeted; the spread of fear of HIV among teens has already been observed, and one author has noted that 79 percent of AIDS cases in young adults are linked to homosexual or bisexual behavior [Nicholas et al. 1989].

Joint Hearing. Foster Care, Child Welfare, and Adoption Reforms. Washington, DC: U.S. Government Printing Office, 1989.

Anderson, Gary. "Children and AIDS: Implications for child welfare." Child Welfare 63 (1) (January 1984): 62–73.

Blanche, Stephane, Rouzioux, Christine, Moscato, Marie-Luce Guihard, et al. "A prospective study of infants born to women seropositive for human immunodeficiency virus type 1." New England Journal of Medicine 320 (25) (June 22, 1989): 1643–1648.

Brandt, A. M. "AIDS in historical perspective: Four lessons from the history of sexually transmitted diseases." American Journal of Public Health 78 (4) (April 1988): 367–376.

Centers for Disease Control. "Kaposi's sarcoma and pneumocystis pneumonia among homosexual men in New York and California." Morbidity and Mortality Weekly Report 30 (July 3, 1981): 305.

Centers for Disease Control. "Unexplained immunodeficiency and opportunistic infections in children." Morbidity and Mortality Weekly Report 31 (December 17, 1982): 665.

Centers for Disease Control. "Classification system for human immunodeficiency virus (HIV) infection in children under 13 years of age." Morbidity and Mortality Weekly Report 36 (1987): 225–236.

Centers for Disease Control. HIV/AIDS Surveillance. Atlanta, GA: CDC, August 1989.

COSSMHO. AIDS: A Guide for Hispanic Leadership. Washington, DC: The National Coalition of Hispanic Health and Human Service Organizations, 1989.

Cutler, J. C., and Arnold, R. C. "Venereal disease control by health departments in the past: Lessons for the present." American Journal of Public Health 78 (4) (April 1988): 372–376.

Darney, Philip, Myhra, Wendie, Atkinson, Elizabeth, and Meier, Jane. "Sero survey of human immunodeficiency virus infection in women at a family planning clinic: Absence of infection in an indigent population in San Francisco." American Journal of Public Health 79 (7) (July 1989): 883–885.

De La Cancela, Victor. "Minority AIDS prevention: Moving beyond cultural perspectives towards sociopolitical empowerment." AIDS Education and Prevention 1 (2) (Summer 1989): 141–153.

Deresiewicz, William. "Against all odds: Grassroots minority groups fight AIDS." Health/PAC Bulletin 18 (1) (Spring 1988): 4–10.

DiClemente, Ralph, Boyer, Cherrie, and Morales, Edward. "Minorities and AIDS: Knowledge, attitudes, and misconceptions among black and Latino adolescents." American Journal of Public Health 78 (1) (January 1988): 55–57.

Falloon, Judith, et al. "Human immunodeficiency virus infection in children." The Journal of Pediatrics 114 (1) (January 1989): 1–30.

Fauci, Anthony. "The human immunodeficiency virus: Infectivity and mechanisms of pathogenesis." Science 239 (4840) (February 5, 1988): 617–622.

Flaskerud, Jacquelyn, and Rush, Cecilia. "AIDS and traditional health beliefs and practices of black women." Nursing Research 38 (4) (July-August 1989): 210–215.

Gentry, Lynn. "AIDS babies—Walls around children?" Colorado's Children 4 (5) (Winter 1985–1986): 4.

Goodman, Elizabeth, and Cohall, Alwyn. "Acquired immunodeficiency syndrome and adolescents: Knowledge, attitudes, beliefs, and behaviors in a New York City adolescent minority population." Pediatrics 84 (1) (July 1989): 36–42.

Hein, Karen. "Commentary on adolescent acquired immunodeficiency syndrome: The next wave of the human immunodeficiency virus epidemic?" Pediatrics 83 (Janaury 1989): 144–149.

Hill, Reuben. "Generic features of families under stress." Social Casework 39 (2–3) (1958).

Institute of Medicine, National Academy of Sciences. Confronting AIDS, Directions for Public Health, Health Care, and Research. Washington, DC: National Academy Press, 1986.

Katz, Samuel, and Wilfert, Catherine. "Human immunodeficiency virus infection of newborns." New England Journal of Medicine 320 (25) (June 22, 1989).

Kegeles, Susan, Adler, Nancy, and Irwin, Charles. "Adolescents and condoms: Associations of beliefs with intentions to use." American Journal of Diseases of Childhood 143 (8) (August 1989).

Koop, C. Everett. Report of the Surgeon General's Workshop on Children with HIV Infection and Their Families. Washington, DC: DHHS, 1987.

Lambert, Bruce. "AIDS legacy: A growing generation of orphans." New York Times (July 16, 1989): A1.

Medina C. "Latino culture and sex education." SIECUS Report 15 (3) (1987): 1–4.

Newberger, Carolyn, Melnicoe, Lora, and Newberger, Eli. "The American family in crisis: Implications for children." Current Problems in Pediatrics 16 (12) (December 1986): 714.

Nicholas, Stephen, Sondheimer, Diane, Willoughby, Anne, Yaffe, Sumner, and Katz, Samuel. "Human immunodeficiency virus infection in childhood, adolescence, and pregnancy: A status report and national research agenda." Pediatrics 83 (2) (February 1989): 300.

Oleske, James. "Natural history of HIV infection II." In Koop, C. Everett, Report of the Surgeon General's Workshop. Washington, DC: DHHS, 1987.

Oleske, James, et al. "Immune deficiency syndrome in children." Journal of the American Medical Association 249 (May 6, 1983): 2345.

Quinn, Thomas, Zacharias, Fernando, and St. John, Ronald. "HIV and HTLV-I infections in the Americas: A regional perspective." Medicine 68 (4) (1989).

Remafedi, Gary. "Preventing the sexual transmission of AIDS during adolescence." Journal of Adolescent Health Care 9 (2) (March 1988): 139–143.

Rickert, Vaughn, Jay, M. Susan, Gottlieb, Anita, and Bridges, Christie. "Adolescents and AIDS: Female attitudes and behaviors toward condom purchase and use." Journal of Adolescent Health Care 10 (1989): 313.

Rubinstein, Arye, et al. "Acquired immunodeficiency with reversed T4/T8 ratios in infants born to promiscuous and drug addicted mothers." Journal of the American Medical Association 249 (May 6, 1983): 2350.

Schilling, Robert, Schinke, Steven, Nichols, Stuart, et al. "Developing strategies for AIDS prevention research with black and Hispanic drug users." Public Health Reports 104 (1) (January-February 1989).

Select Committee on Children, Youth and Families. U.S. House of Representatives, Joint

Hearing. Foster Care, Child Welfare, and Adoption Reforms. Washington, DC: U.S. Government Printing Office, 1989.

Thomas, Patricia. "The epidemic." Medical World News 30 (14) (July 24, 1989).

Yankauer, Alfred. "AIDS and public health." American Journal of Public Health 78 (4) (April 1988): 364–366.

2

Understanding HIV Infection and Its Medical Impact on Children and Youths

VIRGINIA ANDERSON

ACQUIRED IMMUNODEFICIENCY SYNDROME (AIDS) RESULTS FROM A PROgressive destruction of T white blood cells by the human immunodeficiency virus (HIV). T cells protect the body from infectious diseases and, when they reach a critical low level, opportunistic infections or AIDS-related cancer can occur. Opportunistic infections are caused by ubiquitous organisms that do not cause disease in persons with a healthy immune system. Persons with AIDS are especially susceptible to pneumocystis carinii pneumonia (PCP), oral candidiasis, herpesvirus infection, toxoplasmosis, tuberculosis, and a wide range of common bacterial, viral, or fungal infections. In some children, meningitis may result from bacteria, viruses, or the HIV itself. In addition, young children with AIDS suffer from severe, recurrent common childhood illnesses such as ear infections, throat infections, sinusitis, and diarrheal syndromes. Because of the underlying immune deficiency, recurrent or new infections develop, and intermittent illness is superimposed on a chronic debilitative state.

In addition to destroying T helper cells, HIV is carried into the brain by giant cells called macrophages. These cells secrete toxic substances called cytokines, which are toxic to the nervous system and other organs of the body. The progressive destruction of the brain is called HIV encephalopathy. A wide range of clinical symptoms such as forget-fulness, confusion, memory loss, seizures, incontinence, and dementia can occur. Children may lose developmental milestones—for example, the ability to walk or smile—and may suffer a tremendous amount of pain from involvement of the nervous systems. As many as 80 percent of persons with AIDS have evidence of brain damage at autopsy; these findings are more frequent and more severe in children. Most children with AIDS are learning disabled and may require special educational or early childhood intervention programs. In general, the earlier the onset of clinical symptoms in infants or toddlers, the more rapid the pro-gression of the disease and death.

AIDS-related cancers are the consequence of immune dysregula-tion. The T white blood cells may be compared to the conductor of the immune orchestra. Destruction of T cells causes B cells to proliferate unchecked. This autonomous growth eventually leads to an aggressive tumor of the lymphoid tissue, called a lymphoma, which can develop in the brain, lymph glands, or any other organ of the body. Kaposi's sarcoma (KS) is a tumor of blood vessels that occurs primarily in homo-sexual males with AIDS. Children rarely get KS [Anderson 1987].

Unfortunately, therapeutic agents to treat these diseases effectively are sparse. In adult men, death usually occurs within one to two years from the date of diagnosis. Women live half as long as men, and infants frequently die before their second birthdays. The younger the infant at the age of diagnosis of AIDS, the more rapid the progression of the illness. All persons with AIDS eventually die from an infectious disease process. Intensive scientific research is currently under way to identify new drugs to treat both HIV and opportunistic infections.

Transmission

AIDS is not transmitted through any ordinary activity of daily living. Kissing, hugging, sharing the same fork, glass, razor, tooth-brush, or toilet facilities will not spread HIV. There is no evidence to support transmission in a swimming pool, from a mosquito bite, in the classroom, or in the workplace. Sleeping with a person with AIDS will not spread the infection unless sexual intercourse occurs. Since the onset of the AIDS epidemic, no case of transmission through casual contact or the usual activities of daily living has been identified. AIDS is hard to catch. It requires sexual intercourse with an infected individual, sharing infected blood-contaminated drug paraphernalia, or, in the case of an infant, intrauterine exposure to the mother's infected blood—in which case there is a 30 to 50 percent chance that the newborn will develop the disease.

HIV is not transmitted by urine, feces, vomitus, sweat, tears, or saliva from infected persons. Body fluids that contain large numbers of white blood cells, especially blood or semen, are the most dangerous. Body fluids contaminated by blood are potentially infectious. Universal precautions require treating all body fluids as potentially infectious. This technique will provide sufficient protection against HIV and other serious diseases such as hepatitis. Latex gloves, disposable towels, and plastic bags prevent contact with contaminated spills. Lysol, Chlorox, or any other common household cleanser can decontaminate the area. Regularly scheduled educational programs on infection control and the availability of cleaning materials will ensure safety and peace of mind.

HIV infection in adults and older children may be present for a mean period of ten years before the symptoms of AIDS appear. During this time, transmission to an unsuspecting sexual partner is possible. Semen contains white blood cells that may harbor HIV; these cells may be deposited into the body of an uninfected individual during un-protected vaginal, oral, or anal intercourse, and a new case of HIV infection can occur. Anal intercourse is the most risky sexual practice; tears in the lining of the rectum can permit infected white cells from donor semen to enter the recipient's bloodstream. HIV from the infected donor can attach to T white blood cells and initiate a long destructive process that leads to AIDS and overwhelming infection. HIV infection can also be transmitted during penile vaginal intercourse. This route of infection is more efficient if concomitant genital ulcers or other sexually transmitted diseases such as syphilis or herpesvirus are also present. Genital ulcers facilitate access to the blood where the T white blood cells circulate.

HIV is found in vaginal secretions. In the United States, however, transmission of HIV from females to males through sexual intercourse is rare. In all cases, the risk of infection increases with the number of sexual partners, genital ulcers, or drug use.

In the inner city, the AIDs epidemic accompanies the epidemic of illegal drug use. In New York City, more than half of intravenous (IV) drug users carry HIV. Clean needles and avoidance of contaminated syringes can reduce the spread of HIV in this high-risk population. The use of disposable paraphernalia, or flushing the needle and syringe with a 1:10 part chlorine bleach-water solution, will reduce transmission.

A mutual monogamous relationship between two uninfected persons is the best assurance that HIV will not spoil intimate sexual relationships. The risk of HIV infection can be reduced between persons with uncertain sexual history for HIV by the consistent, proper use of latex condoms and water-based spermicidal gel, which provide a physical barrier and chemical destruction of viral-infected white blood cells. Only abstinence from sexual intercourse and intravenous drugs can guarantee an absolutely safe condition for avoiding HIV.

It is understandable that fear of AIDS may be subconsciously confused with fear of persons with AIDS. Fortunately, after nearly a decade of tracking the epidemic, no incident of transmission by casual contact has occurred. Phobias and myths must be replaced by compassion and facts. The empowering message is that AIDS is a preventable disease, and fear of contagion must be correctly associated with certain behaviors, such as unprotected sexual intercourse with persons whose sexual history is unknown or the sharing of blood-contaminated needles or syringes by intravenous substance abusers. Homophobia, or fear of sexual attraction between persons of the same gender, is aroused by the AIDS epidemic because the first cases of AIDS were observed in homosexual men. The virus itself has no sexual preference. New HIV infections are more likely to affect women and children, as the disease enters the heterosexual population through intravenous drug users.

HIV Testing

HIV infection may be clinically silent for many years before AIDS develops. During this period, a person who appears perfectly healthy may infect others through sexual contact or exposure to infected blood. HIV-infected blood can be exchanged during needle sharing by intravenous drug users. Infected blood or blood products can also transmit HIV. This likelihood has been greatly reduced since the introduction of the "AIDS test"; this test for HIV antibodies indicates the presence of HIV. Since the spring of 1985, all blood donations in the United States have been screened for the presence of HIV using the enzyme-linked immunosorbent assay (ELISA) HIV test. The test is extremely sensitive, and it would be rare for an infected unit of blood to escape detection and be transfused into an unsuspecting person. There is no risk whatsoever in volunteering to donate blood. Blood donors are needed now more than ever because of the elimination of many persons who are no longer able to give blood. The AIDS test is also used to detect asymptomatic carriers of HIV infection. When the ELISA method has been positive on two separate occasions, a confirmatory Western blot test is performed before an individual is informed that HIV infection is present. Pre-test and post-test counseling is mandatory because of the serious implications of a positive result.

The Course of the Syndrome

AIDS is a syndrome with many symptoms that mimic other illnesses. Symptoms of HIV infection may include fevers, weight loss, diarrhea, enlarged lymph glands, anemia, memory loss, motor retardation or learning disability, or seizures. Consequently, clinical course and life expectancy vary greatly.

When infected body fluids such as semen, blood, or vaginal secretions are exchanged, the virus attaches to specific sites on T white blood cells. During an approximate six-to-12 week "window" period, an individual may test negative for antibodies to HIV. Seroconversion occurs when detectable antibodies are produced in response to the infection. Because these antibodies are incapable of destroying the virus, a person remains infected and infectious for life. Infected persons may be asymptomatic during a long latency period, which may last for an average of ten years. An infected person may appear perfectly healthy but can spread the disease.

The virus does not proliferate rapidly in the body at all times. It may be activated during exposure to other infections such as the common cold, by additional exposure to HIV-infected persons, or by exposure to persons with other sexually transmitted diseases. As HIV production destroys white cells, there is a gradual weakening of the immune system over time. Many persons develop pre-AIDS or AIDS-related complex (ARC), consisting of fevers, weight loss, and enlarged lymph glands, before full-blown AIDS and opportunistic infections develop.

Since almost all infants with HIV infection acquire the disease in utero, a long incubation period or ARC phase, as seen in older children or adults, usually does not take place. The immature fetal immune system is destroyed before it can develop. The majority of infants with

congenital AIDS become sick and die before age two. They may suc-
cumb to common childhood infections, as well as to opportunistic infections.

AIDS and Children

The primary means of transmission to infants is through intrauterine exposure to virus particles in the infected mother's blood. The
mother's infection most often results from sexual intercourse with an
HIV-infected partner (an intravenous drug user or bisexual man), or
from the mother's own intravenous drug use. Less frequent means of
transmission to infants include blood transfusions or exposure to an
infected mother's milk.

Ninety percent of the children with AIDS acquire their infection
from their mother, who is often a drug user. In one-third of the cases,
the mother is not a drug user herself but has been infected by an HIV-
seropositive sexual partner who was exposed as a result of substance
abuse. Drug use is the most common associated risk behavior, but
bisexual males and hemophiliacs have infected both their spouses and
their children. Nearly all children born to HIV-infected women are
seropositive at birth. The mother's antibody crosses the placenta, resulting in a positive AIDS test in the baby. When the mother transmits HIV
itself, the infant develops AIDS. The Centers for Disease Control define
an indeterminate period when it is uncertain whether the infant will get
AIDS; this interval may be as long as 15 months. Approximately 50 to 70
percent of HIV-positive infants fit this category. These infants have no
clinical signs of infection, such as weight loss, oral thrush, fevers, pneumonia, or diarrhea; they have normal immune function tests and lose
their positive HIV antibody test by 15 months. Babies who go on to
develop AIDS produce their own antibodies beyond 15 months of age,
and therefore the antibody test remains positive. These babies will have
abnormal immune function tests, such as high gamma globulin levels,
low numbers of T helper white blood cells, and clinical symptoms.

The inability to identify an AIDS baby at birth creates serious problems for child welfare agencies concerned with foster care and adoptive
placement. A family is asked to welcome a child into their home not
knowing whether this is a long-term commitment to rear a child, or if
bonding and bereavement counseling are simultaneous concerns. A
foster mother for a baby with AIDS must learn to become a health care

worker if she is to provide day-to-day care. Most foster care programs include provision for respite care to relieve familial stress. Between 30 and 50 percent of infants born to HIV-positive mothers will get AIDS; the remainder will become orphans. It is estimated that 21,500 HIV-infected women will orphan 70,000 noninfected children in New York City in the next five years [Norwood 1989]. These staggering figures will increase as long as women do not know the HIV status of their sexual partners and fail to take risk-reduction precautions. Women must receive assertiveness training to negotiate their sexual arena; some women may end up in the emergency room as battered women if they insist that their partners wear condoms.

Children with AIDS fail to thrive and suffer from multiple common childhood infections that do not respond to usual therapy. Their lymph nodes are enlarged, and they have frequent bouts of diarrhea and fevers. Oral thrush may make eating very difficult. HIV affects the nervous system, and the children exhibit cognitive and motor disability. Expectations for growth, development, and survival must be adjusted to the stage of the illness. Most develop pneumonia and eventually die in respiratory failure. In general, the earlier the onset of clinical symptoms, the more rapid the course of the disease. In congenital AIDS, the long latency period observed in adults is rare. The child with AIDS needs emotional support in a safe and loving home, where medical care can be offered in partnership with a social welfare and health care delivery system.

Latency-Age Children and HIV Infection

Latency-age children have the lowest incidence of HIV infection. Most children with AIDS acquire the disease through perinatal transmission, become symptomatic, and die before school age. Before 1985, when blood donors were not yet screened for HIV, infected latency-age children most often acquired the disease through infected blood products. Very few new cases should develop, since this risk factor is nearly eliminated by use of the HIV antibody test on all blood bank donations. Since transmission by casual contact does not occur, school-age children with HIV infection should be mainstreamed as much as possible. Because learning disabilities are frequent, it is important not to place excessive or unrealistic demands for school performance on HIV-infected children.

The most worrisome latency-age risk group are children who may have been sexually abused by an infected male. HIV transmission as a consequence of child sexual abuse has been reported. It is unknown exactly how many adolescents with AIDS may have contracted HIV as a result of sexual abuse during latency. In geographic areas with high seropositivity, sexual abuse should be considered a high-risk circumstance. Disorganized families on drugs may be unable to protect their young children from incest and sexual exploitation. Drug abuse, incest, and HIV are family problems that affect vulnerable children.

Adolescents and HIV Infection

Teenagers account for fewer than 1 percent of the total number of AIDS cases. Since the disease has an average incubation period of ten years, 20 percent of the persons with AIDS who develop symptomatic illness between ages 20 and 29 were actually infected as adolescents. AIDS in teenagers is similar to that in adults.

Adolescence is a period that may include biologically heightened sexual awareness and initiation into a variety of sexual practices (heterosexual, bisexual, and/or homosexual experimentation). Inexperience in the use of condoms, faulty sex education, lack of appreciation of sexual responsibility, and risk-taking behaviors compound the adolescent's vulnerability to HIV exposure. In geographic areas of high seroprevalence, the additive effects of these cofactors threaten the health of American youths who suffer from ignorance, poor judgment, exploitation, sexual harassment, or bartering their bodies for drugs, money, or the promise of physical or emotional security. Alcohol and drug use reduce inhibitions and may further accentuate age-appropriate experimental and risk-taking behaviors. Hypocrisy, denial, a sense of invulnerability, inadequate school-based sex education and family life programs, and a dearth of health services for adolescents accentuate the risk factor for those who are most vulnerable. Support is needed for young people from abusive homes because their low self-esteem and need for affection make them easy targets for sex and drug traders—an invitation to HIV infection and AIDS. Sexually active teenagers must understand the seriousness of the HIV epidemic and its threat to all sexually active persons. Unprotected sexual activity on the part of an infected individual can have lethal consequences to a partner.

Conclusion

HIV infection will be a challenge for medical and child welfare caregivers for many years to come. It has affected and will continue to affect the most vulnerable members of society: infants, children, youths, women, and minorities. New cases of HIV infection can be prevented. Primary prevention and extensive educational initiatives need to continue and to be intensified. Until AIDS is prevented or cured, great numbers of children and youths will be exposed to HIV, become infected, develop symptoms, and eventually die. They will need compassionate, informed individuals who are consistently devoted to their physical and psychosocial condition.

REFERENCES

Anderson, Virginia. "Comments." In Attention to AIDS: Responding to the Growing Number of Children and Youth with AIDS. Washington, DC: Child Welfare League of America, 1987.

Norwood, Chris. Presentation. Fifth International AIDS Conference, Montreal, Canada, June 1989.

3

The Medical Management of Pediatric AIDS: Intervening in Behalf of Children and Families

JAMES OLESKE

IN 1978 WE SAW OUR FIRST CASE OF PEDIATRIC AIDS. THE CHILD WAS A three-year-old girl who died a year later of hypoxia, complicating lymphocytic interstitial pneumonia, and Salmonella sepsis. At six months, this child had developed chronic diarrhea, anemia, and failure to thrive. By 18 months, she had had her first of several bouts of Salmonella enteritis and sepsis. She was anemic and received several blood transfusions in 1976. When first seen in consultation she was a perplexing case: a three-year-old with lymphocytic interstitial pneumonia and recurrent Salmonella infection. When an immune workup was performed, she demonstrated a low number of total lymphocytes by rosette technique, high B cells, and massive hypergammaglobulinemia. The diagnosis so obvious today was a mystery ten years ago. A serum specimen saved from 1978 has tested positive for HIV antibody. Her mother, still well, had many sexual partners and has had another child, apparently healthy. Because the mother has refused testing, it is unknown if the child acquired the infection perinatally in 1975 or from a blood transfusion in 1976. Regardless, this report demonstrates that sporadic cases of HIV-infected children were occurring in the mid-1970s.

It is just over a decade since our first case of pediatric AIDS, and now our Children's Hospital AIDS program (CHAP) provides ongoing care for more than 180 HIV-infected children. During this time, we have seen 100 additional pediatric AIDS patients die from this frightful viral infection. Based on our experience, we fear that by 1991 there will be between 10,000 and 20,000 HIV-infected children in the United States. If preventive strategies are not developed and implemented, by the new century (the year 2000) there may be over one million HIV-infected women and children.

Epidemiology/Transmission

By February 1989, 1,440 cases of AIDS in children under 13 years of age had been reported to the Centers for Disease Control (CDC). In addition, from March 1987 to March 1988, 416 cases were reported, an increase of 85 percent over the previous year [CDC 1988]. Of all reported children with AIDS, 65 percent have already died.

Most infants and children are infected by perinatal exposure. Theoretically, perinatal transmission can occur (1) in utero, via transplacental infection of the fetus; (2) peripartum, through contact with blood and secretions; or (3) postnatally, via breast milk. The mothers became infected either through intravenous drug use or because a sexual partner was infected, and many became aware of their own infection only after AIDS was diagnosed in the infant. A number of HIV-infected children were exposed before 1985 via transfusion with contaminated blood or blood products. The cohort of infants born between 1978 and 1985 who received blood transfusions are at risk of developing HIV infection and need to be followed for the next five to ten years and beyond [Ammann et al. 1983; Harris et al. 1983; CDC 1982]. The present screening of blood products and treatment of coagulation factors will help to prevent future cases of blood-acquired pediatric AIDS.

Diagnosis and case definition regarding infants are made more difficult due to the presence of passively acquired maternal antibodies early in life. Since passive antibody is thought to persist for as long as 15 months, two age-group criteria have been established. For children older than 15 months (or of any age, if born to a seronegative mother), HIV infection can be documented by (1) virus in blood or tissue, (2) HIV antibody, or (3) symptoms meeting the CDC case definition for AIDS. For infants under 15 months of age suspected of perinatal infection, proof of infection can be established by criterion (1) or (3) above. In the case of an asymptomatic, seropositive infant who is virus-negative (a not uncommon setting), one must also document evidence of both cellular and humoral immune deficiency *and* one or more categories of symptomatic infection (e.g., lymphocytic interstitial pneumonia, secondary infectious disease, or cancer) [CDC 1987].

The growing magnitude of maternal-child transmission of HIV is only recently being appreciated. For instance, in a blinded screening of newborn blood (in an effort to determine seroprevalence among reproductive women), 0.2 percent of samples were positive in Massachusetts and 0.8 percent in New York State [CDC 1988]. In the latter case, 0.2 percent were positive outside of New York City and 1.6 percent within the city. Therefore, in New York City, one in 61 mothers giving birth is seropositive for HIV. In high-risk groups, the seropositive rate becomes extreme, as in Newark, New Jersey, where intravenous drug abusers have a rate of 80 percent and a blinded screening of newborns at University Hospital (Newark, New Jersey) revealed a seroprevalence of 4.3 percent. The transmission rate of virus from mother to infant, although not 100 percent, has been estimated at about 50 percent [Mok et al. 1987; Semprini et al. 1987].

HIV Testing of Women

Never has a clinical screening test been imbued with as many psychosocial issues as that for HIV infection. A crisis has arisen from the paralysis of our public health response to this fatal viral illness. The HIV ELISA assay presently available satisifies all the accepted criteria of an appropriate screening test for a population at risk for HIV infection. This test will identify asymptomatically HIV-infected individuals, and several confirmatory and diagnostic tests are available. Early disease intervention both therapeutically and for education regarding behavior modification satisfy the condition that a screening test result in benefit for the tested individual. In high-prevalence areas, the predictive value of test results is excellent. The availability of appropriate confirmation and diagnostic assays makes testing in low-prevalence areas acceptable under conditions of voluntary testing. The technical and cost aspects of HIV tests are acceptable.

The objection to testing is generated by advocacy groups concerned with issues of confidentiality and scapegoating of identified individuals. Mandatory testing has been an especially objectionable policy but the concept of routine testing has been less so.

HIV infection in women and their perinatally infected children poses significantly different issues than that of other predominantly male risk groups. The vast majority of these women-infant pairs come from minority groups living in urban poverty areas. Only half of the infants born to serologically positive women are truly infected; the remainder are positive by screening tests because of transplacental antibody. The sensitivity and predictive value of HIV tests in infants is thus markedly reduced, compared to such tests in adults. Infants identified as HIV-positive at birth may require other assays—in particular, immune function assays. Abnormalities identified at the onset of clinical disease compatible with HIV infection further identify infants who are actually infected. There are HIV diagnostic assays in development, such as polymerase chain reaction (PCR), that may provide definitive diagnoses for positive HIV-screened infants. The objection to routine testing of pregnant women or infants centers chiefly on the issue of what available prophylactic and therapeutic programs would truly benefit identified infants and mothers.

Confidentiality issues may be of less concern for identified infants but become predominant for HIV-infected children when they approach school age. Unfortunately, there are no effective advocacy groups who adequately represent the needs of minority women who are infected and have infants and children infected with HIV. Poverty-associated high levels of intravenous drug abuse are major promoters of perinatal HIV infection. Since the identification of pediatric AIDS in Newark, New Jersey, before 1984, 14 percent of perinatal infection occurred in women whose only risk factor was heterosexual contact. Data since 1984 demonstrate that this number has increased to 43 percent. Many of this group of heterosexually exposed women first become aware of their HIV status after the diagnosis had been made in their infants. Access to the health care system is already limited for women at greatest risk of HIV infection; the occurrence of AIDS in this group is frequently perceived as just another problem in a life situation already overwhelmed by preexisting problems related to poverty. Simplistic approaches recommending avoidance of pregnancy do not take into consideration cultural-social pressures for such women to bear children as an expression of self-worth. Confidentiality issues thus become less important in this group of women compared to other, more immediate and overwhelming issues. Given the multiple problems and concerns of this group and the lack of appropriate advocacy groups, an ever greater burden is placed on their health care providers to guard aggressively their patients' confidentiality while providing the increasingly sophisticated care available for HIV patients.

Clinicians, usually a priori, feel that early identification improves their ability to intervene more appropriately in a disease. Several specific issues related to perinatal HIV infection support the belief that early identification of HIV-infected (or potentially infected) infants promotes provision of medical benefits that outweigh the psychosocial disadvantages of testing. Models for the comprehensive case management provision of service to HIV-infected families improve the quality of life by a number of factors. Potentially HIV-infected infants and children receive appropriate prophylactic and therapeutic intervention. Resources for nutritional, educational, and neurodevelopmental intervention can be appropriately focused, and families at risk for future infected children can be more appropriately counseled. Decisions on breast feeding and immunization programs would also benefit HIV-identified infants. Access to the increasing number of investigational drugs (such as AZT) requires HIV testing, and, without routine testing, high-risk untested infants would suffer delayed participation in such programs.

Although there are still controversies regarding the public health value of HIV testing in low-prevalence populations, and a paucity of controlled data on the absolute benefits of intervention therapies, there are cogent arguments for routine testing for HIV in high-prevalence areas. From a public health perspective, HIV testing should be routinely performed for women in high-risk areas. Adverse psychosocial effects of testing need to be addressed, but these should not paralyze the development of available testing and counseling services linked to appropriate medical care.

Guidelines for HIV Testing of Sexually Abused Children

The question has been asked whether sexually abused children and adolescents should be screened for HIV antibody, and, if so, what studies should be performed and when should they be repeated. Conservative estimates indicate that over 200,000 children are sexually abused each year in the United States, and that over 20 percent of all children may be sexually abused before they reach adulthood. Similar projections of high numbers are expected for the prevalence of HIV infection in the United States. By 1991, there may be from three million to 13 million HIV-infected individuals (one to five percent of the total U.S. population). Our experience in Newark, New Jersey, supports an increase in the heterosexual spread of HIV, including transmission through sexual abuse.

Of 15 children and adolescents sexually abused by a known HIV-positive attacker who had HIV testing in our program, three became positive. There are no prospective data, however, to document the actual risk of transmission of HIV by sexual abuse. Exposure of the abused individual to semen (rectal, vaginal, or oral) would be a prerequisite for HIV transmission. The greater the trauma, the more likely would be the transmission if the attacker were HIV-infected. Accurate information on the details of a sexual attack is frequently not obtained. The presence of risky behavior in the attacker is also difficult to determine with confidence.

In light of these facts, I would recommend that every sexually abused child or adolescent, as well as the attacker, have an HIV screening antibody assay performed at the time of the attack and again three months and six months afterward. I would also test after six months if any signs or symptoms of HIV infection are noted. Presently constituted sexual abuse clinics usually have the appropriately trained medical and social service staff to add HIV testing and counseling economically to those tests now being performed on abused children and adolescents. Multi-center prospective studies should be funded to define the exact magnitude of HIV infection in sexually abused children and adolescents.

Clinical Manifestations

The average age of diagnosis for pediatric AIDS patients is six months, with the majority of children being of toddler and preschool age. A significant number are diagnosed because of a predisposing family/social setting and are not necessarily symptomatic. Most, however, present with a wide range of signs and symptom complexes.

Since it is felt that HIV can be transmitted in utero, it is not surprising that some infants are born with classical signs of congenital infection [Oleske 1983; Rubinstein 1983]. These signs include low birth weight, small size for gestational age, hepatosplenomegaly, thrombocytopenia, jaundice, anemia, and elevated liver function tests. In addition, dysmorphic features have been described in affected newborns, including microcephaly and craniofacial abnormalities, although a definitive cause-and-effect relationship has not been established [Nicholas 1988].

Outside the newborn period, many infants present with a non-specific symptom complex that may include failure to thrive, recurrent fever, thrush, diarrhea, and lymphadenopathy. The nonspecificity mandates a thorough workup to rule out other disease entities, but, in urban areas in the United States, AIDS has become the predominant diagnosis for this presentation.

The most frequently affected organ system in children with AIDS has been the lungs. Tachypnea with fever, cough, and even hypoxia are often the hallmark of pneumocystis carinii pneumonia (PCP) or lymphocytic interstitial pneumonia (LIP). PCP tends to develop as an acute disease with more pronounced fever and diminished breath sounds and rhonchi on physical examination. LIP develops more slowly and chronically, with generalized lymphadenopathy, salivary gland enlargement, and nodular and interstitial infiltrates evident on chest radiograph. With experience, a clinician can make the diagnosis without invasive procedures, but the definitive test is microscopic examination of lung tissue. LIP reveals diffuse mononuclear infiltration of the alveolar septa and peribronchiolar areas [Joshi 1985]. Culture in some cases has yielded HIV, and in situ hybridization has revealed the presence of both HIV and Epstein-Barr virus (EBV) [Andiman et al. 1985; Rubinstein et al. 1986]. The role EBV plays in the pathogenesis of LIP, and whether it is a primary or a secondary agent, is not known.

Severe, recurrent infections caused by pyogenic bacteria, such as *Hemophilus influenzae, Streptococcus pneumoniae,* and *Staphylococcus aureus,* are quite common. Immunizations with antigens from encapsulated bacteria also are less successful than in otherwise normal children. As in adults with AIDS, opportunistic infections are a serious problem and frequently the immediate cause of death. Table 1 lists the incidence of such infections in the first 316 children reported to the CDC.

Common to all of these infectious agents is the fact that they are ubiquitous; that is, most of us are infected/colonized with these agents, which are held in check (latent) by a normal immune system. Pneumocystic carinii and chronic interstitial pneumonia (LIP) are the most common, with the pathogenesis of the latter being poorly understood, as discussed above. The herpesviruses as a group cause a significant amount of morbidity and mortality. Disseminated cytomegalovirus (CMV) with multi-organ involvement, especially diffuse pneumonitis, is

Table 1

Opportunistic Infection in 316 Children with HIV
Infection Reported to the CDC

Infection	n	%
Pneumocystic carinii	167	53
Chronic interstitial pneumonia	155	49
Disseminated cytomegalovirus	55	17
Candida esophagitis	48	15
Disseminated mycobacterium	26	8
Cryptosporidiosis	16	5
Epstein-Barr virus	14	4
Others	20	6

the most common. While EBV was seen in 4 percent, it can be difficult to diagnose serologically and may cause generalized disease as well as specific organ dysfunction in a higher proportion of cases. Mycobacteria, especially avium intracellulare, which can be difficult to diagnose, cause disseminated disease in some children and pose therapeutic problems, since there are few effective non-toxic drugs.

The gastrointestinal (GI) tract is frequently involved, and malnutrition cachexia is a serious problem in a significant number of children. Candida can invade all or part of the GI mucosa, but esophagitis is especially troublesome. Many of these children are unable, as a result, to swallow their own secretions or to ingest nutrition orally. Infectious enterocolitis caused by CMV, mycobacterium avium intracellulare, salmonella, and cryptosporidium all can contribute to malabsorption. In addition, some children who malabsorb have nonspecific villus atrophy on biopsy. The end result of these multiple GI pathologies is that young AIDS patients frequently have a serious nutrition problem that requires fastidious attention.

An all-too-common clinical manifestation in children with AIDS is progressive encephalopathy [Epstein et al. 1985]. Clinically, this condition presents as either loss of developmental milestones or failure in development altogether. Microcephaly and cortical atrophy can be documented, and in pathological specimens microglial nodules and neuronal loss are demonstrated. HIV has been cultured from brain tissue in such cases, and HIV antigen and antibody are detected in the cerebrospinal fluid (CSF). In situ hybridization has revealed the presence of HIV nucleic acid. The course of HIV encephalopathy is generally persistent and progressive and frequently occurs in the absence of other opportunistic infections.

It is clear that all organ systems can be involved primarily or secondarily in children with AIDS. Anemia and thrombocytopenia are common. Similar immunologic abnormalities, as seen in adults, are observed in children—hypergammaglobulinemia, reversed helper/suppressor lymphocyte ratios with decreased numbers of helper T lymphocytes, depressed lymphocyte response to mitogen stimulation, and impaired humoral immunity. Some children also experience cardiovascular disease in the form of congestive cardiomyopathy and AIDS arteriopathy. Nephrotic syndrome has been observed in some children with focal glomerulitis and glomerulosclerosis depicted by biopsy. It is now clear that all organ systems can be adversely affected by HIV, and infection with HIV is a chronic multi-organ system disease.

Management of Pediatric HIV Infection

Supportive Care

Those professionals who regularly care for children with AIDS realize the complex challenge and the need for a comprehensive, multidisciplinary treatment program. Dedicated teams of medical, nursing, and social service personnel are essential for success. Table 2 supplies an outline of supportive care provided in our program for HIV-infected children.

Table 2

Supportive Care of HIV-Infected Infants
and Children

---

1. Nutritional support
2. Treatment and prophylaxis of HIV-related infection
3. Treatment of lymphocytic interstitial pneumonia
4. Immune support with intravenous gamma globulin
5. Treatment of tumors, end organ failure, and chronic pain
6. Psychosocial support of the child and family
7. Education
8. Advocacy

Nutritional support is a key element in childhood AIDS care but can be difficult to achieve because of the frequently poor or difficult social environment and overwhelming infectious complications/GI disease. Over 35 broviac catheters have been utilized for parenteral alimentation at the Childrens' Hospital of New Jersey. Of these, 12 were inserted for a successful home use program in selected patients. Infectious complications occurred in about 10 percent overall. Ongoing nutritional assessment of all children is an important facet of the therapeutic program.

Another important feature is a high index of suspicion and aggressive management of frequent infectious complications. Presentation with pulmonary symptoms is most common, requiring hospitalization and institution of broad-spectrum antibiotics and trimethoprim-sulfamethoxazole (tmp-smx) for potential bacterial and parasitic (PCP) disease. Chest x-rays and cultures should guide ultimate therapy. Some patients with PCP will not respond to tmp-smx or may develop troublesome side effects necessitating pentamidine. Trimetrexate is an investigational drug that needs to be studied in both children and adults with PCP. Prophylaxis with tmp-smx (10 mg/kg/day tmp divided twice a day orally) is recommended for patients with a past episode of PCP or when T-lymphocyte counts fall below 400 cells/μ.

Disseminated as well as severe mucocutaneous candidiasis usually responds to amphotericin b therapy and is well tolerated. Recurrences are frequent once therapy is stopped, however, in which case ketoconazole should be considered for persistent thrush and esophagitis. Ketoconazole is not effective for the more serious, invasive cases of candidiasis.

Troublesome mucocutaneous herpes simplex virus (HSV) or varicella zoster (VZ) infections will respond to treatment with acyclovir. There is no established therapy for CMV, although the investigational drug gancyclovir (DHPG) offers some hope. Gancyclovir can be lifesaving but does not eradicate the virus (recrudescence is common on cessation of therapy), and hematologic toxicity frequently occurs. Although a substantial number of adult AIDS patients with CMV have been treated with DHPG, experience with this drug has been limited to only a few children.

Lymphocytic interstitial pneumonitis (LIP) is an indolent, chronic process with intermittent exacerbations causing significant hypoxia and shortness of breath. Sporadic or chronic administration of supplemental oxygen may be necessary. Although not an established therapy, some investigators have used steroids for LIP and found patients to respond favorably. Studies are needed to document efficacy and establish guidelines for the potential use of steroids in this common condition among pediatric patients.

Many centers are now providing their patients with immune support by administering intravenous gamma globulin (IVGG). Preliminary observations and clinical experience have suggested that IVGG dramatically reduces the incidence of secondary bacterial infections. Indeed, between 1984 and 1986, there were 30 episodes of systemic bacterial infections in patients followed by our CHAP program (20 *Streptococcus*, four *Salmonella*, three *H. influenza* type B, two *Staphylococcus aureus*, and one *P. aeruginosa*). All but two of these occurred before institution of IVGG therapy. Since the introduction of prophylactic IVGG in 1983, the incidence of bacterial sepsis has fallen from a high of 45 percent to 2.5 percent. The promise of observations like these and others is being pursued by a collaborative trial being sponsored by the National Institutes of Health. It is clear that despite the presence of hypergammaglobulinemia, HIV-infected children have an abnormal antibody/B-lymphocyte response to polysaccharide (pneumococcal, Hib) antigens, both during natural exposure and immunization.

Specific Therapy for HIV Infection

The ultimate goal for researchers and (potential) victims of AIDS is treatment and prevention of the viral infection itself. More progress has been made with specific antiviral therapy, although only limited Phase I data are available in children with regard to two drugs—ribavirin and azidodeoxythymidine (AZT). Phase I trials establish pharmacokinetic data; although efficacy was not tested in these trails, AZT was felt to hold more promise and therefore is being pursued in Phase II efficacy trials in symptomatic HIV-infected children. Future trials should include less symptomatic infected infants, asymptomatic newborns/infants, and even HIV-infected women, in an effort to prevent the symptomatic and more advanced stages of AIDS. Other antiviral agents that are being considered for trials in humans include DDC, DDA/DDI, and soluble CD4 antigen (helper T-cell receptor). In addition, biological response modifiers may have some role in the future: alpha-interferon, granulocyte/macrophage colony-stimulating factor, and interleukin 2. Unfortunately, progress in prevention/immunization has been very slow. Marked strain variation, privileged status within host lymphocytes, monocytes, and CNS, and the fact that retroviral DNA integrates into host cell chromosomes and can remain latent (inactive), all contribute to making the development of a vaccine appear many years in the future. In the meantime, we must depend on social and educational programs to prevent the transmission of this virus in the human community.

The Burden of Care for HIV-Infected Children

We have found that infants and children infected with HIV have one to three hospitalizations per year, each lasting ten to 12 days. The average hospital cost for each child is $50,000 per year. Based on current estimates, by 1991 one of every ten pediatric beds will be occupied by a child with HIV infection (there are more than 40,000 pediatric hospital beds in the United States), costing almost one billion dollars. At present, 90 percent of the hospital costs for most pediatric HIV-infected children are covered by Medicaid. This program at best covers only half the real cost of hospitalization.

The outpatient care requirements of HIV-infected children are extensive and are projected to exceed 100 million dollars by 1991. Care of such a chronically ill child often requires skills that are beyond the capabilities of a mother who may also be sick. Effective care must not only provide medical services to the infected child but provide the child's mother and family with a wide range of psychosocial support services in addition. Training and support programs must be available for parents, foster parents (more than 40 percent of pediatric AIDS cases are in foster care), and caregivers to prepare them to meet the extensive services the HIV-infected child requires. Each HIV-infected child requires two to three outpatient visits per month. The cost of each visit is often high ($600 per month per child) because of the intensity of the medical services provided, and only part of that cost is covered by Medicaid. For these patients, physician reimbursement schedules will discourage private patient care and further burden hospital facilities. Pediatric AIDS has to date been an illness that has occurred in economically depressed minority populations. Continued spread of the AIDS virus among intravenous drug abusers and by heterosexual contact will ensure the tragic increase in cases expected throughout the country. The major burden of pediatric AIDS for the next decade will, however, continue to fall on the already overtaxed urban public health care system.

The burden of care for adolescents with HIV infection is just being recognized. Issues regarding preventive education of adolescents in high-risk areas and behavior groups, although not addressed here, need to be confronted by those providing services to this group. The risk to our adolescent population is an all-too-real crisis that must be confronted.

Most younger children will die within two years of diagnosis, although examples of longer survival are not rare. The factors governing length and quality of survival are not understood. Worrisome prognostic factors include presentation in the first year of life, presentation with PCP, and presentation with HIV encephalopathy. Patients with LIP as the only manifestation have, in general, longer survival rates. As physicians become more knowledgeable and adept at providing health care for children with AIDS, we are documenting a marked decrease in hospitalization time. Part of this phenomenon is due to preventive care (prophylactic antibiotics, IVGG), part to home-based therapy (TPN, parenteral antibiotics), and in large part to the development of sophisticated social services and educational networks.

REFERENCES

Ammann, A. J., Wara, D. J., Dritz, S., et al. "Acquired immunodeficiency in an infant: Possible transmission by means of blood products." Lancet i (1983): 956.

Andiman, W. A., Eastman, R., Martin, K., et al. "Opportunistic lymphoproliferations associated with Epstein-Barr viral DNA in infants and children with AIDS." Lancet i (1985): 1390.

Centers for Disease Control. "Unexplained immunodeficiency and opportunistic infections in infants—New York, New Jersey, California." Morbidity and Mortality Weekly Report 31 (December 19, 1982): 665.

Centers for Disease Control. "Classification system for human immunodeficiency virus (HIV) infection in children under 13 years of age." Morbidity and Mortality Weekly Report 36 (15) (April 24, 1987): 225.

Centers for Disease Control. "Quarterly report to the domestic policy council on the prevalence and rate of spread of HIV and AIDS in the United States." Morbidity and Mortality Weekly Report 37 (14) (April 15, 1988): 223.

Epstein, L. G., Sharer, L. R., Joshi, V. V., et al. "Progressive encephalopathy in children with acquired immune deficiency syndrome." Annuals of Neurology 17 (1985): 488.

Harris, C., Butkus Small, C., et al. "Immunodeficiency in female sexual partners of men with the acquired immunodeficiency syndrome." New England Journal of Medicine 308 (1983): 1181.

Joshi, V. V., Oleske, J., Minnefor, A. B., et al. "Pathologic pulmonary findings in children with the acquired immunodeficiency syndrome: A study of ten cases." Human Pathology 6 (1985): 241.

Mok, J. Q., Giaquinto, C., DeRossi, A., et al. "Infants born to mothers seropositive for the acquired immunodeficiency virus." Lancet i (1987): 1164.

Nicholas, S. W. Pediatric Annuals 17 (May 1988): 353.

Oleske, J. M., and Minnefor, A. B. "Acquired immunodeficiency syndrome in children." Pediatric Infectious Disease 2 (March-April 1983): 85.

Rubinstein, A. "Acquired immunodeficiency syndrome in infants." American Journal of Disease of Children 137 (1983): 825.

Rubinstein, A., Morecki, R., Silverman, B., et al. "Pulmonary disease in children with acquired immune deficiency and AIDS Related Complex." Journal of Pediatrics 108 (1986): 498.

Semprini, E. A., Vucetich, A., Pardi, G., et al. "HIV infection and AIDS in newborn babies of mothers positive for HIV antibody." British Medical Journal 294 (1987): 610.

4

Creating Programs To Care for Children with HIV/AIDS

GARY R. ANDERSON[1]

IN THE LATE 1980S, A NUMBER OF INDIVIDUALS AND ORGANIZATIONS RE-sponded to the crisis of children with AIDS by initiating or recasting a variety of services to help children and families. Some programs developed independently of traditional agencies serving children, while others were part of a number of services provided by a child welfare or health care agency. Some were new; others were modifications of existing services. In all the programs, new or modified, familiar service delivery issues have been accompanied by unexpected and sometimes unprecedented challenges that have required creative and innovative responses.

These developments, some noted here and others described in greater detail in ensuing chapters, reveal a continuum of services for children with HIV encompassing family-based, in-home supports to help families with these children; residential settings for short-term, transitional, or sometimes longer-term care of children; and family foster home care.

[1] The author wishes to acknowledge the significant contributions of Stefanie Held, Open Arms, Inc., Dallas, Texas; and Rachel Rossow of Connecticut; as well as Nancy Winestock, Grandma's House, Washington, DC; Fred Weaver, Bethana, Philadelphia, Pennsylvania; Sue Van Alstine, Farano Center, Albany, New York; and Sisters Kathy and Mary Patricia, Houston, Texas.

Supporting Families

The majority of children with HIV infection are living with their families in the community and are cared for by family members. Supporting families in their caregiving is essential to enhance the quality of life for the family and to help the family continue to care for their child. Some of this assistance is currently offered by medical clinics and health departments involved in the family's health care, but the need for more comprehensive, community-based services is urgent.

The Center for Attitudinal Healing, in California, is an example of an organization that has modified its program to include children with HIV. Established in 1975, this organization began a range of activities to provide a positive environment for children and adults facing life-threatening illnesses. To enhance the quality of life, support groups were formed for people dealing with catastrophic or long-term illnesses, specific illnesses such as breast cancer, and bereaved persons. Helping persons with HIV/AIDS began in the 1980s. A special program for children with HIV/AIDS, and their families offers (1) a Hot Line for Kids (415-435-5022) providing information about services, referrals, and support available nationwide; (2) support groups throughout the San Francisco area; (3) a Phone Pal/Pen Pal Program that links families together for emotional support; (4) training for people working with children and families, specifically in principles of Attitudinal Healing;[2] (5) educational outreach services for community agencies, schools, and organizations; (6) the creation of posters for educational outreach; and (7) advocacy for policies concerning children with HIV/AIDS.

Efforts to educate the community and children's caregivers, to reduce the social isolation of families and increase their involvement with a network of helpers and service providers, and to assist with concrete and psychosocial problems of families are often a function of child welfare and health care agencies. Assistance to biological families may not receive the priority it deserves, owing to an emphasis on substitute care for children and the difficulty of locating or engaging some families. Pursuing the child's best interests may have to be balanced with parental rights and informed by an assessment of the child's bond to the biological family.

[2]"Love is the most important healing force in the world. Attitudinal healing is the process of letting go of painful, fearful attitudes. When we release fear, only love remains. At the Center our definition of health is inner peace, and healing is the process of letting go of fear" [The Center for Attitudinal Healing, pamphlet].

Services to Families: The Role
of a Residence

Examples of how work with families developed into a range of services for children are afforded by Open Arms, Inc., and Bryan's House, in Dallas, Texas. In the summer of 1987, the AIDS Interfaith Network of Dallas organized a support group for women affected in some way by AIDS. Lydia Allen, a psychiatric nurse, and Stefanie Held, a hospital chaplain and director of pastoral services for Temple Emanu-El, co-facilitated the group, which met at the Temple. Although the disease had spread beyond the homosexual community, few people acknowledged the number of women and children who were infected; the support group provided the only assistance for women with AIDS in the Dallas area.

At first the group consisted of four women: *(1)* Ms. S. had been infected by a blood transfusion during childbirth four years earlier. Before she knew she had AIDS, she had given birth to a second child, who lived only seven months. She had recently moved to the Dallas area after being forced to move from another state by the isolation and fear created by community prejudice and ignorance. *(2)* Ms. L, in her late twenties, had contracted AIDS while she was between marriages. She had two healthy children and a third who was HIV-positive. Her primary concern was "Who will care for my children after I die?" *(3)* Ms. E. was a young, single mother who had originally planned to give up her child for adoption. After she was informed that she was HIV-positive, she could not give up the baby and could not return to the maternity home where she had been living. Uneducated and alone, she was ill-equipped for parenthood, particularly for the medical needs of her child while she was facing her own terminal illness. *(4)* Ms. J., who had raised nine children, was presented with a granddaughter abandoned by one of Ms. J.'s daughters, who was an HIV-infected drug abuser. Ms. J. chose to raise the child as her daughter and soon lost her job, was asked to leave her church, and was shunned by her family due to fear and ignorance associated with AIDS.

It was clear that special services for these families were required. The group leaders tried to help by taking children temporarily into their homes when parents could not care for them. It was soon apparent, however, that families' needs would outstrip the resources of the support group.

After considerable thought, the group facilitators created a home for children and mothers with AIDS. On a first-come first-serve basis, day care for children with AIDS, respite care for HIV-infected parents, and residential care for children without parents were proposed. In January 1988, Open Arms was incorporated with the support of religious leaders, the two pediatricians in North Texas whose practices centered upon HIV-infected children, several attorneys, and the leaders and members of Temple Emanu-El.

The process of obtaining a state license was difficult; there were standards for day care and standards for foster care but no category for a facility that provided day care, overnight respite care, and foster/residential care. In addition, Texas Department of Human Services reimbursement procedures did not encompass the primarily medical needs of this population.

By the spring of 1988, with small grants from the Women's Foundation of Dallas and from the Design Industry Foundation for AIDS, the search for a facility began. In a Dallas neighborhood near the Children's Medical Center and other AIDS services, a dilapidated four-bedroom house on a quiet residential street was rented. Volunteers cleaned, painted, refurbished, installed heating and air conditioning, and donated necessary materials. Named for the first Dallas/Fort Worth child to die from perinatally acquired AIDS, Bryan's House celebrated its November 1988 opening stocked with food, formula, diapers, toys, and games in brightly painted and nicely decorated rooms.

There was space for nine children, but in the two years since the support group had begun, the number of adults seeking help had risen to 118, with at least 83 children needing some level of care. Although volunteers continued to play a substantial role in running the house, a paid staff was necessary: (1) a part-time volunteer coordinator; (2) a pediatric nurse-practitioner; (3) part-time (eight-hour shift) child-care workers—the first was Ms. J., a member of the original support group; and (4) eventually a Project Director for Bryan's House, as Mrs. Held became more involved in administrative, fund-raising, and planning functions. Staff members and volunteers were initially trained by an interdisciplinary team of experts experienced with AIDS or children.

Open Arms helps families affected by AIDS by providing community-based, family-centered support services at no charge to the clients. It increases the time that families can remain intact; increases the time that a parent can work after diagnosis; decreases the number of children abandoned by families, reducing the number of children unnecessarily hospitalized; and decreases the number of perinatal transmissions of AIDS through prevention education and counseling. Services include concrete assistance, information and referral, and advocacy and education, in addition to day care, respite care, and residential care. Intake decisions are based on a priority-needs determination by a team evaluation. Children can receive care as long as they need it and space allows. Children served have been newborn to age 11.

One year after opening, Bryan's House is home to four residents:

1. A four-and-a-half-month-old girl, born to an intravenous drug abuser who abandoned her in the hospital; the baby weighed two pounds at birth, was microcephalic, had syphilis of the brain, and was HIV-positive. A relative tried to care for her but was overburdened and returned the child to the hospital.

2. A newborn girl delivered by a drug-abusing, HIV-positive mother who was already caring for an 18-month-old infant.

3. A newborn girl delivered by a teenage intravenous drug abuser with AIDS, who abandoned her in the hospital.

4. A four-year-old girl born with multiple handicaps—impaired vision, deafness, and retardation, who, during surgery at the age of two, had received a blood transfusion that contained the HIV virus. For two years she had remained in pediatric isolation because all hospital personnel wore surgical masks, gloves, and gowns when they entered the room where she was kept in a covered crib to prevent her from climbing out. When discharged to Bryan's House, she was unable to communicate and constantly thrashed about uncontrollably. After five months of consistent attention and care, she had made considerable progress, enough to attend a class for handicapped children in a public elementary school.

The remaining five spaces are used on a priority-needs basis for any of the 48 children associated with Open Arms. For example, a two-year-old HIV-infected girl whose father died of AIDS is brought for day care so her mother can continue employment, and a ten-month-old boy whose mother died of AIDS is brought for overnight periodic respite care to relieve his HIV-infected symptomatic father.

Bryan's House/Open Arms is not part of a larger agency. It participates in area AIDS coalitions and with the Children's Medical Center and Visiting Nurse Association. The budget covers salaries, rent, and utilities; everything else is donated.

Several lessons have been learned from this experience:

Staff members must be highly dedicated and motivated individuals who can turn obstacles into creative challenges.

Planning must be flexible and expansive.

Bridges must be solidly built between different populations afflicted with the same disease.

If the founders had known how much red tape and wrangling they would face, they might have thought twice before giving reality to their vision; it would not have been possible without the steady support of friends and family.

Across the country, small residences for children with HIV infection have been created and provide a range of services. Three are described here in some detail.

The Children's Home (Houston, Texas)

This residence for six children from birth to six years was opened in November 1986 and was originally planned as a hospice—a loving environment in which children with AIDS could be cared for until their expected deaths. The staff members soon discovered, however, that these children were not so close to death; in fact, none of them died. The residence's mission was transformed into helping children and their families live with HIV infection.

Affiliated with Casa De Esperanza—a child care agency—and operated by the Sisters of St. Mary of Namur, the agency now maintains two residences for children who are HIV-positive or have AIDS. These residences provide long-term care for some children whose parents cannot care for them or respite care for families faced with temporary crises. The children are cared for by staff members and volunteers. The children's medical supervision is done at a residence-operated medical clinic staffed by a volunteer pediatrician; the city's children's hospital makes itself available for more extensive services or hospitalization. Two volunteer psychologists meet with staff members and volunteers monthly to discuss the children and their families.

The Children's Home provides assistance to family members with children in residence and to family members caring for their own children in the community. A family worker visits families in their homes and provides counseling, concrete assistance, information and referrals, and advocacy for services. This worker reaches out to pregnant women in the county jail, a number of whom are HIV-positive, to begin assisting them and establishing a supportive dialogue that will continue after their deliveries or release.

A foster home program will soon be started for children who cannot be cared for by their parents.

Grandma's House (Washington, DC)

With five beds, Grandma's House opened as a transitional residence for HIV-positive children in January 1988. With the District Department of Human Services, Grandma's House works to return children to biological parents or to placement in foster homes, a sometimes slow and difficult task. In almost two years of operation, one child has returned to her parent, one baby was adopted, one was placed in foster care, and two have died. The five children, age eight to 28 months, in the home currently are HIV-positive, nonsymptomatic, and awaiting placement.

As work with families continues, children are provided a warm, loving, and lively home. Staff members include two nurses (L.P.N. and R.N.), child-care workers, an administrator, a clinical director, and a large number of trained volunteers. Choosing, training, and supporting staff members is a significant key to the quality of a transitional residence.

The staff members work as a team with the community hospital and other pertinent community groups. The children have a number of problems, including developmental delays and complications from other conditions such as drug addiction and neglect, requiring physical therapy, speech therapy, and nutrition control in addition to medical and social service practitioners. Because involvement with multiple agencies and helping people is commonplace—one worker estimated that each child is involved with ten different persons—case management is an important function for staff members.

Grandma's House is part of an organization called Terrific, Inc. Another Terrific program, called PEER, recruits and trains teenagers to be community AIDS educators, speaking at schools and churches.

Farano Center for Children (Albany, New York)

In December 1987, the Community Maternity Services of Albany opened the Farano Center for Children, a residence licensed for six infants, to provide a transition from being a boarder baby in a New York City hospital to being placed with a foster care family. The infants are cared for by a staff that includes a registered nurse, child-care workers, a social worker, a community educational coordinator, and volunteers. Additional medical needs are attended to by the Albany Medical Center, which has a specialized pediatric AIDS clinic, partly funded by the Robert Wood Johnson Foundation.

Over 20 children have passed through Farano Center to area foster homes that are part of the Community Maternity Services program. The center remains involved with the foster homes and provides respite care. Through its community educational coordinator, the center offers consultation and AIDS educational services to a 14-county region. Besides serving HIV-positive children, Farano Center has opened its doors to special-needs children with other handicapping conditions.

In addition to these residences and to St. Clare's homes (described in a later chapter), residences have been opened in several other cities, including Childkind outside of Atlanta, Georgia; the Children's AIDS Program in Boston, Massachusetts; and The Children's Place, scheduled to open in Chicago, Illinois, in August 1990.

Pioneering group home efforts for homosexual, lesbian, HIV-positive, and high-risk adolescents is the Gay and Lesbian Adolescent Social Services (GLASS) of Los Angeles. The executive director, Teresa DeCrescenzo, reported that they opened their first home for homosexual and lesbian adolescents in 1984; their second residence opened in 1987, for HIV-positive teens; and a third group home (six beds) has recently opened. In addition to the group homes, which serve 22 adolescents and young adults, the agency has begun a mobile outreach unit and a specialized foster care program for HIV-positive infants, toddlers, and adolescents.[3]

[3]The GLASS residences, organized for adolescents at high risk or already HIV-positive, are an example of a specialized program, as are HIV-specialized foster care programs described here and in later chapters. Often, however, foster parents or group home providers in regular programs are surprised to discover that a young person in their care is HIV-infected. For an example, see a residential center's experience (Bellefaire, Cleveland, Ohio) by Patrick McWeeny in *Attention to AIDS*, published by the Child Welfare League of America, 1987.

Family Foster Home Care

In the United States, the large majority of children needing out-of-home care are placed with foster families. In some states the foster parents may be relatives—kinship foster homes—but usually the foster parents are not related to the children. Foster parents are recruited, licensed, and trained to provide a home and family environment for children whose parents cannot provide care for them for a variety of reasons, including the serious, debilitating illness or the death of the parent. When children are placed in foster care, they are typically encouraged to maintain contact with their biological families. Connecticut has had some foster parents taking not only children with HIV but also the ill parents of the children into their homes.

Department of Children and Youth Services
(Hartford, Connecticut)

"Tell Mama I love her" was the message from the terminally ill mother in the intensive care unit to the nurse on the telephone with the foster mother of the dying woman's daughter. Mrs. B., the foster parent, had originally been assigned as a parent aide to the mother when Tina was born HIV-positive. As the relationship between the two women grew, the mother asked Mrs. B. to be Tina's godmother. And, as the mother's health deteriorated, Mrs. B. became Tina's foster mother. In time, Mrs. B. became the foster parent to the mother and Tina. Now, after the mother's death, Mrs. B. is in the process of adopting Tina.

Certain characteristics can emerge from this bridging of two families: a deeply humanistic or spiritual motivation, which may or may not be expressed religiously; fulfillment of the receiving family's need to parent in more ways than caring for a young child; and an uncanny ability for all the adults to focus on the children who will be surviving the death of a parent and/or sibling. Not all of these relationships have been successful. A negative situation occurred when the biological mother's AIDS-related encephalopathy resulted in paranoid thinking. She lost all memory of having voluntarily placed her child in the foster home where she too was living. She believed the foster mother was stealing her children, kidnapping them, and no one would help.

A strong philosophical and historical base for taking care of HIV-positive children and their families in foster care existed in Connecticut. For 20 years the Department of Children and Youth Services (DCYS) had been finding family placements for seriously disabled, medically fragile, and terminally ill children in place of long-term hospitalizations or institutionalization. Despite this commitment, however, in April 1984, a toddler, Ray, at Yale–New Haven Hospital was suspected of having AIDS, probably congenital. Born intellectually normal, he was able to walk, talk, learn, and play. Ray was under the care of DCYS, but, despite extensive efforts for foster home placement, Ray remained in the hospital for one year, until his death. His experience became a motivating force compelling DCYS to ensure that all future children exposed to the AIDS virus would receive the consistent, loving, nurturing care of a family.

In March of 1987, Dr. Amy B. Wheaton was appointed Commissioner of DCYS. She crystallized the agency's mission for all children in the state to develop as healthy, productive, caring persons, experiencing enduring, nurturing relationships as members of permanent families, receiving services responsive to their individual and developmental needs and sensitive to their race/heritage. This aim included the fundamental right of all children to grow up as members of a family. By the winter of 1989, DCYS had a caseload of 60 children with suspected exposure to the AIDS virus who were being cared for in 30 foster homes.

A foster parent support group is central to the ability to care for children in foster homes. On October 1, 1987, the first group was convened in New Haven at the home of one of the foster mothers. Babysitting was provided. An instant excitement and harmony occurred as each person arrived. Parents brought pictures, clothes to exchange, and an anticipated freedom to share their compassion, concern, grief, and anger over what had happened and was happening to their foster children. The majority of these parents had not told relatives, neighbors, or even their own adult children that their foster child had been exposed to AIDS. With a common sense of isolation and loneliness replaced by attachment and freedom, the group focused upon its greatest concern— the very real possibility, or experience, of critical illness and potential death of their children. A cohesiveness and identification developed around one mother's description of her foster son, who was at that time in a coma due to an opportunistic infection characteristic of AIDS. Grief and anger emerged. Two mothers told how their pastors had stated that their children were not allowed in church. The support group became and continues to be a vital part of enabling families to bond with a child who is dying. Later meetings incorporated various professionals to help the group in working through their feelings.

To enhance service provision to children who are HIV-positive and to bring consistency to decisions regarding medical care for all children under the legal guardianship of the commissioner, a Medical Review Board will begin work in 1990. This six-member interdisciplinary board will establish uniform policy and practice in HIV testing, experimental drug trials, isolations, immunizations and prophylactic treatments, autopsies, and other decisions with medical, legal, or ethical ramifications.

In addition to public child welfare responses to children and families, a number of private child welfare agencies have created specialized programs for children with HIV.

Best Nest (Philadelphia, Pennsylvania)

When Philadelphia was confronted with its first child identified as having AIDS and needing to be placed in a foster home or residence, no placement could be found. With support from Bethana, a 50-year-old child-care agency, a new agency was created—Best Nest—and recruitment of nurses and social workers to be foster parents for children with AIDS was begun. The prospective foster parents would be given a sufficient stipend for their foster parenting to be considered a full-time occupation. A Bethana board member recruited a nurse to be the first foster parent, and the first child was placed in November 1988; a second foster parent was recruited from Alaska and relocated to Pennsylvania. Recruitment was bolstered, paradoxically, by vocal community opposition to the proposed creation of a group home for three infants with AIDS. The ensuing publicity resulted in the recruitment of a number of foster parents, making the opening of a group home unnecessary.

In addition to placing children with AIDS, Best Nest found foster homes for infants born addicted to cocaine. Due to the severe medical problems of children with drug addiction and drug-related illnesses, the program has experienced five infant deaths. Consequently, an important part of this foster care program is a bereavement group for foster parents who know their child is dying or who have lost a foster child. There are special events for grieving foster parents, including planting trees on Arbor Day and the creation of a Children's Quilt. Foster parents have experienced emotionally wrenching experiences—such as when a biological parent insisted on all efforts being used to maintain her infant's life despite the great pain inflicted on the child. Planning with foster parents and support for foster parents by staff members and the support group are truly vital. With its expanded program, Best Nest has 30 children in placement; eight have AIDS.

Conclusion

Organized efforts in behalf of children with HIV have arisen in areas with the highest rates of infection but have, and will continue to, spread throughout the country. After programs begin, they often assume a variety of actions and educational and case management functions, resulting in their becoming small, multi-purpose agencies trying to provide a range of services for women and children. These pioneering efforts can act as encouragement for others; they demonstrate that it is possible to help these children and families. They are also examples to learn from, to copy, or to modify in accordance with local needs and resources. The next chapters describe a number of programs and the ways that these have evolved.

5

Caring for Children with AIDS in a Day Care Setting

CAROLYN LELYVELD

IN 1986, THE BRONX MUNICIPAL HOSPITAL CENTER (BMHC) IN NEW YORK City opened a day care center for children infected with the human immunodeficiency virus (HIV).[1] The task of planning for this population was complex, and the setting assured even at the beginning that the center was positioned to respond to the growing needs of the Bronx community. The project is funded by the New York City Health and Hospitals Corporation (HHC); BMHC is an HHC facility. Bronx Municipal Hospital and individual and corporate donors have provided additional resources to enhance the program. The center is licensed by the New York City Department of Health, Bureau of Child Care.

The center is housed in a renovated ward in Van Etten Hospital on the grounds of the Bronx Municipal Hospital Center and was designed to provide day care of a high standard for children from six months to seven years of age. The enrollment capacity is 25, consisting of a preschool group of 17 divided into two sub-groups, and an infant/toddler group of eight children. The center has been allowed complete freedom to invent and reinvent its program so that it can continue to respond adequately to the needs of the children and parents it serves.

When people learn that the center exists and what the staff mem-

---

[1] The center has a staff of 21. It is not possible to list them here by name, but each of them makes an essential contribution to the larger team effort.

bers have taken on as their daily work, they somehow expect that the center itself will reflect the unusual nature of the task, that it will be a depressing place. When they visit they are surprised by the liveliness of the center—it speaks best for itself. The walls are dotted with children's artwork and their own way of describing the life around them. A sheet of computer paper is posted each day to serve as the center's newspaper. This paper records the small and large triumphs of early learning: R. can write the first letter of his name; J. visited her mother in the hospital; E. went to visit big school today; L. bought his birthday in the store. Children are learning to read and write, but, more significantly, they are learning that what they think is important. The words they learn are words they have chosen for themselves.

A Typical Day

The school day can start as early as 7:30 A.M. when the first child is picked up by the school bus. The school day begins as soon as the children board the bus. The bus trip is made a part of the school day and necessary information is given to both shifts of bus escorts, who then move into the classrooms with the children because they also serve as teacher's aides. When children arrive at the center, they are met by their teachers, and the work of the day begins with each group meeting over a full, and sometimes hot, breakfast. These meetings are a time to encourage children to talk about anything on their minds. An activity period follows, which might mean a short painting or play dough exploration for the youngest children or a reading readiness activity for the preschool groups. In the latter, the meeting itself sparks off an activity that the group will use as its work for the morning, such as when the children decide to write a letter to a classmate who is in the hospital. These impromptu lessons are often more important than what had been planned.

A morning snack comes after the activities, and, if the weather permits, the children will go outside. If they must stay inside, each age group also has the use of an activity room outfitted with tumbling mats and climbing equipment. The groups then return to their rooms and prepare for lunch and nap time, which is followed by a snack and story or circle time—a children's meeting time. Some of the older children will skip the nap and use the library for individual math or reading activities. Attention is given to the needs of each child, including special nutrition and adequate rest. In general, the day proceeds like a normal day in a good day care center. This year the program was enriched by the participation of both a drama therapist and a music therapist.

Staff Members

The center is a team effort. The staff comprises a team of seven teachers under the supervision of the director. It also includes a medical director, a social worker who also functions as assistant director, a nurse, an office associate with significant responsibilities for dealing with hospital personnel and parents, housekeeping and dietary aides, two bus drivers, and the four bus escorts who serve as aides in the classrooms.

The school buses are essential to the life of the center. Few of the families have the means to bring their children to the center daily, and the children live throughout the Bronx. The buses transport children to school and home again and bring parents to the center; they are also used for group trips and for taking children to scheduled medical appointments. These buses are supplied with radios so that drivers can stay in contact with the center while on the road.

Initial Questions

Important questions were provoked by the plan for a day care program. It was not clear at the start, for example, whether grouping these children in a day care environment might compromise their health even further because of exposure to more infections. The center has formulated a number of procedures, however, that have adequately protected them. The nurse is not only available at all times, but she knows each child well and is sensitive to any change in a child's condition. This knowledge often enables her to detect minor changes and to prevent more serious developments. She examines each child weekly, reporting problems to the medical director. These procedures interfere as little as possible with the children's school day. No invasive procedures are allowed at the center except in emergencies; in fact, in the first three years of operation no such emergency has ever arisen.

Another question is raised continually by visitors to the center: How does the knowledge of the children's disease and their shorter life expectancies affect the program and the staff members? To sustain staff members, a variety of support strategies are necessary, ranging from group discussions over lunch to sessions with a psychiatrist. Originally it was difficult for staff members to understand how they would respond to the deaths of children either as individuals or as members of a group. In the three years that the center has been open, five children have died. It was hard at first to see whether the center would resemble a hospice or a school, but it is now clear that we are a school. For some of the children, we will be their only school. For others we will be just the first step; four have already gone off to public schools.

Working with Parents

The center has often been the first place where families can feel comfortable talking about AIDS. Both the biological families and foster families are often afraid to talk about AIDS because they fear discrimination. The center becomes like "home free all" in the game hide and seek. Families served by the center keep many secrets, which often leads them to lie and fabricate stories. One day in the group, some parents were discussing what they tell their neighbors when the bus pulls up. They all said that people got very excited when they knew there was a day care center that picked children up. One mother said that she told everyone that the center costs $125 a week; then she added that she always tells them the bus is extra. When the audience looks dumbfounded, she simply replies that she has her ways to raise such a large amount. Another mother says that her sister arranged everything for her; on her block, it is sufficient to say that it costs $145 a week; the bus still remains extra. These conversations started a group ritual—we keep a chair at our group meetings for the "noseybody," the person who is always on the verge of finding out.

We do not suggest that these secrets be kept, but we understand the difficulties that the families face in communities where knowledge might lead to discrimination and isolation. The center provides a place for these families to find anchor. Many have a number of regular agency appointments, necessary to maintain their welfare status or their ties with foster care agencies and for regular appointments for the children and their treatment. Some parents who are ill themselves have yet another set of appointments for their own treatment. The social worker and the nurse help them to link up with these other agencies.

Because these families lead complicated lives, we try to keep their relations with the center uncomplicated. The rules are kept simple, and the intake procedure, handled initially by the social worker, reflects this concern. It is important to enable the parents or caregivers to visit the center as soon as they feel they might want to enroll a child there. Often a parent requires some time to move from this initial phone call to the first visit. So much can happen between these two points! One parent lost her housing; another was hospitalized. It is hard for people to imagine what the center might be like. Parents have told us that they thought they would see something that resembled a hospital ward, filled with very sick children attached to intravenous lines. When we discovered this supposition, we revised our brochure so that it now shows children painting and building with blocks. A visit to the center reduces anxiety and replaces the parent's image of it with the picture of an active learning environment. This fact does not mean that the initial visit is easy; often it proves difficult for parents to see and understand that they have brought their child to a community of children united by the common denominator of the AIDS virus. Parents can feel that they are telling highly personal details of their lives when they discuss their child's diagnosis.

This first visit is made as comfortable as possible for parents and caregivers. The parent or caregiver and child are met by the social worker and the director and are taken on a tour of the center. Most of this first morning is spent in a room equipped as a small playroom, talking to the parent and describing the center and its activities to them. An informal assessment of the child is done through play. The parent is encouraged to ask questions, and the pace is slow. The meeting is not a formal fact-finding session; only the most basic information is taken. There is time for a longer interview when the child's medical papers are completed and the child is brought in to begin at the center. Although this information is important and would help us to understand this child and family, delaying it does allow a better exchange of information.

Two types of children have not received the medical clearance necessary to enter the program: one, a child who was too severely handicapped to participate in the program; the other, a child who had an active infection that would be contagious to other children.

At the end of the initial visit, when we determine what group seems appropriate, the child and the parent or caregiver are taken into the classroom for a brief visit to see what a part of the day is like. The director acts as guide, so that the classroom routine can be explained and the child can be introduced to the teachers by someone who has learned something about the child's strengths through playing with him or her. The visit enables the teachers to see the child in the group setting, and the mother or caregiver to learn some features of the classroom that make it easier to talk to the child when it is time to begin. It is much easier to be able to say, "We are going to the place where we played with the yellow school bus" or "where you played with water and made bubbles" than to speak of going to the center.

Food also plays a part in this early introduction to the center. As we walk down the hall to the room we will use for our meeting, we pass the kitchen, which has become central to the program. Coffee and tea are always available for visiting parents as well as staff members. There is often bread or cake, and parents are invited to help themselves, which conveys the message that they are invited to share the resources of the center. Because people with AIDS are so often made to feel like outcasts, concealing the fact that they have the disease frequently becomes a major preoccupation of their lives. At the center they can acknowledge their condition and still feel confident that they will be treated with respect. The kitchen delivers a strong message of concern; it functions, in essence, as a refuge. We have been fortunate to receive from private donors money that allows us to invite parents in for breakfast or lunch at the center. The staff members believe that it is important for families to be invited to school to see their child at work and to savor their child's experiencing normal learning and growth.

When this first visit is over, parents generally express surprise and relief. Nothing seems to prepare them adequately for what they have observed. They have seen the whole center and met a number of staff members; they have had the attention of both the director and the assistant director-social worker. We have talked together, admired the child together, eaten snacks together, and played. They have seen the classroom and the teachers' sensitive handling of their child, which focuses on the child's strengths rather than the disease. They have also seen children hugged and cuddled.

When a child is accepted by the program, the parent or caregiver usually spends a week at the center learning about us, meeting all the people who will help to care for the child and helping the child to ease into the program. Much of this week is spent with the child in the classroom, where teachers make it clear that they are asking for guidance from the parent or caregiver in what works best for this child. By the time that parents or caregivers meet either with the nurse to develop a fuller picture of the child's medical history, or with the social worker to complete the family history, they have had time to ask a good many questions themselves.

Dealing with Separations

This whole first experience is treated with enormous respect. It carries within it all the elements of initiation that are raised by entry to school. Many of our children are all too familiar with separation. Some were initially raised in hospitals, have faced adapting to and losing mothers, foster mothers, and homes. They have also lost siblings to AIDS or to placement in foster care, which is certainly sufficient reason to move both child and caregiver through their early days at the center with great concern. There is also a shadow over this early learning, this first chore of separating from a parent at school. We hope, when we work with children in other early childhood settings, that an early understanding of separation will be handled with solicitude as the child grows and gradually learns to trust people outside the home. What children at the center are helped to learn and build within themselves about trust is often tested too soon—when they are hospitalized, when they face a parent's hospitalization or death, or when in fact they face their own deaths.

In many ways this looking ahead is always a consideration present when a child begins at the center. The child's choice of a "transitional object" will be respected; it may be called into service again and again. In the progress of children toward autonomy and separation from parents, they will often choose some object that will both represent those early feelings of mother and stand in for her when she is not present. In this role, the blanket or teddy bear or cloth with mother's smell will represent both her and the loss of her. For the children at the center, that loss can be sudden and unplanned (when mother is hospitalized) or final (when she dies). Every support or strength a child has will be called upon to encourage the child's stability. After the death of her mother, one child brought her mother's woolen hat to school and kept it with her all day for comfort and a sense of continued connection.

Teaching these children the curriculum of early childhood remains essential, especially when it enhances their own ability to make and do and express their feelings. The power that independence brings is of enormous value. The children with mothers who are ill will be testing their newfound abilities with what is for them a final separation, the deaths of their mothers.

Some of these mothers and caregivers join the center's weekly support group meeting. Run jointly by the social worker and the director, the meetings have known good attendance and have been striking in the variety of concerns that are voiced. Beyond the ordinary concerns of parents about their children's eating habits, schooling, and toilet training, the meetings also provide a forum for struggling collectively with the complications of living with HIV infection. Aside from coping with "keeping the secret" (i.e., the necessity they feel to keep neighbors from knowing about the health crises in their families), the group discusses how to talk with children about topics such as illness, the deaths of friends and of parents, and even the child's own death. Most recently the group has talked much about moving the older children into public school. One of the parents asked if she could still come to the meetings after her child moved out of the program and was assured that she could come back to her chair whenever she wanted, that she was still in the group. The meetings have helped staff members understand the particularly complex issues and concerns of the group; staff members have often used what was learned to revise or change the center's procedures.

When a Parent Dies

Early in the author's first month as director at the center, the mother of one of the children died. The staff members decided to have a meeting in the preschool room to tell the children. We not only decided who would tell the children but how we would comfort particular children in the group who we knew would need the most help. We also knew that it was important to say that she had been very sick and that her child, their friend, was all right. Even with a plan, this was a difficult meeting. We made sure that the children had enough time in the circle, and then we asked if they would like to phone their friend. They lined up to take turns at the speakerphone in the classroom. One little boy asked her if her mother was dead; she said yes. Then he asked if she had been very sick. Again, she said yes. Next he asked if he was still her friend. She said yes. That was not the end of the questioning, and the entire staff knew that it needed to be ready for more such questions without warning.

When the parents' group met, they were told about the death. After a few minutes, the social worker and the author described in detail how the children were told, to the point of saying which teacher held each child. At this point, one of the mothers raised her hands to her face and said, "Not my child." She meant she did not want her child told. We spent the rest of that session and many more that followed explaining how we could not let people disappear without comment. These discussions roamed far and wide. Parents sometimes found themselves searching out their early childhood memories of death or thinking back on mourning that was not given space to happen. Later, when the mother who had covered her face experienced the death of her child, she came to the center the next day to be there when we told the children. She wanted to be where her child had been in life, and she wanted to allow the children to see that she was all right. She made a courageous journey.

Sustaining Staff Members

Support for the staff is crucial for maintaining morale at the center. Staff members are tested in a variety of ways. Their first task is to understand their own reactions to working with children who have a terminal disease. When the center first opened, the staff was given an extensive orientation that included numerous lectures on AIDS and its effects on children and families. Staff members joining the center more recently receive a basic introduction from the nurse and learn from her the precautions to take in working with children at the center. These are not complicated: rubber gloves when changing diapers, or when helping a child bleeding from an injury (a scraped knee or a bloody nose); washing hands frequently. They learn that wearing gloves is not a substitute for washing the hands—the center's protocol calls for washing the hands after gloves are removed. All staff members keep a pair of rubber gloves in their pockets to make sure that these will be easily available; people in early childhood programs should be able to go directly to the aid of a child without searching for supplies. Careful disposal of waste is also necessary.

Newspaper articles about AIDS are clipped daily so that staff members can keep in touch with recent developments. The nurse and the medical director are always available to answer questions. Every month the medical director comes to a staff meeting to answer staff questions about AIDS. For the past two years, the center has had help from a psychiatrist who has met with the staff weekly to discuss the rich but difficult work experiences at the center.

At meetings, we have considered how children understand death, how they react to the deaths of their friends and family members, and how they express their feelings about their own illnesses and their sense of diminishing energy. We also discuss the past week's trials and tribulations. How do we start work with a child who has been living in a hospital for three years and has never been outside? Can we keep a child in the classroom who is so weak that she needs to rest on the outskirts of the classroom and only get up for her favorite activity? Obviously, staff members have also had to examine their own feelings and those of co-workers. How long should staff people remain at the center? How can one learn to tell the difference between feeling the kinds of stress and sadness that accompany this work and feeling the unbearable stress that might signal one is giving more than one has? Some teachers have left this year, and each time someone leaves we all are forced in a most healthy way to reassess our feelings about the center.

The center should be a comfortable place to work, but the staff is faced with the impotence that is a natural part of working in this field. One kind of help is eliminating and reducing other sources of impotence. This year, the center has been working with a psychologist who observes and tests the children, and who has been helpful to teachers in developing individual teaching strategies for each child. Many children arrive with a range of developmental deficits and delays. They have emotional problems related to their illness and to the disruptive nature of their early lives, often characterized by institutionalization or loss of family members. Some children have neurological impairment related to AIDS and experience difficulty with motor function and cognition. The children also change both physically and emotionally as their disease progresses.

Money from the Children's Hope Foundation has enabled us to send emergency food home to families who, at the end of the month, often have little left. We select items that are easy to prepare and that children will eat. Very often we send food home to be cooked by a sick mother for her sick child. Donations of children's clothing from the hospital community enable us to send home clothes when needed.

The support strategies for staff members constantly change; we are always adding things that feel good. A friend asked how we are "able to maintain responsiveness without pathos, how we can remain cool without being overly matter-of-fact?" This is a hard but important question. As a group, we try to provide more society for one another than is usually required at work. We try to be together in less formal ways than just the organized support meetings or staff meetings. Two years ago, there was always a jigsaw puzzle going. This year our Thursday staff lunches were cooked in our own kitchen. Some staff members talk more easily when they are performing small tasks like sorting "Legos" or washing dishes than in formal settings; a certain closeness is necessary both for support and for communication. There is little warning when matters become difficult, when a child or mother becomes critically ill, or when a child has to be removed from home and placed in foster care. Good teaching must have some of the elements of good soccer playing: plans and strategies are necessary but one doesn't know when the ball will come one's way. The constant readiness to handle the most difficult problems does create tension, however, which can be lessened if we understand how staff members feel in their own lives.

The center's staff members are an unusually varied group. Most have chosen to be involved in community service work. For example, one had been in the Peace Corps, and another had worked with emotionally disturbed children. Each staff member brings experience in working with children. For some, there is an important connection between their work and their religious commitments; one, for instance, had been in a religious order, and another preaches regularly.

More and more it seems to be necessary to find staff members who have a rich life outside the center so that the often difficult, roller-coaster days can be balanced by something more reliable. The center itself must include within its procedures opportunities for teaching staff members to step outside the classroom and relieve the pressure. Each room is given some choice in planning and varying the hour that staff members arrive, as long as coverage is good. Sometimes a day working away from the center or visiting other programs is necessary. Sometimes it is important to know when someone needs "out" to clean a closet or wash toys—to be by oneself.

The most significant development in the evolution of this day care program is that it has become a center for families. The array of problems concerning housing, public assistance, adequate home care, agency red tape, and the strain on family relationships in households with AIDS, give rise to many needs for all types of support. The assistant director is available to all family members for individual counseling and assistance; she is also available for individual play therapy with children. These sessions have been extremely important to children who come to the center with complex emotional problems as well as for children who need help as they face the death of a parent or sibling. This year, for the first time, the center had a social work student who assisted in this task, supervised by the social worker.

It has been the day care center's policy, albeit taxing at times, to accommodate scheduled visitors and to make staff members available to answer questions. Since it is a new service arena, the center has experienced visits from a large number and wide range of groups making plans for children who are HIV positive. Some members of the staff have participated in conferences on children with AIDS or have spoken to professional groups about their work.

Conclusion

There is a bittersweet feeling that always accompanies bringing another child into our group. We are pleased to make the center available to another child and family because that is why the center is here, but that feeling is coupled with great sadness at facing another life or group of lives that have been foreshortened. Once a child is accepted, the staff understands that the center will hold that child until the child is ready to go off to school. If a child becomes seriously ill, we are committed to hold that child for as long as it makes sense for that child and for the children at the center. This policy has often been difficult for staff members, but when we invest so much in getting to know a child and discovering the child's learning style, we should not let go when we are needed most.

Each time it is necessary to decide about separating a child from the center there is a long discussion, and the effect on the center as a whole is carefully weighed. Although it is never demanded of them, teachers have worked with their children not only in the classroom but when they became very ill in the emergency room, on the ward in the hospital, and in the hospital's intensive care unit. Their devotion to the children is remarkable. Very often mothers will ask early in the process of getting to know the center if the children graduate in caps and gowns. This poignant question imparts an even greater sense of how precious these early years are for these children and their mothers. Through working with children with AIDS, we have all developed a reverence for learning and growth.

6

Supporting Families Caring for Children with HIV Infection

MARY G. BOLAND

THE CHILDREN'S HOSPITAL AIDS PROGRAM (CHAP), OF CHILDREN'S HOS-
pital of New Jersey (CHNJ), has provided care for children and their
families since the first cases of HIV infection were treated at the institution in 1981. Although HIV infection may present as an acute process, it
also manifests with a spectrum of symptoms from mild to severe. The
majority of children acquire the infection perinatally. Mothers have a
history of intravenous drug use or were the sexual partners of drug
users. The families in the program are involved with multiple agencies
and suffer from poverty, inadequate housing, and poor or inadequate
health care. To be successful in reaching these families and serving the
children, CHAP had to move beyond the traditional hospital boundaries.

As the number of infected children increased, it became obvious
that care based on the traditional medical model would be inadequate.
HIV infection is a chronic illness with biological, behavioral, and social
manifestations for the entire family, which must be considered when
planning services for the child. Although the program grew informally
at first, a chronic illness model of care was adopted, and CHAP emerged
as a comprehensive program with a point of view that care must be
community-based, child-centered, family-focused, comprehensive, and
coordinated. The goals established for the program are described in
Table 1.

Table 1

Goals and Strategies of a Multidisciplinary Treatment Program

Treat the illness/symptoms of HIV infection:
  Prevent/treat infections
  Monitor growth and development
  Provide nutritional support
  Treat chronic lung disease
  Provide antiviral therapy

Prevent the disease process and treatment regimen from interfering with the development of the child:
  Provide parents with information on the effect of illness on development
  Provide periodic comprehensive evaluation of development
  Provide therapeutic intervention when delays are identified
  Provide access to appropriate educational services
  Help the child to cope with and understand the illness at an age-appropriate level

Prevent the disease process and treatment regimen from disrupting the family unit:
  Help the family to understand and manage the illness
  Teach parents their rights within the system
  Assist parents to identify and use resources
  Provide grief/bereavement support when needed
  Help parents to meet the needs of all family members
  Support the efforts of the family to focus on continuing their lives

The CHAP program provides service on a continuum-of-care model. Children receive coordinated service from a consistent team of physicians, nurses, and social workers and have access to all forms of care, including ambulatory, inpatient, home health, psychosocial, and psychiatric, legal and financial assistance, and, as appropriate, home-based hospice service and residential placement. Since the child's family members may be HIV-infected, the entire family must be considered when planning services to the child. To meet the program's goals, the multidisciplinary team provides care from the time of testing/diagnosis in both acute and ambulatory settings and in the home, using a case-management approach. Parents are considered an integral part of the team and are encouraged to participate in decision making at all stages of the illness, including decisions about resuscitation efforts. Through CHNJ, families have access to the full range of medical subspecialists and ancillary services, as well as an early intervention program and specialized day care center. Each family is helped to find a primary care provider in the community, if they do not already have one.

Since many children and families are under the supervision of child protective services, a formal relationship has been developed for maximizing collaboration between the human services and health care delivery systems. The CHAP staff maintains close communication with community-based services available to families, such as community nursing services, hospice care, home care vendors, and social service agencies. These services have enabled families to keep children at home even in terminal stages of the illness or when "high tech" interventions were needed.

Since 1984, CHAP has worked with 250 HIV-infected children. By including families in making decisions about their children and fostering mutual trust and respect, the families acquire the knowledge and services necessary to cope with this devastating illness. Despite obvious difficulties in working with this hard-to-reach population, no child has ever been lost to follow-up; parents may miss appointments, move away, or disappear for short periods, but eventually they will contact someone from CHAP and reestablish the relationship.

Family Involvement

The CHAP goal of minimizing the disruption that illness causes in a family provides a focus for helping families to choose treatment options throughout the course of the illness. Counseling sessions with families of newly diagnosed children provide basic knowledge about the disease and its management while providing families with a safe, nonjudgmental setting for asking questions and expressing feelings. The same information must often be repeated a number of times before parents master it. Mothers often learn of their own infection for the first time when they learn their child's diagnosis. Coming to terms with the diagnosis of HIV infection requires time for individuals and families to deal with alternating periods of disbelief and denial, as well as anxiety and guilt. A variety of techniques, including the development of printed and video information, are used to help caregivers deal with the diagnosis. Because of the stigma associated with AIDS and HIV infection, families frequently do not tell the diagnosis to extended family members or friends. CHAP often provides the only place where families feel comfortable about openly discussing their child's illness.

Families actively participate in making decisions throughout the course of the child's illness. Open, honest communication with consistent care providers helps to establish trust between the family and the CHAP team. Formal and informal parent and staff conferences, initiated by either, discuss diagnosis, prognosis, and treatment options.

CHAP is involved in research related to the management and treatment of HIV infection, and the distinction between research and care is not always clear to parents and guardians. Parents are informed of all research efforts through informal staff interaction, meetings, and a written newsletter. Program staff members involved in research are separate from the case managers and those providing direct medical care. The separation of these functions helps parents to understand the distinction between research and care. A particular effort is made to explain the implications of participation in research and to obtain informed consent. Parents are assured that a decision not to participate in research will not affect the care of their child, which is particularly important because many poor people of color distrust and fear experimentation by institutions that have a history of insensitivity to them.

During the terminal stages of the disease, the relationship between the family and the CHAP team becomes crucial for decisions about treatment options. In a retrospective study of 35 children who died, families and health care providers were in agreement about the plan of care in the majority of the cases. Seven children received care at home until they died, and seven others received palliative care while hospitalized. The majority of families wanted the child to receive the maximum care possible, including life-support devices [Rudolph 1988]. Offering families options supports the parents' need for control. Sensitivity to the wishes of the family and the availability of services to support the family's choices can help families to cope during this difficult period.

Case Management

CHAP defines case management as a proactive system through which assessment, planning, procurement, delivery, coordination, and monitoring of services take place. A nurse-social worker team provides case management for a designated group of children. The majority of service delivery is ambulatory and community-based. The delivery of specific health care services is separate and distinct from case management. Although a nurse or social worker may provide both types of services, the case-management responsibilities are clearly distinguishable. The case-management team is responsible for assuring delivery of services throughout the course of the child's illness and is assisted by other providers within CHAP and the community.

The case managers make home visits to families as needed, targeted especially to families new to the program and families in periods of transition, such as hospital discharge. The case managers work closely with the families and community health care agencies to facilitate the delivery of quality nursing care to the children and support to the families. With the assistance of the CHAP staff and community nursing services, many families have cared, at home, for children who require oxygen, hyperalimentation, intravenous gamma globulin, intravenous antibiotics, and other treatments.

Structure

The CHAP approach to HIV infection has four distinct components, outlined in Table 2: direct care, education, research, and advocacy.

Table 2

Children's Hospitals AIDS Program

Direct care:
  Comprehensive, family-focused, child-centered, community-based

Education:
  Child, family
  Health care providers
  Community

Research:
  Medical treatment (supportive, clinical trials)
  Nursing
  Psychosocial

Advocacy:
  Lay and professional community
  AIDS service organizations
  State and federal governments
  Public policy (funding, legislation, antidiscrimination)

Direct care provides the foundation for the program and serves as the focus for other activities. When a young patient is hospitalized, the child is admitted under the care of CHAP physicians, who provide inpatient medical management in collaboration with the house staff. There is no designated AIDS unit; children are placed on the various units as determined by their need for nursing care. Universal precautions are maintained, and the children can participate in all hospital activities, including the playroom and schoolroom. The clinical nurse specialist works closely with the family and case managers to assure discharge planning and continuity of services from hospital to home. HIV-related illness accounts for approximately 10 percent of all admissions to the hospital.

Ambulatory services are provided for children in clinics organized to facilitate quality health care and continuity of services. One clinic session serves children and families who are being tested for HIV infection. Counseling begins with the initial phone contact to the nurse. Intensive post-test counseling is done by members of the team, two of whom meet with the family to explain HIV results and to begin teaching and counseling. Once the guardian has been told the child is infected, case management is initiated. Particular care is taken to protect client confidentiality and to respect a family's wishes as to what and how the child is to be told concerning his or her HIV status.

In another clinic session, symptomatic HIV-positive children receive outpatient treatment, which may include infusion of intravenous gamma globulin. Each child is examined by the physician or nurse practitioner and seen by the social worker. Children are also regularly evaluated by the neurologist, nutritionist, speech pathologist, and child development specialist. Consultation with other medical subspecialists is also available. The ambulatory nurse coordinator maintains a tracking system for each child to be sure that appropriate baseline and follow-up lab work, x-rays, and CAT scans, as well as consultations, are arranged.

The management of each patient is discussed at a multidisciplinary team meeting held at the end of each clinic. Children who fail to keep the scheduled appointment are also discussed, and a plan for contact and follow-up is developed.

CHAP is involved in many activities related to HIV infection, including education of health providers, and is designated as the National Pediatric HIV Resource Center by the Bureau of Maternal and Child Health and Resource Development. These activities encourage the use of a comprehensive chronic illness approach to care, as well as supporting advocacy for children and families at both a local and a national level. In cooperation with the New Jersey Department of Health, and supported by a Pediatric AIDS Demonstration Project grant, CHAP is assisting in the development of a statewide network of regionalized pediatric HIV centers throughout New Jersey.

The complete CHAP program is charted in Figure 1.

Community-Based Services

To facilitate community-based care for HIV-infected children and their families, the CHAP team has established working relationships with a broad range of community agencies. Before diagnosis, the State Child Protective Services Agency, New Jersey Department of Human Services, Division of Youth and Family Services (DYFS), was involved with many of the families. Approximately 50 percent of these children are in some type of foster care placement, often with an extended family member.

A task force of DYFS workers identified access to generic and specialized social services for HIV-infected children and their families as the major obstacle to fulfilling their casework responsibilities. Because of the limited amount of time that child welfare workers have to spend on individual cases and the extensive amount of time many HIV-positive families require, workers were asking for assistance. Four major issues were set forth: *(1)* the responsibilities of direct service staff members, *(2)* testing and confidentiality, *(3)* custody, and *(4)* the responsibilities of collateral agencies to provide services to HIV-infected children and families [Boland 1988]. The findings and recommendations of the task force resulted in a suggested continuum of child welfare and pediatric services developed by Ted Allen, the DYFS regional administrator (Table 3), which began as a collaborative effort between DYFS and CHAP. Each agency recognized that HIV infection is a medical and social problem requiring specialized services that demand a high level of expertise and knowledge. Since 1987, CHAP has contracted with DYFS to serve as a resource and to assist in the development of pediatric HIV/AIDS services, including access to physicians, nurses, and social workers experienced in the care of children with HIV infection; training and education; medical consultation; and the identification of health-related or specialized social services. In 1988, the contract was expanded to provide health and social work services to a DYFS-supported day care center for symptomatic HIV-infected children who cannot be mainstreamed.

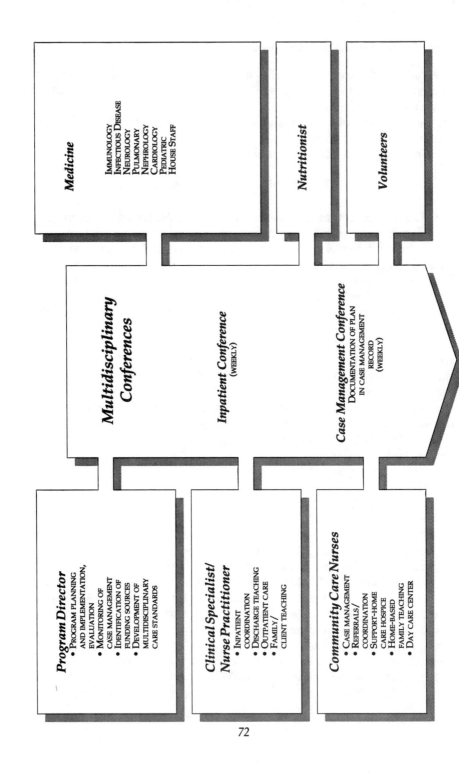

Medicine

IMMUNOLOGY
INFECTIOUS DISEASE
NEUROLOGY
PULMONARY
NEPHROLOGY
CARDIOLOGY
PEDIATRIC
HOUSE STAFF

Nutritionist

Volunteers

**Multidisciplinary
Conferences**

Inpatient Conference
(WEEKLY)

Case Management Conference
DOCUMENTATION OF PLAN
IN CASE MANAGEMENT
RECORD
(WEEKLY)

Program Director
• PROGRAM PLANNING
AND IMPLEMENTATION,
EVALUATION
• MONITORING OF
CASE MANAGEMENT
• IDENTIFICATION OF
FUNDING SOURCES
• DEVELOPMENT OF
MULTIDISCIPLINARY
CARE STANDARDS

**Clinical Specialist/
Nurse Practitioner**
• INPATIENT
COORDINATION
• DISCHARGE TEACHING
• OUTPATIENT CARE
• FAMILY/
CLIENT TEACHING

Community Care Nurses
• CASE MANAGEMENT
• REFERRALS/
COORDINATION
• SUPPORT-HOME
CARE HOSPICE
• HOME-BASED
FAMILY TEACHING
• DAY CARE CENTER

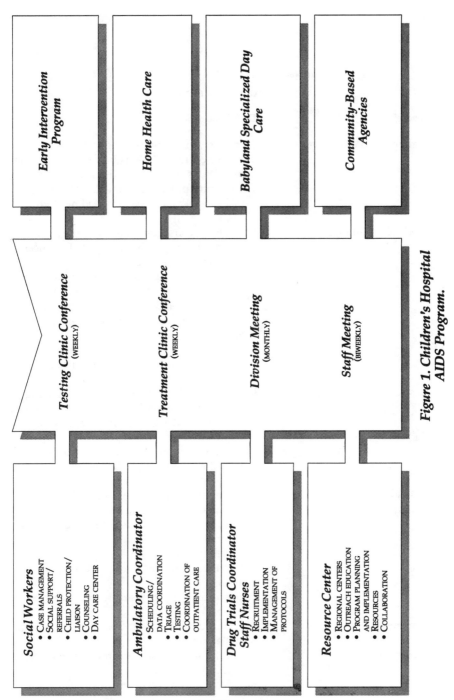

Social Workers
- CASE MANAGEMENT
- SOCIAL SUPPORT/
  REFERRALS
- CHILD PROTECTION/
  LIAISON
- COUNSELING
- DAY CARE CENTER

Ambulatory Coordinator
- SCHEDULING/
  DATA COORDINATION
- TRIAGE
- TESTING
- COORDINATION OF
  OUTPATIENT CARE

**Drug Trials Coordinator
Staff Nurses**
- RECRUITMENT
- IMPLEMENTATION
- MANAGEMENT OF
  PROTOCOLS

Resource Center
- REGIONAL CENTERS
- OUTREACH EDUCATION
- PROGRAM PLANNING
  AND IMPLEMENTATION
- RESOURCES
- COLLABORATION

Testing Clinic Conference
(WEEKLY)

Treatment Clinic Conference
(WEEKLY)

Division Meeting
(MONTHLY)

Staff Meeting
(BIWEEKLY)

*Early Intervention
Program*

Home Health Care

*Babyland Specialized Day
Care*

*Community-Based
Agencies*

*Figure 1. Children's Hospital
AIDS Program.*

73

Table 3

Continuum of Essential Services for HIV-Infected Children and Their Families

Types of Service	Description of Services
Training and education	Protective service workers: general facts; modes of transmission and safeguards; case practice issues (when and where to get help) Community providers: same as above plus assistance that can be provided by state agency
Medical consultation	Emergency consultation: understand diagnosis, prognosis, and related medical and social service needs Regular case consultation: assistance in making decisions based on facts (such as when to test siblings) and ensuring that proper services (for example, visiting nurse, home health aides) are provided Medical case monitoring: regular reviews (for example, quarterly) to ensure consistency of medical and social service plan
Case advocacy	Individual: helping to arrange homemaking and transportation, and coordinating income assistance; advocating with agencies for client services Program development: where service is not available, work with state agency and community to develop
Individual and group supports	Information groups: for protective service workers and biological and foster parents (such as what agency is available and is able to provide services) Counseling groups: address significant emotional concerns (such as death and dying) Policy forum: update workers and receive feedback
Homemaking	Specialized homemaker: training in care, plus higher remuneration
Transportation	Medical transportation: to and from medical appointment Regular: visiting and so on

Table 3

Continuum of Essential Services for HIV-Infected Children and Their Families

Types of Service	*Description of Services*
Placement	Placements with relatives: most desired Foster care: emergency, regular, and respite Group home: Short-term, family-like, awaiting placement with relatives or foster parents

In addition to the essential social services listed, many other services are helpful.

Reprinted with permission from Boland, M., Allen, T., Long, G., Tasker, M., "Children with HIV infection: Collaborative responsibilities of the child welfare and medical communities." Social Work 36 (6) (November-December 1988): 504–509.

A number of children followed by CHAP receive case-management services through county-based case-management units of the Special Child Health Services (SCHS), New Jersey Department of Health, serving chronically ill children. Ongoing consultation between SCHS case managers, CHAP staff members, and the families ensures that needed services are made available to families without duplication of efforts. This service is especially useful for children outside the Newark area because the county-based case managers are knowledgeable about available community services and provide a bridge between CHAP and the home.

Children and families often receive services from visiting nurse agencies, hospice, mental health centers, and agencies providing support to persons with AIDS. CHAP makes a concerted effort to inform other agencies and has invited them to attend case-management meetings but has found that participation is minimal. When staff members from other agencies attend, however, they report that it was helpful to meet with others providing services to the families.

Summary

The HIV epidemic has been much discussed both in the public policy arena and the media. Although it is impossible to predict the extent of the HIV epidemic, it is clear that the inner-city communities, such as Newark, have yet to feel its full effect. Devastated urban communities already struggling with crime, violence, widespread drug use, and inadequate health care resources are now dealing with an epidemic of tragic proportions that will weaken if not destroy an entire generation.

The use of a family-focused, community-based model for the care of children with HIV infection has proved to be an effective approach to their care. CHAP staff members develop relationships with families that have resulted in increased utilization of ambulatory services, compliance with health care appointments, and a decreased level of inappropriate and prolonged hospitalizations.

The challenge for programs serving persons with HIV infection, such as CHAP, is to deliver comprehensive care in an existing health care environment that promotes fragmentation and competition, where those most in need of care are least able to obtain it. CHAP is able to provide comprehensive service through a patchwork of grants that support various program activities. In the absence of such support, the program would cease to exist and families would be forced to rely on the traditional medical model, because existing reimbursement mechanisms do not support a comprehensive approach to care. Despite public attention to HIV and numerous reports and policy recommendations, little responsive action has facilitated guaranteed access to care or support for service delivery.

Advances in both supportive and symptomatic treatment will continue to improve prognosis and lengthen the life span of infected children. As a consequence, the familial and social concerns will provide the greater challenge, since the societal conditions that support the epidemic of HIV infection defy easy solution.

REFERENCES

Boland, M., Allen, T., Long, G., Tasker, M. "Children with HIV infection: Collaborative responsibilities of the child welfare and medical communities." Social Work 33 (6) (November–December 1988): 504–509.

Rudolph, P., Boland, M., Connor, E., Evans, P. Children with AIDS: Acute Care at the Terminal Stage. Presented at the IV International Conference on AIDS, Stockholm, Sweden, June 1988.

7

The Development of an Early Intervention Model for HIV-Infected Women and Their Infants

TONI CABAT[1]

MODELS OF INTERVENTION FOR HUMAN IMMUNODEFICIENCY VIRUS (HIV)-infected infants and children have moved from biopsychosocial management of the acutely and terminally ill to case finding through aggressive community education and outreach aimed at early identification. The initial reports of HIV infection and acquired immune deficiency syndrome (AIDS) in the pediatric population were brought to the attention of the health care and child welfare community once children displayed symptoms and signs of HIV infection; many of these children fulfilled the initially established Centers for Disease Control (CDC) criteria for AIDS or AIDS-related complex (ARC) [CDC 1985]. These classifications

[1] The author would like to thank Arye Rubinstein, M.D., Albert Einstein College of Medicine; Anne Willoughby, M.D., National Institute of Child Health and Human Development (Contract NO1-HD-8-2913); James J. Goedert, M.D., National Cancer Institute; Paul Jellinek, Ph.D., Robert Wood Johnson Foundation (Grant 10810); Elaine Erhlich, M.S.W., New York State Department of Health, AIDS Institute (Contract CO-03620); Phyllis Gurdin, M.S.W., and Monte Gray, M.S.W., Leake and Watts Children's Home, Inc., for the support they offered in the development of this early intervention model; special thanks are extended to the Albert Einstein College of Medicine AIDS Team and secretarial staff for contributing in every way possible.

have since been revised by CDC [1987]. Infants and children were often diagnosed during hospitalization or through an extensive evaluation when a physician was suspicious of the etiology of the presenting symptoms. Many of these children were in foster care, and biological family history was absent or limited. The models of interventions developed by major medical centers around the country, where pediatric HIV infection was on the rise, responded to infants or children largely infected perinatally. These models (see Figure 1) were interdisciplinary

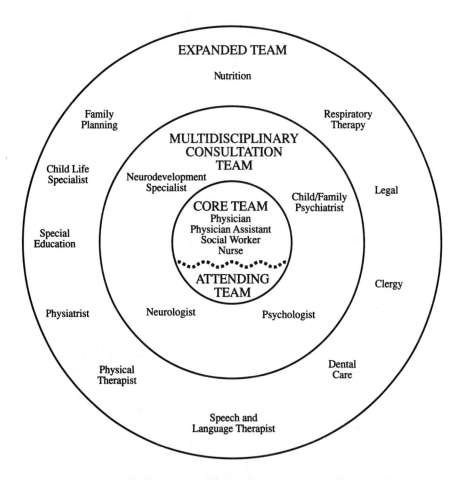

Figure 1. Interdisciplinary Model for Care of Pediatric AIDS.

in nature [Cabat 1988; Cohen 1986]. They included physicians, (pediatricians, immunologists, infectious disease specialists), social workers, nurses, and a neurological/neurodevelopmental component addressing the reported high incidence of developmental delay [Ultman 1987]. These infants and children were infected perinatally as a result of their mothers' infection, caused by intravenous drug use (shared infected needles) or heterosexual transmission from an HIV-infected partner. The models of intervention therefore were family-oriented, with expertise in assisting substance abusing family systems.

Background

With the encouragement of federal agencies, research scientists were interested in developing a data bank and a specimen pool of blood samples from pregnant women at risk for HIV infection and from their offspring after birth. A prospective study would shed further light on the routes of transmission and the outcome for women and infants. In 1987, a study designed by the National Cancer Institute (NCI) and National Institute of Child Health and Human Development (NICHD), under the National Institutes of Health (NIH), in contract with the Division of Allergy and Immunology at Albert Einstein College of Medicine (AECOM), Yeshiva University (Bronx, New York), enrolled pregnant women at risk for HIV infection. Two target populations were sought: *(1)* HIV-infected pregnant women, and *(2)* pregnant women at high risk for HIV infection who tested HIV-seronegative upon enrollment. The initial commitment was for a two-year postpartum follow-up. A study of this nature would result in moving clinicians from initiating treatment/interventions when young patients were frequently at an advanced disease stage, to prevention of opportunistic infections because infants at risk would be identified by the mother's status.

The study would offer free of charge to high-risk pregnant women *(a)* pre- and post-HIV test counseling, with on-site HIV test laboratory facilities to ensure testing procedures, and *(b)* obstetrical care and two-year postpartum enrollment for adult (women) and pediatric immunological assessment and medical care. Enrollment, with informed consent, included: *(1)* a 32-page questionnaire on basic epidemiological data, health status, pregnancy history, drug, alcohol, and tobacco history, and sexual practices; *(2)* a brief eight-month pregnancy questionnaire on drug, tobacco, alcohol data, and sexual practices; and *(3)* three or four scheduled examinations and blood sample collections during pregnancy and subsequent second, sixth, twelfth, eighteenth, and twenty-fourth months postpartum for the women. Women who opted for abortion followed the same schedule. Infants were seen monthly for the first six months and every three months thereafter until the eighteenth month, and then again at the twenty-fourth month for the final examination. Within one year, the study was extended to provide data points for four years postpartum for women and infants; a neurological and neurodevelopmental component for the infants was also incorporated. After the twenty-fourth month, both women and infants were seen every six months until four years postpartum.

Federal funds allowed the medical college to offer obstetrical, epidemiological, immunological, neurological, neurodevelopmental, nursing, and laboratory services; study coordination and administration were provided by a master-level social worker.

The research scientists' interest in obtaining data regarding perinatal transmission coincided with increasing rates of perinatal transmission nationwide. On January 6, 1986, CDC reported 229 pediatric AIDS cases; on January 5, 1987, 410 cases were reported. (A steady increase of 44 to 45 percent has been reported annually; 1,346 cases were reported by January 1989.)

New York City has led the nation in CDC-defined pediatric AIDS cases. The Bronx, where AECOM is located, fluctuates between the highest and the second highest borough for CDC-defined pediatric AIDS; 30 percent of all New York City-reported cases live in the Bronx. In November/December 1987, a NYC/NYS Department of Health Study of 19,157 newborns revealed that one of 61 were HIV-seropositive in New York City; one of 43 were seropositive in the Bronx [Lambert 1988]. At the same time, women were being diagnosed at an increasing rate; in New York City the leading cause of death for women 25 to 34 years old is AIDS. Whereas in the early 1980s most HIV-infected women who used the immunology facilities affiliated with AECOM reported a history of intravenous drug use, by the late 1980s as many as 40 percent of the HIV-infected women reported no history of intravenous drug use but reported heterosexual transmission as their risk factor.

With the impetus of research inquiry and the social alarm regarding perinatal transmission, an early intervention model was developed at AECOM. Early intervention would allow clinicians to treat prophylactically and give the support staff an opportunity to offer counseling before onset of the devastating disease process. Drug trials were not available to adults or children when this model was developed.

Initial Phase

The initial phase of program development involved the integration of research, clinical management, and psychosocial components, which allowed for complementary funding. The Robert Wood Johnson Foundation, in July 1986, awarded a three-year demonstration project grant to AECOM to develop a comprehensive AIDS Family Care Center; this grant provided support for physicians, social worker/administrator, nursing, and secretarial services. Since 1984, the AIDS Institute of the New York State Department of Health has funded a pediatric community service project that includes physicians, social workers, nurse/health educators, and administrative support.

These principal funding sources and the NIH-NICHD research funding provided the financial assistance, technical assistance, and direction to our early phase of development. The partnership of public and private sector supports is essential for such project development, since no single source has sufficient funding or scope to provide all of the initial elements for program development; as this project grew in size and scope, it became clear that these three significant sources of support and guidance were not sufficient.

Outreach and Inter-Agency Collaboration

To intervene before the presentation of symptomatology for the purposes of gathering valuable prenatal data, increasing compliance with prenatal care, and stabilizing the family system prior to the onset of disease manifestation, it is necessary for the program to establish outreach methodology via inter-agency collaboration. Within the AECOM community there were several vectors of services to pregnant women at high risk for HIV infection. The two principal vectors were the Department of Obstetrics and Gynecology (OB/GYN) and the Division of Substance Abuse. The Department of OB/GYN, through its affiliate contracts, delivered 10,052 pregnant women in 1988. The municipal hospital serves primarily the indigent minority community, where there is a significant incidence of intravenous drug use. The Division of Substance Abuse is the second largest methadone maintenance program in New York City, with seven clinics throughout the borough serving 2,800 clients, of whom 800 are women; approximately 1,200 children under 18 are identified with this client population. The seroprevalence rates among intravenous drug users in New York City range from 30 to 60 percent.

Outreach services in collaboration with these two departments/divisions were initiated through the exchange or complement of services with mutual funding of projects. The Department of OB/GYN established a specialized clinic to receive referrals from a central prenatal screening clinic. An interdepartmental interdisciplinary team comprising obstetricians, a nurse, an epidemiologist, and a social worker/administrator was established to offer pre- and post-HIV test counseling, risk reduction counseling, crisis intervention, and obstetrical care and to gather study data and specimens. Pregnant women at risk for HIV infection were offered culturally sensitive HIV information, literature, and the opportunity for on-site confidential HIV screening. The initial referrals were primarily asymptomatic women.

This was a somewhat controversial aspect of the project in early 1987, since no drug treatment trials were available. We could test but not provide active intervention. The mental health community also feared that test results would lead pregnant women diagnosed as seropositive into a psychiatric crisis. There was little previous literature or experience of HIV counseling with pregnant women. It was clear that the HIV counseling staff must have a level of comfort in (1) how they would impart diagnosis, and (2) the medical and psychosocial supports they and their clients would need following diagnosis of HIV status. The staff must also believe that early diagnosis would improve outcome through preventive medical care and early access to newly developing drugs and other interventions.

This point must be emphasized because the early intervention team members must serve both as a support to clients during the crisis of HIV diagnosis and as a support to other health care professionals, who will be identifying clients at risk and making the necessary referrals. This team is pivotal in the development of an early-intervention model.

Building and sustaining the team are essential elements of outreach and collaboration. Each member must know the others' areas of expertise and rely upon the collective strength of team membership. No one team member can carry the burden of outreach and HIV test counseling. It is best if HIV test counseling is provided by two team members simultaneously; if this method is not possible, the two functions should be shared and reinforced by all team members.

One major meeting of all key Division of Substance Abuse personnel was organized in order to establish a referral procedure based upon mutual trust. The Division of Allergy and Immunology followed with an on-site field visit to each of the seven clinics throughout the borough. This approach enabled each division to experience each other's particular area and all of its ramifications, as well as to establish personal connections among representatives of the various divisions to ensure commitment to follow-up. For all child-bearing women and pregnant women at risk a referral mechanism was established that featured, once again, (1) one-site pre-HIV test counseling and sample collection, (2) highly skilled team intervention in terms of post-HIV test counseling, and (3) immunological and psychosocial follow-up for all HIV-positive women. Pregnant women were offered enrollment in the perinatal study.

Middle Phase

The middle phase of the development of an early intervention model is represented by the establishment of an ongoing clinical setting conducive to family participation, since timely care to women and infants in the community is the principal psychosocial goal. The second goal is reducing foster care placement of children because of parental abandonment or death. The setting's receptivity toward the HIV-infected family dyad or triad must be continually demonstrated and reinforced, concretely and symbolically, by all team members. It should be clearly recognized at the outset that parents are anxious about attending a clinical setting for fear of confirming the diagnosis for themselves and their infants, of being identified in the community as HIV-seropositive, and of confronting deterioration. Avoidance of clinical visits is often related to the level of anxiety regarding acknowledgment of the diagnosis, previous negative experiences with the health care and social service systems, and a different time orientation and perspective. Bonding with health care professionals is essential in altering families' perspectives and obtaining compliance with medical care and intervention.

To combat the avoidance that many families display early in the process of diagnosis, the program must demonstrate the tenacity and concern of health care professionals. Repeated one-to-one contact with families via telephone, letters, and home visits, where possible, is one way; many families have never experienced this kind of reaching out in the past from traditional health care facilities. The setting that they confront once they attend clinic should offer a blend of professional competence and human acceptance by (1) welcoming patients warmly and informally; (2) providing breakfast snacks for morning clinics or light lunch snacks for afternoon sessions; (3) augmenting the staff with a dependable volunteer program that assists families in registration, oversees distribution of snacks, and provides babysitting and play activities while parents attend to their medical appointment; and (4) by arranging for staff members and families to celebrate holidays and milestones together, reducing impediments erected by differences in lifestyle and social status.

To achieve this milieu, the health care community finds itself appealing to a divergent group of local religious and community organizations; they are willing and interested in contributing food, toys, and gifts: this is an opportunity for expressions of concern and support for HIV-infected families from the community. Specific AIDS-related organizations are available to provide trained volunteers. Volunteerism has been resurrected with the onset of AIDS; changes in society have relegated the traditional hospital candystriper to the wayside. Women, students, and the aged are no longer available to volunteer, especially at facilities in high-crime areas. The AIDS-related volunteer organizations in most major cities throughout the United States have found new pools of volunteers that include minorities and working adults committed to assisting innovatively in the AIDS crisis. A unique bond develops between families, including young children, and the volunteers who faithfully staff the clinics. The families understand the meaning of volunteerism and will often confide their anxieties and fears to volunteers, who must be free to tell the health care providers about the families' concerns and to learn appropriate responses.

The overall goal of acceptance is reinforced when staff members, families, volunteers, and, at times, community organization members join in celebrating holidays and milestones. Clinic attendance is optimal with good weather conditions and at holiday times. It is not only the receiving of Christmas gifts, flowers for Valentine's Day, or Easter baskets, but the opportunity for an expression of happiness while confronting the sadness of ill health. Physicians, nurses, and social workers are no longer viewed only as pronouncing diagnosis and inflicting pain related to testing, but as people celebrating the birthdays of young families, who should be celebrating life rather than facing chronic illness and death.

Compliance should also be sought through (1) understanding a difference in time orientation between nonworking families and the medical community, (2) rewards for attending clinic, and (3) constant reminders of appointments directly and through collaterals. Future versus present-time orientation is a major obstacle to compliance. The health care system has a future-oriented perspective; appointments are scheduled weeks or months in advance. Health care professionals come from a social milieu where their lives are scheduled well in advance. Clinics begin at eight or nine A.M. Our HIV-infected families function on a more present-oriented time frame; they don't have the resources to plan for the future. All families have infants, and many have school-age children; most travel by public transportation. Those who work or must be home early for young school-age children are scheduled for the early appointments; the remainder don't arrive until 10 A.M. or so. The staff is understanding, but limits have to be set if we are to accomplish many goals.

The clinic combines all health care specialties, to minimize the number of visits for the families and to reinforce the health care plan. Mothers and infants are seen at the same visit by the immunologist; the infant or child receives most of the neurological and neurodevelopmental testing at the same time. Support staff members are available for crisis counseling, risk reduction counseling, concrete services, and collateral referrals. Provision for transportation is essential in order to help families keep appointments. Public transportation or cab fare is sufficient when family members are healthy; once they experience deterioration, additional assistance in arranging transportation is required.

Collaboration with Children's Service Agencies

In 1984, the health care community was confronted with the boarder-baby crisis in New York City. When perinatally transmitted HIV infection was identified and the number of infants born with evidence of illegal drugs in their systems increased, foster care agencies could not locate suitable and sufficient placements within their existing structures. A specialized child welfare demonstration project was needed to establish the criteria for recruiting and retaining suitable foster care placements for HIV-seropositive children, many of whom were abandoned [Boland 1988]. Leake and Watts Children's Home in Yonkers, New York, took the lead, working closely with major New York City medical centers to provide proper discharge from the hospital to foster care and medical follow-up to this initial group of boarder babies [Gurdin and Anderson 1987]. In 1985, CDC published guidelines for educational and foster care agencies [CDC 1985]. The Leake and Watts agency was able to recruit foster homes with the assurance that medical centers, such as AECOM, would provide medical care to the HIV-seropositive children, support the foster parents through an educational program about HIV precautions, and reinforce understanding of routes of transmission. Foster families were offered ongong support groups and participation in other specialized programs such as Make-a-Wish Foundation and Starlight Foundation, and bereavement counseling upon the death of a foster child.

An early intervention model requires a close relationship between the child welfare community and the health care community. AECOM identified 45 HIV-seropositive mothers in their Women and Infants Project by 1988. Their serostatus was known before delivery. All of the mothers infected heterosexually (38 percent) have taken their infants home from the hospital. Of those infected who have intravenous drug use as a risk factor (62 percent), placement of the infant in unrelated foster care has taken place only when the mother was actively using drugs. Five infants of 28 (18 percent) have, at this writing, been placed in unrelated foster homes; three (11 percent) are in the custody of relatives. Either these mothers abandoned their infants or the infants were removed from their mothers' custody through a child welfare investigation. To facilitate proper placement, the medical center, with the mother's signed consent to reveal her HIV status, works closely with the child welfare agencies, offering the foster parents full discussion about HIV precautions and providing comprehensive health care to the infants on a preventive (to prevent opportunistic infections) as well as an acute care basis. The relationship between the medical community and the child welfare sector ensures continuity of care for the infant, with linkage to the mother's health status. Biological mothers are offered ongoing participation in the study project, regardless of need for placement of their infants. Coordination between the agencies reinforces medical and child welfare-centered planning. Thus the mothers' health care is not jeopardized by placement.

Both the child welfare sector and the health care sector have maintained a preventive modality ever since Leake and Watts obtained demonstration funding to prevent placement of infants and children of HIV-seropositive families. Families are assessed through the medical center's interdisciplinary team model. Families that (1) are actively engaging in substance abuse, (2) have limited or poor coping skills due to the HIV diagnosis or long-standing emotional or cognitive limitations; and (3) are suspected of neglect, are referred by the medical center. These families are asked to participate in a referral meeting. The Brown family was one of the first referred to preventive services. Ms. Brown was a single-parent head of a household with two children. She was diagnosed as having HIV infection during her second pregnancy. Her oldest daughter, Aisha, five years old, was healthy, bright, and vibrant. The mother had a history of polysubstance abuse, including intravenous drugs, and was bisexual, with multiple male partners who used intravenous drugs. She was treated psychiatrically with antidepressants and was maintained on methadone for her heroin addiction. Under stress, she abused alcohol. She had minimal family supports; the one sister in whom she could confide had a serious cardiac condition requiring home health services. The fathers of her two children were not reliable sources of support. Even though she was asymptomatic at the time of referral to preventive services and her youngest child's status was still indeterminate, she was referred because of her history of polysubstance abuse, lack of family supports, and history of depression. It was feared that once she or her young daughter became symptomatic she would be unable to provide support to her family.

Enrollment in the study is in no way jeopardized by a woman's decision to accept referral to the preventive program. Of four high-risk families referred for prevention, two have been active recipients of preventive services that included home-based counseling, placement of a homemaker/health aid, case advocacy, and other concrete supports. The third family refused preventive services; when later investigated by the municipal child welfare agency, their infant was placed on the basis of neglect. The fourth family has employed other supports.

The interrelationship between preventive child welfare services and the medical center staff focuses on preventing placement, reinforcing medical care, providing case advocacy, identifying gaps in service, and assisting in long-range planning and support during bereavement of either child or parent (refer to Table 1).

The final significant component in an early intervention model, which is anchored in the health care system but is linked to community-

Table 1

Summary of Preventive Services

Home-based counseling and support
Placement of homemakers/home health aides
Infant clothing allowance
Emergency food referrals
Referral for day care for infected and noninfected infants and siblings
Referral for alcohol and drug detoxification
Referral for psychiatric evaluation
Referral for visiting nurse services

based services, is that of habilitation of developmentally delayed HIV-infected infants/young children. Our neurological/neurodevelopment assessments begin at birth and are followed at specific intervals with Einstein and Bailey examinations and neurological assessment. Appropriate services are delivered by a health care team specializing in the education, habilitation, and psychosocial needs of developmentally delayed or impaired infants and young children. Services range from physical, speech and language, and occupational therapy that are hospital-based or community-based, to placement in special day care facilities.

Future Trends for Early Intervention

The development of a model of early intervention for HIV-infected children was an evolving process of complementing research, clinical management, and psychosocial components. This model has allowed us to offer a continuum of services to HIV-infected families with infants at risk. It provides services and alternatives to placement of seropositive infants while stabilizing the family system before the onset of disease manifestations. Future trends should involve reaching out to pregnant teen mothers to determine their risk status so as to provide early intervention for HIV-positive teen mothers, to incarcerated women at risk for HIV who deliver during incarceration and keep their infants with them in prison during the first or second year of life, and to homeless pregnant women at risk for HIV. This task would mean collaboration among a wider variety of social service and correction agencies. The child welfare system should develop its preventive services to HIV-infected families along the lines demonstrated by Leake and Watts in its prevention model, as intervening before placement is necessary.

At the same time, major medical centers should work more collaboratively with diverse community-based groups such as churches, community organizations, and specialized AIDS service agencies to identify their complementary roles in sustaining the HIV-infected family in the community.

REFERENCES

Boland, M.G., Allen, T., Long, G., and Tasker, M. "Children with HIV infection: Collaborative responsibilities of the child welfare and medical communities." Social Work 33 (6) (November-December 1988): 504–509.

Cabat, T.L., Novick, B., and Rubinstein, A. "A preschool model for symptomatic HIV infected children." In Schinazi, R., and Nahimas, A. (editors) AIDS in Children, Adolescents, and Heterosexual Adults. New York: Elsevier Science Pub. Co., 1988.

Cohen, M.A., and Weisman, H.W. "A biopsychosocial approach to AIDS." Psychosomatic 27 (4) (April 1986).

CDC. "Revisions of the case definition of acquired immunodeficiency syndrome for national reporting—United States." Morbidity and Mortality Weekly Report 34 (1985): 373–375.

CDC. "Education and foster care of children infected with human T-lymphotrophic virus type III/lymphedenopathy-associated virus." Morbidity and Mortality Weekly Report 34 (1985): 517–521.

CDC. "The classification system for HIV-infection in children under 13 years of age." Morbidity and Mortality Weekly Report 36 (1987): 225–236.

Gurdin, P., and Anderson, G. "Quality care for ill children: AIDS-specialized foster family homes." Child Welfare 66 (4) (July-August 1987): 291–302.

Lambert, B. "One in 61 babies in New York City has AIDS antibodies, study says." New York Times (January 13, 1988): A1.

Ultmann, M.H., Diamond, G., et al. "Developmental abnormalities in children with acquired immunodeficiency syndrome (AIDS): A follow-up study." International Journal of Neuroscience 32 (1987): 661–667.

8

Caring for HIV-Infected Children and Their Families: Psychosocial Ramifications

ANITA SEPTIMUS[1]

WOMEN AND CHILDREN WITH HIV INFECTION HAVE A RANGE OF COMPLEX psychosocial needs that affect every aspect of their lives. Women are reportedly more likely than men to contract AIDS heterosexually, with high-risk partners who are intravenous drug users or bisexual [Friedland and Klein 1987]. In addition, in New York City there are an estimated 200,000 intravenous drug abusers, 50,000 of whom are women, 50 to 80 percent of whom are believed to be HIV-infected. Women may unknowingly be sexually involved with HIV-infected intravenous drug-abusing partners. These factors present alarming future implications for pediatric AIDS.[2] As infected women have infected children, they struggle with medical, psychosocial, and basic care issues. In response to these needs, Albert Einstein College of Medicine in the Bronx, New York, established an AIDS Comprehensive Family Program in January 1984.

The Comprehensive AIDS Family Center has served over 250 Bronx

---

[1] Several sections of this chapter are adapted from the author's article from Seminars in Perinatology 13(1) (February 1989). Used with permission.

[2] In January 1988, a New York City survey concluded that one of 61 newborns tested positive for HIV infection at birth; in the Bronx, the prevalence was one of 43. Based on such results, 1,000 seropositive infants were born in 1987 [NYSDOH 1987].

families, 90 percent of whom are headed by single mothers. Sixty percent of these 250 families are extended family members, such as grandmothers and aunts, or foster mothers or adoptive mothers; 40 percent are single-parent biological mothers ranging in age from 20 to 40 years. Sixty percent are Hispanic, 30 percent are black, and 10 percent are white families. Ninety percent of these families receive public assistance.

The multidisciplinary program provides a range of responses to family needs, including mental health services [Septimus 1989]. These mental health services address the social and psychological needs of children and women through several means of intervention:

1. *Information and Referral:* To assist and advocate for persons needing appropriate medical/dental assistance, mental health, financial/economic entitlements, social services, AIDS-related outreach. The center also operates a medical information hot line concerning HIV infection/AIDS.

2. *Psychosocial Assessments:* To evaluate the type and number of mental health services that can be delivered to women and children by this facility or other cooperating agencies.

3. *Crisis Intervention:* To assist caregivers, particularly when they first learn the diagnosis or at times of hospitalization, when it may be difficult to focus on the child's immediate needs and plan for the future. Referrals to inpatient psychiatric hospital units may take place when suicide risk is high.

4. *Group Involvement:* To provide mothers and caregivers of children (such as relatives and foster parents) with a weekly forum for problem solving and support.

5. *Family Therapy:* To help members of a family function better, enhancing communication between couples and providing therapeutic intervention.

6. *Grief Counseling:* To respond to family members who are anticipating losing or have lost a loved one due to HIV infection, through individual counseling or family sessions.

7. *Case Management and Coordination of Treatment:* To survey and monitor services provided to a family, to provide continuing psychological support, and to encourage and facilitate compliance with medical appointments and follow-up instructions.

Case Example

Adam, a bright and handsome four-year-old, was in a number of ways typical of children served by the center. He acquired HIV infection from his mother. His father had been an intravenous drug abuser; he had died of AIDS in March 1986, while in prison. Adam's mother was not a drug abuser. She had become HIV-infected through her infected husband. Adam was first diagnosed as having AIDS in December 1986, after three relatively asymptomatic years during which his HIV infection was unknown. Adam's mother was pregnant with her third child when she learned of Adam's illness. There was also an eight-year-old daughter.

Team intervention began with Mrs. M. as soon as Adam was tested and she was informed of the seriousness of his illness, as well as her own HIV status. She was also tactfully informed of the serious risks posed by her pregnancy—the risk of infection to her unborn child and the higher health risks for her. She reacted with profound shock and panic to the double blow of Adam's diagnosis and the risky pregnancy. Overwhelmed by the situation, she was paralyzed with fear and incapable of making decisions, particularly with regard to her pregnancy.

The team maintained contact with her, and at an interview two weeks after she had been given the initial information she reported feeling depressed but capable of making some decisions, including terminating her pregnancy in view of the multiple health traumas. On Christmas Eve, Mrs. M. knew that Adam was terminally ill and her pregnancy was over.

In early January 1987, Adam was hospitalized at Albert Einstein College of Medicine for a series of complex tests. His first tests showed atypical tuberculosis, which does not respond to medical treatment. He subsequently developed pneumocystis carinii pneumonia, a life-threatening opportunistic infection that ended his life. Throughout his hospitalization, Adam was exceptionally bright and verbal, understood in his own way the nature of his illness, and hung on to his fragile life. Throughout his suffering, he fought illness stoically, inspiring the staff with his love and courage and comforting his desolate mother. His wish to live and awareness of his own impending death heightened the grief for the staff. He died April 13, 1987. Mrs. M. stayed with her son throughout his hospitalization, rarely leaving him. She was sustained through these difficult months by a sense of hope, prayer, and supportive counseling.

A year later Mrs. M. was still in individual and group counseling to help her deal with her losses. She was still depressed, missed Adam, and had difficulty sleeping and carrying out routine tasks. She was also preoccupied with her own increasing AIDS symptoms and concerned about her only surviving child, her daughter. With staff help, she was fighting the disease while searching for an existential meaning in her ordeal [Septimus 1989].

In December 1988, Mrs. M.'s medical condition took a dreadful turn. She had a series of hospitalizations for pneumocystis carinii pneumonia (PCP) and central nervous system (CNS) involvement and severe vomiting. The last weeks of her life were tragic both to her family and to the staff because she suffered from progressive encephalopathy with dementia.

When Mrs. M. died on April 12, 1989, her mother was torn by feelings of intense grief as well as relief. She could not bear to see her young daughter going through such a slow and painful death. Mrs. M.'s mother is a survivor, a single mother of six children. She lost three children and one grandchild to the complications of drug addiction and AIDS. She has now been called upon to raise her eight-year-old granddaughter and is using counseling at the center.

The granddaughter, on the surface, seems resigned to her multiple losses. Her recurring dreams, however, point to intense unresolved grief, pervasive anxiety over her own possible death, and the death of the few survivors in her family.

Psychosocial Implications of Pediatric AIDS

The psychological and social issues confronting families with an AIDS-infected child are far more complex than those of other childhood chronic and life-threatening illnesses such as cancer. As observed at the center and, reportedly, throughout the nation in similar institutions, AIDS is experienced chiefly in the context of extreme poverty, lack of social networks, lack of psychological support, often a premorbid history of depression, and stigma and rejection. These burdens overwhelm already weak coping capacities, pushing vulnerable families into disorganization and crisis.

A child diagnosed with HIV infection causes chaos, disrupts family balance, and upsets the operational structure of the family at almost all levels. Families find themselves challenged with multiple powerful stresses by the medical diagnosis, the treatment, the course of the disease, and the possible outcome of life or death. Although the initial shock, anger, and chaos occur with the diagnosis, parents experience continuous fear, disbelief, anxiety, pain, stress, and feelings of being on an emotional roller coaster.

> Linda's mother, 39-year-old Jenny, was stunned by the news of HIV infection in her family. She questioned, "Why me? I have done no drugs, I was faithful in my married life, I was a hardworking mother, my husband isn't gay!" She felt numb. Then, for months all she could do was cry. She left her job, shut herself away at home with her sick child and a ten-year-old uninfected son. Friends and neighbors deserted her. When she mustered up the courage to tell her family, they also deserted her. Her mother said she wouldn't "set foot in her house." Yet Jenny lamented, "I love motherhood; it is terrible for me to live knowing I have given this to my daughter. 'Who will die first' runs through my mind constantly. Some days I want Linda to die first, but then I feel it is wrong. I worry about who will take care of her. I wish I could choose her foster mom now."

Many clients report that the effect of the child's disease on the family continues throughout life, even after the death of the child. Recurring themes include social isolation, depression and grief, guilt, and disruption and disorientation.

Social Isolation

Most families report that they are not willing to share their child's diagnosis with friends and relatives. The reasons for not informing the natural sources of social supports are a parental sense of guilt and shame associated with the behaviors that result in HIV infection, a fear of community disapproval/stigma, and withdrawal or denial of services to the infected child and the entire family. Many families are also unwilling to share the diagnosis with the ill child and find themselves further burdened by a lack of candor within the home at a time and place where they might benefit from being able to talk about the situation. The child is caught in a conspiracy of silence. The loss of social support results in isolation, which contributes to depression and to difficulty in accomplishing family tasks.

Mothers with HIV infection or with infected children need constant support from helping professionals. If abandoned by professionals and friends, they may quickly decompensate psychologically, particularly during the acute illness or death of a child. This response may result in hospitalization or disappearing homeless into the streets. Agency or institutional contact and work with families should not cease when the child dies. Because of the extreme social isolation and stigma of the disease, mothers have tended to come back and maintain contact with the accepting and trusting environment of the center.

Depression and Grief

In addition to the reactive depression resulting from learning about their own or their child's HIV infection, parents may have a complicated chronic depressive state triggered by a multitude of problems that contributed to the single parent's initial resort to intravenous drug abuse or other substance abuse. The socioeconomic problems in these families further contribute to depression. They experience the most serious traumatic life events—loss of jobs or permanent unemployment, illness, criminal involvement, disabling accidents, and other catastrophes. Although they are barely coping with or recovering from earlier blows, AIDS introduces a new and staggering set of conditions. Without savings, insurance, employment or income, legal counsel, and medical support, there are few if any supports, particularly in the context of social isolation, to break a vicious cycle that drains psychic and physical resources and deepens the vulnerability to and the experience of depression [DesJarlais et al. 1986].

Studies on depression in women conducted in London show that the main precipitating cause is not grief itself but the hopelessness that precedes the grief. This finding is consistent with our observations of poverty-stricken single mothers [Brown and Harris 1978]. In pediatric AIDS, this perception of hopelessness precedes the acquisition of AIDS and is compounded by the suffering and fatality of AIDS.

> Mrs. G. discovered that she was HIV-positive when her nine-month-old baby was diagnosed with AIDS. At age 26, she had known little happiness or stability. She could remember only years of trauma, losses, poverty, drug addiction, violence, abuse, and now AIDS. She had lived accustomed to the idea that she would die young and possibly violently. She felt that she did not deserve to live longer than her mother, who had died at age 28 and left her and her three sisters orphaned. Yet the idea of dying a painful, slow death was unacceptable to her, and she said obsessively that she would "smother her baby and then put a gun to her head." Out of her rage, despair, and guilt

she refused to care for her baby. A two-week emergency psychiatric hospitalization and follow-up therapy sessions proved beneficial; she was able to care for her child until the child's death at age two. She is still in counseling.

Guilt

Contributing to shame and depression is the parent's sense of guilt. A helping person must be aware that parents feel personal guilt over the illness of their child and their own HIV infection. They blame themselves for their behavior or for failing to protect their children from behavior that could lead to AIDS and the death of everyone involved.

Working with Families

Families feel a loss of control when facing an irreversible, fatal illness. This reaction is similar to drug users' perceptions of lack of control (and many families with children with AIDS have been involved with drug use), resulting in a fatalistic approach to life. The hopelessness of the family with HIV infection can evoke a hopelessness in the worker attempting to serve the family. Consequently, the heart of the therapeutic task and challenge for the worker is to infuse hope into the family while helping them to find sufficient strength to cope with multiple problems.

Infusing hope in the context of AIDS is the most effective way of imparting coping skills, through the worker's ability to maintain personal hopefulness in the midst of apparently hopeless situations, to maintain a sense of optimism that transcends the most despairing of life situations. Family members refer to this approach as a positive attitude. To the extent that the same strengths and intrapsychic processes become parallel and interactive in the professional relationship, a pattern of mutual trust, strength, and hope is established that in turn generates more positive attitudes and nurturance.

The infusion of hope begins in the parents' role with their children. Although the parents are faced from the outset with the fatal outcome of the child's illness, the focus is not on a "dying child" but on the "child living with AIDS." Medical treatment, community resources, educational and recreational programs, and other services are explored and mobilized to strengthen family equilibrium and enhance the quality of the child's life.

Although children with AIDS are often quite ill and experience painful medical treatment, the center tries to alleviate pain to the extent possible and to introduce experiences of joy, love, and care. The Clown Care Unit (CCU) comes weekly to the center to cheer the children during intravenous gamma globulin treatment and on the pediatric floor of the hospital. Over 40 of our children have gone to Walt Disney World in Florida with the Make-A-Wish Foundation and Starlight Foundation, with noticeable results in lifting the depression of both children and parents. Camp Sunburst in California has been host to a number of our children. Visitors to the program may at first be overwhelmed with sadness at the sight of such young children experiencing so much pain, but they often leave comforted by the celebration of life that goes on.

Children who are loved are likely to fight the illness and survive longer. Children who appear to be forgotten in hospitals often die of abandonment and loss of hope before dying of AIDS. Dr. Elisabeth Kubler-Ross, in her 1987 Riverside Church address, said that children are not afraid of death; they are afraid of abandonment. When surrounded with love, joy, and hope, children hang on fiercely to their fragile lives.

Imparting hope begins at intake and permeates all services. Parents are often confused about AIDS, having conflicting or incomplete information gained from the media. Through compassionate, careful education about the illness, precise facts, and current statistics, much anxiety and despair can be alleviated. Almost all our mothers respond to the HIV/AIDS diagnosis with total panic. Within four to six weeks of counseling sessions and supportive information, they gradually move from panic to acceptance of the diagnosis and the use of coping skills. This work is done with openness, empathy, compassion, and patience in a non-judgmental fashion. Understanding the spectrum of HIV infection/AIDS and knowing precisely one's prognosis reduces fear and enables the patient to organize her life in a more future-oriented manner. The implicit message imparted to the mother is, "There is life after HIV infection."

Intervention continues with a range of services, family counseling, crisis intervention, and groupwork.

Service Provision

Beginning with an initial assessment of family needs and resources, important issues are providing emergency food, emergency housing, facilitating proper medical care, and helping mothers place their children in day care or other educational settings. Exploring educational and employment possibilities for HIV-infected mothers is critical in raising self-esteem, satisfaction, providing income and independence, and keeping them, one hopes, from the drug scene. Socialization is crucial but difficult to achieve in view of the societal rejection and isolation of AIDS patients.

A number of difficult, delicate subjects are addressed:

> Family planning and decisions about future pregnancies
> The complexity of sexual involvement in relation to AIDS and enabling the person to make an educated decision concerning sexual intimacy
> Helping parents express their denial, fear of death, and anger, and allowing them to prepare for death by setting conditions, discussing burial, and arranging for eventual foster care for their children

Parents are anxious about the progression of their own infection as it parallels their child's. The almost obsessive questions, "Will I die before my child?" and "Who will care for my child?" are understandably and universally expressed. Careful discussion of these topics triggers deep emotions and often leads to a sense of liberation and increased hopefulness.

Family Counseling

Family interventions, involving as many family members as possible, aim at restructuring the family in a realistic way that respects the kinship system, sibling system, and a three- to four-generational hierarchy. This process does not necessarily follow traditional family restructuring, but these systems can be effectively reorganized with realistic expectations and families strengthened at a most crucial point in life. Couples need informed, educated reassurance in continuing intimate relations, since they often react to HIV infection by completely withdrawing from each other.

The assessment of family functioning and needs is assisted by using genograms, which point out family dysfunctional patterns such as alcohol and substance abuse, and family-transmitted diseases such as diabetes and AIDS (see Figures 1 and 2). A genogram may answer at a

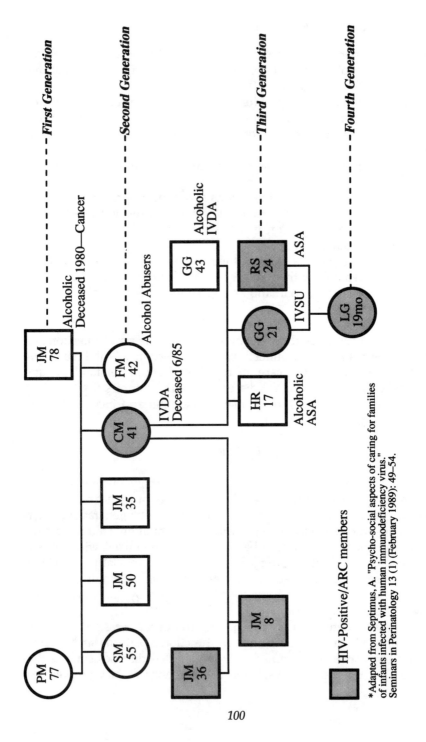

*Figure 1. A Four-Generational Genogram of an HIV/AIDS Family.**

*Adapted from Septimus, A. "Psycho-social aspects of caring for families of infants infected with human immunodeficiency virus." Seminars in Perinatology 13 (1) (February 1989): 49–54.

First Generation

Second Generation

Third Generation

Fourth Generation

JM 78
Alcoholic
Deceased 1980—Cancer

FM 42
Alcohol Abusers

CM 41
IVDA
Deceased 6/85

JM 35

JM 50

SM 55

PM 77

GG 43
Alcoholic
IVDA

RS 24
ASA

GG 21
IVSU

LG 19mo

HR 17
Alcoholic
ASA

JM 36

JM 8

HIV-Positive/ARC members

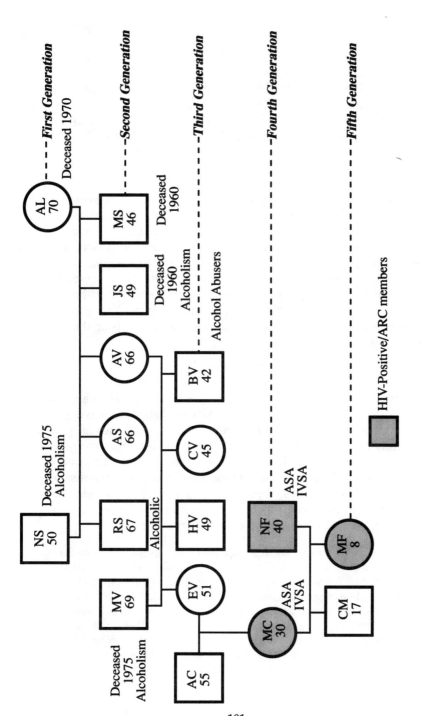

Figure 2. A Five-Generational Genogram of an HIV/AIDS Family.

101

glance such basic questions as sudden losses by young infants of their young parents or unavailability of parents due to intravenous drug abuse (IVDA) or incarceration. Numerous and varied losses, often the result of circumstances beyond individual control, may establish patterns of unresolved grief and predispose family members to a state of chronic depression [Coleman 1980; Coleman et al. 1986].

Crisis Intervention

With targeted and timely interventions—such as supportive counseling to individuals and families, psychiatric referral for suicidal patients, and grief counseling for parents who have lost a child—parents are able to express their despair, their unbearable isolation, and their multiple fears. They can mourn their multiple losses, talk about their fears of sexual involvements, their intense guilt about contracting the disease and infecting their loved ones. To the extent that these young, dying adults who are losing their young children can express their emotions, they can be gradually helped to find an existential meaning to their ordeal.

Groupwork

Group support is a most effective way to turn persons around from despair to optimism. Dr. Victor Frankl established effective groups in concentration camps for a similar purpose, to tap sources of hope in an environment of despair [Frankl 1976]. Groups also diminish the individual's sense of isolation. They provide a safe, supportive environment that participants believe in and respond to through mutual disclosure of emotions and experiences. Typically, the group is perceived as the surrogate family, much needed in time of crisis and isolation. Groups have become an essential component of AIDS programs.

> Mrs. A., a foster mother, reported, "My attitude towards family has changed. I have a new picture of family now." Having been deserted by friends and family because she cared for AIDS children, Mrs. A., like others, sought other concerned adults to fill the roles of grandparents, aunts, and uncles for their AIDS children. Stressing the importance of joining a support group, she said, "This is not a support group, this is a family." Transcending the limits of agencies and programs, families in the support group were available to each other 24 hours a day if the need arose.

Groups meet weekly at Albert Einstein Hospital, include five to 12 members (foster mothers, biological mothers, grandmothers, and aunts), and are led by the pediatric AIDS team social worker. Although fathers are routinely invited, they have chosen not to participate. Children are cared for by a regular hospital volunteer. Groups have been open-ended, with no time limits for length of involvement.

Initially these groups began with foster mothers who had difficulties and unanswered questions in caring for AIDS children. During the initial phase of the group, foster mothers expressed intense anger at biological mothers. As an experiment and a challenge, some biological mothers were included in the group—the result was encouraging. Foster mothers emerged as teachers, supporters, and nurturers to biological mothers, and the latter felt comfort in meeting the persons who would someday care for their own children. The biological mothers also shared valuable information about their drug addiction and, in general, each increased their knowledge of the other. Both parties used their strength in reaching out to each other in time of crisis. It has been extremely difficult, however, to get biological mothers still involved in drug use to attend support group sessions.

The support group experience normalizes caregivers' crises, teaches them new social skills, and taps new sources of strength and hope. Recurrent group themes include "Do what needs to be done to meet the challenge"; "Take one day at a time"; and "Love, give, nurture, and enjoy the child today, because tomorrow is never guaranteed."

Based on four years of experience with parent/relative/foster parent groups, several coping strategies have noticably emerged [Septimus 1988]:

> *Denial:* Some level of denial is necessary for parents and professionals caring for HIV-infected children. This reaction reduces the negative effect of the illness and enables parents to mobilize their strengths for the difficult course of the illness. The reaction becomes problematic when it interferes with getting required treatments and medications for the child. Although all mothers and caregivers know of the impending death of their children, they all express the need to be hopeful and to feel that the hope is shared by the health care professional. Mothers unanimously declare that they cannot, will not, and do not want to be prepared for their child's death: "It will be

soon enough when the child has died; every day that my child wakes up and smiles, to me, my hope is alive."

Resignation: Parents confronted with the inevitable fatality of AIDS may react by accepting this fate and facing the illness with courage and reality. The emphasis is on caring, because there is no cure. Resignation should be monitored, because positive resignation may enable the family to care for the child, but negative resignation could lead to undue passivity and the surrender of active involvement, leading to neglect of the child. A balance between denial and resignation has seemed to result in effective family coping.

Comfort in Religion: Most mothers caring for HIV/AIDS children have strengthened their coping through religion. Many express their increasing closeness to God as a source of emotional support and protection against depression. Religious convictions provide an explanation for the suffering, giving some meaning to the illness and reinforcing their belief in eternal life. Some mothers describe how their children prepared them for dying. Their children told them they were "going to Heaven and that they should not cry." Many mothers find comfort in their children going to God "where their suffering and tears have finally ended."

Education: Searching for knowledge and understanding of the illness is an effective way of reducing stress. It helps patients to focus appropriately on their emotional reactions and lessens their anxiety and fear of impending death. Mothers can establish a sense of control and plan for the future because of their extensive knowledge of the illness and how it affects children.

Problem Solving: Mothers in group sessions enthusiastically share solutions, suggestions, more effective ways of raising children in the context of their illness, nutrition information, school issues, and how to be of help in the child's medical treatment. After a child's death, mothers find consolation in having been actively involved in caring for and fighting for their children.

Expression of Strong Emotion: The recognition and expression of anger are adaptive and reduce the emotional burden of caregivers. Anger may be directed at individuals (the person who infected them, physicians, God, the social service system, and so on) or turned inward as self-hatred. It may be undirected, inappropriately focused, or directed toward the ill child. The expression of these feelings in the groups has a beneficial, almost liberating effect.

Mrs. C.'s expression of anger and stress surfaced repeatedly in group sessions. She is a middle-class, educated woman in her thirties. She adopted Melissa at birth only to discover that the child was HIV-positive at age 17 months. Melissa was now seven years old, had full-blown AIDS, multiple hospitalizations and medical problems, and was bravely fighting the illness. Mrs. C. was "wiped out" by her daughter's illness and crushed with guilt—wanting Melissa to die so she could "get on with her life." She felt as if she was on an "emotional roller coaster," either elated by the idea that her child would "lick this terrible disease" or totally hopeless. Her anger often took her to such extremes that she left her husband in charge of the children and spent her time with friends to disconnect herself from the reality. In individual and group sessions, Mrs. C. was supported in pursuing her career and social goals. She became able to attend to herself while strengthening her family's emotional stability.

Foster parents are more likely than biological mothers to seek help in group sessions to prepare for the eventual loss of the child. Biological mothers are generally less willing or not emotionally strong enough to withstand the prospect of a child's death for a variety of reasons, including their complicated feelings of guilt and of having to face their own illness as well. This difference should not be interpreted as implying that foster parents care less for a child, nor should the complexity of the challenge to cope for the biological mother be underestimated. It is, however, crucial for biological mothers to be present at such discussions since it may give them the necessary courage to deal with the issue in individual sessions. It is also important for them to hear the foster mothers' expression of deep commitment, love, and grief at the eventual loss of their foster children. It will comfort the biological mothers with the knowledge that, in the event they die first, their children will continue to be loved, nurtured, and cherished.

Conclusion

The challenges facing professionals caring for HIV-infected children are enormous. In this time of crisis, struggles to cope are further complicated by social isolation, and, for many biological parents, the fearful prospect of their own illness and mortality. The sensitive intervention and commitment of caring professionals is crucial to assist families by means of education, connections to community resources, and therapeutic support. In addition, caregivers have found tremendous strength and comfort from one another through formal and informal contact and encounters. These resources play a crucial role in enabling families to endure and to provide the love required to ensure a certain quality of life for their children. Enabling families to find meaning in life, praising their survival skills, tapping new sources of psychic strength, self-healing, courage, and resiliency are the heart of this demanding yet rewarding work.

REFERENCES

Brown, G., and Harris, T. Social Origins of Depression: A Study of Psychiatric Disorder in Women. New York: Free Press, 1978.

Coleman, S. "Incomplete mourning and addict family transactions: A theory for understanding heroin abuse." In Lettieri, D. (editor), Theories of Drug Abuse. Washington, D.C.: U.S. Government Printing Office, 1980.

Coleman, S., Kaplan, J.D., and Downing, R. "Life cycle and loss—The spiritual vacuum of heroin addiction." Family Process 25 (1986): 5–23.

Des Jarlais, D.C., Friedman, S.R., and Strug, David. "AIDS and needle sharing within the IV-drug use subculture." In Feldman, D.A., and Johnson, T. M. (editors), The Social Dimension of AIDS. New York: Praeger, 1986: 121–126.

Frankl, Victor. Man's Search for Meaning. An Introduction to Logotherapy—From Death Camp to Existentialism. New York: Beacon, 1976.

Friedland, G., and Klein, R. "Transmission of the human immunodeficiency virus." New England Journal of Medicine 317 (1987): 1123–1135.

New York State Department of Health (NYSDOH). Report (November-December 1987).

Septimus, Anita. "Coping patterns and stress management of HIV/AIDS caretakers." Unpublished paper, 1988.

Septimus, Anita. "Psycho-social aspects of caring for families of infants infected with human immunodeficiency virus." Seminars in Perinatology 13 (1) (February 1989): 49–54.

9

Quality Care for Children: A Specialized Foster Care Program

PHYLLIS GURDIN

A BOARDER BABY CRISIS IN NEW YORK CITY IN 1985, COMPLICATED BY THE discovery of infants with HIV infection, led to a request by the city for a child welfare agency to begin a special program to provide foster homes for HIV-infected infants. At that point these children were experiencing long hospital stays, beyond medical necessity, due to an insufficient number of foster parents in general and fears concerning AIDS. In fact, a number of infants who had been placed in foster homes were abandoned to hospitals by fearful caregivers when they learned that the illnesses their foster children displayed were symptomatic of HIV infection.

At approximately the same time, a number of board members at Leake and Watts Children's Home, a child welfare agency with programs in foster care, adoption, group homes, and residential treatment, became informed and concerned about children with AIDS and urged the agency to respond to the city's appeal. Under the direction of the board, with the active support of the administration, and with the encouragement of the state and city, the agency applied for city approval and began a specialized program for AIDS children.

First lessons in organizing the program included (1) the value of an informed and committed board that would champion an AIDS outreach program and commit agency resources to the task; *(2)* the importance of enthusiastic support from an administration committed to caring for children in need—a motive that would steer the program through the objections, risks, and obstacles that would emerge in the days and months ahead; and *(3)* the crucial role of a child welfare agency—in this case, the Child Welfare Administration (formerly Special Services to Children) of New York City and the New York State Department of Social Services—willing and able to commit funds and administrative support to facilitate the program and to provide oversight and flexibility in responding to a new need. This significant crisis posed an opportunity to create a truly useful program and bring together agencies and organizations in response to the suffering of children and their families.

Getting Started

The foster care program began with the hiring of a project director, who experienced some skepticism and fear from colleagues within and outside the agency. Some expressed a general fear of AIDS and its transmission. Others expressed concern that the agency would become known as an "AIDS agency" and be stigmatized by professionals and the community, complicating the agency's ability to carry on its more extensive child welfare services. Would other biological parents and foster parents be upset? Finally, some warned that the director had committed herself to an impossible project that was doomed to failure. There were no precedents for recruiting and serving a large corps of foster parents to care for children with HIV infection.

The program also experienced some solid early encouragement. In addition to board, administration, and city and state support, the program received assistance from several important quarters: *(1)* a strong relationship with a nearby medical center that possessed the expertise and willingness to treat the medical needs of the children and the ability to marshal specialists, both medical and social service providers; *(2)* the educational assistance and encouragement of New York City's Gay Men's Health Crisis (GMHC), a large and effective agency responding to the AIDS crisis; and *(3)* additional financial support from the AIDS Institute of New York's Health Department to bridge the period between launching the program and placing the first children in foster homes.

Foster Parent Recruitment

The first priority was to recruit foster parents. It was recognized that finding a sufficient number of qualified foster parents capable of meeting the specialized needs of these children might be the most difficult aspect of this program, both in the beginning and as a continuing challenge. A foster parent recruiter was hired.

The program director and foster parent recruiter set out to (1) learn everything they could about AIDS and keep abreast of emerging information; (2) alert agencies, institutions, and community groups that the project had been established and was recruiting foster parents; (3) explore relationships with relevant health care and social service providers who might be a potential resource for children with HIV infection and foster parents; and (4) establish a network with other programs serving persons with AIDS.

A number of recruiting strategies were undertaken. First, the program sought and received local publicity describing its mission and desire to recruit foster parents. The director responded to requests to speak before professional and community groups when they became aware of the program. There were also city-supported mass appeals for foster parents through citywide television stations and radio. In general, these actions gained attention for, and interest in, the program even if only a few foster parents were initially recruited by these means.

The first recruits were developed from the program director's personal approach to foster parents already affiliated with Leake and Watts Children's Home. She visited a number of existing foster homes and discussed AIDS and the needs of children infected with HIV. She described the benefits that foster parents would receive in caring for these children, both the emotional rewards and the tangible benefits—the support and intensive commitment of the foster care worker, the availability of respite care through babysitting/day care, the provision of necessary supplies, and an exceptional board rate. Veteran foster parents were asked to suggest friends and relatives who might consider caring for an HIV-infected child with the help of this package of agency supports. The first foster home for the program was recruited by a Leake and Watts foster parent.

Recruitment of foster parents has been a continual challenge. From the recruitment of the first foster parents, this group of individuals have been transformed into the most effective recruiters of all. They have also served as role models and spokespersons for fostering children with

AIDS. Recruitment has also required a willingness to look to less traditional persons to be foster parents, such as single men and the elderly. Once recruited, foster parents are carefully screened and receive both initial AIDS education and training and ongoing formal and informal education.

In summary, the key to recruitment has been use of a foster parent network. Prospective parents have been attracted by the exceptional board rate offered for caring for these children. In addition, they have appreciated the intensive involvement and support provided by program staff members. The availability of day care, babysitters, or homemakers providing a respite function has increased the attractiveness of the package offered to these foster parents.

Homefinding

The counseling and educational role in homefinding is often expanded when working with families considering special-needs children. When a potential applicant for foster parenting contacts the agency and indicates an interest in caring for a seropositive child, a home visit by the homefinder is immediately scheduled. This initial visit is described as an educational meeting rather than a formal part of the application process. The foster parent and homefinder discuss HIV infection and children and the agency's service. This discussion is preliminary to formal submission of an application [Gurdin 1989].

During early contacts, foster parents ask a number of questions about the symptoms and medical condition of the potential foster child. It is important to avoid highly specific answers because each case is different. A typical response to a prospective foster parent considering an infant for placement might be the following:

You would be getting a young child who tests positive for antibodies to the HIV virus. At the time of placement, nobody knows if the child is actually infected with the virus. Even if the child is not infected and has picked up the antibodies from the mother's blood, the child may still start out more sickly than normal.

If it turns out that the child is infected, nobody knows how the disease is going to progress in his or her particular case.

The homefinder poses a number of questions for the prospective parent:

> What will happen when the child gets ill? Are you going to be able to stay up in the middle of the night when the child has a high fever or a bad cough and chest infection? Are you going to be able to take the child to the hospital that night, and back and forth to the doctor over the next week or so? These are the kinds of things you must consider before proceeding with the application.

Since the reactions of family and friends often shapes a family's willingness or ability to provide care for an HIV-infected child, these relationships are explored. Confidentiality is addressed:

> We are not discouraging you from revealing the child's condition, but only those persons who need to know should be told about the child. The real issue is what persons should know either because they are going to be physically handling the child or because you need the emotional support of your best friends and close relatives. You shouldn't just tell anybody; some people won't understand, and it violates the child's confidentiality, which is against the law. You must carefully consider two questions before you disclose this information. First, can you trust this person not to reject you and the child; second, will he or she keep the knowledge confidential and not violate the child's rights and the law?

Certain qualifications and qualities are assessed in the homefinding process: (1) there should be no other non-seropositive foster children[1] in the home and preferably no children under the age of six, to reduce potential exposure to infections; (2) family members must believe with absolute conviction that they cannot become infected with the AIDS virus by means of casual contact with a foster child in their home; (3) family members must understand that the foster child may often be sick and require many medical visits, may demonstrate developmental delays, failing to reach developmental milestones or regress from levels once achieved, and, in some cases, the child will die; (4) a responsible family member must be available in the home almost all of the time and employed foster parents must give evidence of a proven support system;

---

[1] This requirement is because of a New York State confidentiality law that does not permit the agency to tell the biological parents of the uninfected child that there is an HIV-positive child living in the home.

(5) caring for the child must be a top priority of the family such that schedules are rearranged to meet the child's needs; and (6) the family must demonstrate an ability to respond to emergencies by the way they have responded to past challenges and emergencies. Some medical knowledge by at least one family member is often helpful.

If the applicant seems appropriate and wants to be licensed for this special care, additional home visits are scheduled (as many as three more). Homefinders must adhere to state regulations governing foster parent certification. These standards typically state:

> Foster parents must be able to provide for the physical, emotional, social, and educational needs of a child who may be placed in their home, as well as being willing to facilitate visiting by, and promote a positive relationship with, the child's biological parents.

Although recruitment is a continuing, major challenge for a foster care program, lowering standards in homefinding is not the solution to licensing homes. In fact, home studies of foster parent applicants for children with special needs require a particular educational component with prospective foster parents, reality testing concerning the challenges of caring for potentially ill children, and extensive visits and interviews. This care will lessen the likelihood of overwhelming underprepared applicants or discouraging applicants with unrealistic expectations and will go far to assure quality care for these special children.

Case Example

Mrs. S. is a single woman who is trained as a licensed practical nurse. She has two biological children ages 12 and 14. She is the sole support of the family; her husband deserted her when the children were toddlers. Mrs. S. worked as a nurse on the night shift in a large general hospital. Often her assignment was to care for AIDS patients. She decided to leave her job and applied to be a foster parent for two HIV-infected children. In the hospital she was unable to provide the level of care she felt her patients needed. She believed that in her home she could make a difference in the lives of two children. As a foster parent of HIV-infected children, she would be provided with the same income she had been earning at the hospital.

A 15-month-old girl was placed in her home. The child had been hospitalized during most of her life. Her mother was an intravenous drug user, HIV-infected, and could not care for her daughter. In the hospital the child had numerous illnesses, such as thrush, ear infections, and diarrhea.

She has neurological damage and is developmentally delayed. The child exhibited highly disturbed behavior in the hospital and in the foster home. She had violent temper tantrums that did not respond to intervention by a caring person. She was sullen, moody, and most of the time did not interact with another person.

After ten months in the foster home, she is making progress in meeting developmental milestones, although speech development and fine motor coordination are still delayed. She continues to be a sullen, cranky, and difficult child, although her temper tantrums have decreased. She is in the process of receiving a full neurological workup to determine to what extent her symptoms are related to the progression of the disease.

Six weeks after placement of the first child a second child was placed with Mrs. S., a seven-month-old girl who was born prematurely and who had lived in the hospital all of her life because no home could be found for her. Her mother was an intravenous drug user who was unable to care for her. At placement the child weighed seven pounds. She could not smile or turn over. It was considered that the child's prognosis would be greatly improved if she had a consistent maternal caregiver.

Ten months after placement (at the time of this writing), her weight has more than doubled. She has had infections and illnesses, but none have required hospitalization. She has made remarkable developmental progress: she is able to walk and say simple words, and is friendly, cheerful, and responsive.

Mrs. S. knows that AIDS is a fatal disease. The fact that the children have done so well in her home has convinced her that, in spite of the prognosis, they will survive. She focuses on the present for the children, provides them with an excellent quality of life, and feels she can handle their illnesses and even their deaths [Anderson et al. 1989].

Child Placement

The placement process usually begins with a telephone call from the public agency worker who is responsible for children in public guardianship. The initial call may also come from a hospital social worker notifying the director that a child is in the hospital with a positive HIV antibody test, whose parent(s) cannot care for him or her, and who is in need of a foster home because medical discharge will soon be possible.

At the referral stage a number of questions are asked. From the hospital social worker the child's demographics (age, gender, race) and medical condition (what level of sickness is present and what medical problems have been observed) are ascertained. The next program question—"Do we have a home that can handle this child?"—may result in an immediate rejection.

Certain types of children do not do well in foster care. Some medical conditions are so far advanced that a foster home placement may not be advisable. For example, an unresponsive child was placed in a foster home and did not change, despite the valiant efforts of the foster mother, because the child's brain had been infected. Both the child's medical condition and the foster mother's feeling that she had failed depressed the foster mother. In a short time the child died, further upsetting her. It is difficult to assess unresponsiveness because of the complicating effects of the previous home or hospital environment, but workers should be alert to this problem when monitoring and talking with the foster parent soon after placement. This difficulty should be assessed on a case-by-case basis with respect to the child's condition and to the foster parent's expectations.

If an appropriate foster home is possible, a staff member will arrange an appointment to see the child in the hospital and to gather additional information. Ideally, this visit is conducted by a staff nurse and social worker, with the nurse gathering medical information and the social worker seeking information about the family. Written referral information is also requested.

After this visit, the staff member will alert the program homefinder, who discusses the case with the prospective foster parent, who then visits the child in the hospital. After a conference with the foster parent and a discussion of the child's medical condition, the placement is accepted if the foster parent agrees. The foster parent is provided with necessary equipment to care for the incoming child.

The two program staff members go to the hospital and transport the child to the foster home, rather than requesting that the foster parent make the transfer. This method allows the foster parent time to prepare for the entry of the child into the home. The child's medical care responsibility and records are transferred to the hospital that will now care for the child, and medical appointments are set up.

While that transfer is taking place, efforts are being made to locate and assess the condition of the child's parents. When this program began, there was a general sense that children would be dying and parents would be unavailable because they were either dead or had abandonded their child in the hospital. This situation did not prove to be the case: the children have not been dying, a number of parents have been located, and some have maintained contact with the agency and their children.

The location effort includes sending mailgrams and letters and making telephone calls. Often it involves a diligent search to find a parent who has not been present since the child's birth and who may be involved in the urban drug culture. The search may result in steps to terminate the parent's guardianship or in the establishment of ongoing ties to the parent, including encouraging parent-child visiting at the program office site.

With the child placed in the foster home, a social worker and a nurse are assigned to each home. The nurse makes home visits to monitor the medical condition of the child and helps supervise medication or other medical treatment procedures; the nurse also makes medical appointments with the foster parent for the child and attends the appointments with the foster parent. The social worker initiates steady contact with the foster parent. Although a monthly visit in the home is mandated, the worker may visit more frequently, particularly during the beginning of placement, during times of stress, or at the foster parent's request. Frequent telephone contact is maintained. Both staff members educate, support, and advocate for the foster parent; both are also available to the foster parent around the clock.

This attention from staff members is crucial to recruiting and maintaining foster homes. It requires a low caseload size (ten to 12 children) for the staff, so that supportive work can be maintained as well as responding to those homes that are experiencing a crisis. This low staff member-foster parent ratio may be expensive, but it is essential for a successful program. The concern is not only to support foster parents who are caring for the children but also to support staff members so that they do not become overly frustrated or burned out by the unrealistic demands of high caseloads. Recruiting staff is a challenge for this program; it is difficult to recruit for child welfare in general, and AIDS adds an extra challenge to the task of finding competent, sensitive personnel.

Program Description

Staff

The program began with a director, a foster parent recruiter, and a nurse, but it has grown steadily as the number of children coming into care expanded from ten to over 60. At the time of writing, the staff consisted of the program director, the assistant program director, six social workers, four nurses, and two secretaries.

The director's role has changed dramatically. In the first years of the program, it included many of the duties of the social worker and extensive contact with foster parents, including homefinding responsibilities. The director's function currently is primarily administrative, involved with consultations, fund-raising, professional education, interagency collaboration, and public relations.

Foster Parents

As of June 1989, 33 foster parents were caring for 61 children. The number of children in care may vary according to medical status. Foster parents range in age from 27 to 59. The oldest foster parent, age 75, recently retired. As to marital status, foster parents are single, separated, divorced, and married. They are black, Hispanic, and white, predominantly from the New York City metropolitan area, primarily the Bronx, the city borough closest to Leake and Watts' Yonkers office. Most of the foster parents are not employed outside their homes. Several single parents are employed and have arranged babysitting and day care services for their foster children. Many of the foster parents have had some experience with illness or medical issues; some are nurses or medical personnel [Gurdin and Anderson 1987].

The children in care, who are predominantly black or Hispanic, have a range of diagnoses and medical conditions. Approximately ten have full-blown AIDS; 20 are symptomatic; and 20 are HIV-positive without symptoms. Although a number of children have seroconverted to negative status after initially testing positive, it was surprising to see that children who have seroconverted still pose health problems and developmental delays such that some of them appear to be more ill than some HIV-positive children. Because of recent medical research in which seven seronegative children were shown to have the virus in their blood, this group of children will be followed and retested.

The children range in age from six weeks to nine years; most are male. The older preschool children are often the sickest but stay in placement the longest. Five children have died; they were all under the age of two, and all but one were quite ill at the time of placement.

Generally there are one or two children in each foster home, with occasional exceptions allowing three in one home. Twenty-five percent of the children are classified as preadoptive, and several are being considered or are in the early stages of adoption. Very few foster homes have withdrawn or been closed. In four years, two homes have been closed because they were unable to maintain sufficient quality of care for the children in the homes.

Services

From the beginning of the specialized program, a variety of services have been provided that are consistent with a foster care program of high quality. Foster parents have received the highest board rate granted in New York, approximately $1,200 per month per child. The agency has supplied necessary child-care equipment (carriages, cribs, play equipment), clothes, and, if necessary, washing machines. Funds for recreation have been provided. Foster parents have also been assisted with medical insurance. Day care, babysitting, and respite care are arranged by foster parents in cooperation with the agency and reimbursed to the extent possible [Rendon et al. 1989].

In addition to these concrete services, frequent home visits are made by the social worker and the nurse. The nurse usually accompanies the foster parent to doctor, clinic, or hospital. There is 24-hour coverage for emergencies—a support to foster parents, although it has not been heavily used. Frequent contact with the foster parents and child supplements and enriches regularly scheduled foster parent training and small support-group sessions. Foster parents report that their own informal and formal networking is one of the most helpful resources available.

When the program began, as noted earlier, it was thought that all the children would die, that their parents had abandoned them, and that there would not be much work with parents. These impressions have not been borne out. Although some parents are unavailable or do not want to be involved with their child's care, and others have died, a number have come forward and shown interest in their children. In some cases, parents have not been involved, but extended family members who were unable to provide a home for a child have maintained contact by visiting. In one case a child did go home to live with an extended family member, and several more may return to their families. No children have as yet returned home to their parents. The social worker's role has therefore come to encompass locating, involving, and supporting the families, or, when appropriate, involvement in the work of terminating parental rights or seeking parental surrenders to plan for adoption for their children.

The program's relationships to medical centers with pediatric AIDS services have been a key component. These centers have provided medical education, medical treatment, counseling, and medical specialty referrals for foster families. They have also made possible continual care by well-informed and compassionate medical personnel who understand the child welfare system.

As the program has progressed, a number of additional services and activities have been added. With the support of the City of New York public child welfare agency, a foster parent appreciation dinner is held annually. A foster parent/foster care worker hot line has been established to provide information or referrals to foster families served by the Leake and Watts program as well as by other New York City agencies.[2] In June 1989, a newsletter for caregivers and foster care agencies was inaugurated. Agency staff members are also involved in consultations with other agencies and citywide and national educational and professional conferences to exchange information on serving HIV-infected children.

Conclusion

Children with HIV infection can be cared for in family homes. It is a challenge and, often, hard work. Foster parents report that their love for the children, the support of the agency, and financial compensation by the state make it possible for them to undertake the care of these children. Foster parents need the support and assistance of a qualified and committed staff and the occasional relief of respite care services. Such care in foster homes is considerably less expensive than inappropriate hospital or residential settings. More important, it provides all of the children with what they need most: a caring home environment with persons who are devoted to them and dedicated to providing for them a life of acceptance, concern, and dignity.

REFERENCES

Anderson, G., Gurdin, P., and Thomas A. "Dual disenfranchisement." In Ken Doka (editor), Disenfranchised Grief. Lexington, MA: Lexington Press, 1989.

[2] A range of new services have been possible due to a 1988 grant from the Office of Human Development Services, U.S. Department of Health and Human Services.

Gurdin, Phyllis. "Homefinding guidelines for HIV-seropositive children." Unpublished paper. Leake and Watts Children's Home: Yonkers, New York, Spring 1989. (The section "Homefinding" has been adapted from these draft guidelines.)

Gurdin, Phyllis, and Anderson, Gary. "Quality care for ill children: AIDS-specialized foster family homes." Child Welfare 66 (1987): 291–302.

Rendon, M., Gurdin, P., Bassi, J., and Weston, M. "Foster care for children with AIDS: A psychosocial perspective." Child Psychiatry and Human Development 19 (4) (Summer 1989): 256–269.

10

Kaleidoscope-Chicago's STAR Program

SANDRA M. STEHNO

KARL W. DENNIS

MARIANNE WEST[1]

ILLINOIS IS A "PRIVATE AGENCY" STATE; WITH THE EXCEPTION OF SOME preventive services and some foster family homes supervised directly by the public agency, child welfare services are delivered via state contracts with agencies in the private sector. Specialized services for difficult-to-serve populations are almost exclusively the province of the private sector, and yet the private sector has often been unable or unwilling to accept these children into care. As a result, out-of-state placements and the unnecessary use of shelters and hospitals have been the lot of behaviorally disturbed, dual-diagnosed, and other difficult children and youths. Not surprisingly, the first HIV-infected babies coming into state care in the mid-1980s received hospital care instead of child welfare services, for want of foster homes or private agencies willing to accept them.

Kaleidoscope is a comprehensive child welfare agency that was founded in 1973 to serve unserved children and youths. Over the years, its typical clients have been seriously emotionally disturbed adolescents, but they have also included teen parents and their children, psychotic

[1]The authors wish to acknowledge the contributions of Olivia Dundich and Doug Stevens to this paper.

children, and multi-problem families whose children have been placed in state care. The agency's policies of "inclusive admission" (no one is denied admission because of the severity of his or her problems) and "no punitive discharges" (no one is discharged from care because of failure to adjust to the program) are distinctive. Although there are three basic program structures—therapeutic foster family care, supervised independent living, and intensive family-based services—Kaleidoscope seeks to fit the program to the child and thus supplements basic program services with individualized services.

Program Genesis

The Illinois Department of Children and Family Services (DCFS) recently has been trying to increase the number and size of programs it operates directly. Its first response, therefore, to the need for child welfare services for HIV-infected infants languishing in hospitals was to develop its own specialized foster family care program. Two problems quickly appeared that were to prove this initial program response inadequate to meet an obviously growing need: first, the public agency, DCFS, like other area agencies, was already having difficulty in recruiting a sufficient number of qualified people to foster children without special service needs, and, second, DCFS had no experience in providing specialized (or therapeutic, or professional) foster family care.

Early in 1986, senior DCFS officials asked Kaleidoscope-Chicago to consider adding a program for this population. To provide this service was consistent with the agency's mission and supported by its experience in providing therapeutic foster family care. Although the proposal met resistance from the senior staff, who cited the strains of program expansion, the lack of resources for rigorous foster parent recruitment, and the legal and political volatility of the AIDS disease, executive persuasiveness won them over and cleared the path to developing the STAR program (Specialized Team for AIDS Relief).

Although the basic program framework for STAR was already in place with the Therapeutic Foster Families Program, several months were spent reviewing the literature, talking with other pediatric AIDS child welfare programs around the country, and with legal and medical experts, to design the policies and services appropriate to this population. The design work and the pre-service training of STAR team staff members were financed by the agency; despite the eagerness of DCFS to have the program, it could not figure out a funding mechanism that would support the extensive start-up work. The carefully conceived program plan was transposed into a purchase-of-service contract with the state in July 1987, and the program opened its doors.

A Case History

Joy was referred to Kaleidoscope by DCFS when she was one month old. The department had taken protective custody one week earlier, when Joy's mother left her overnight at the shelter for homeless women and children where they had been staying. The mother said that she had been arrested on her way to the store and that she had not willfully neglected her child. She had become aware of her own HIV-positive status when she was tested after a prostitution arrest in another state. She also admitted to using cocaine throughout her pregnancy with Joy.

DCFS placed Joy in a hospital-based emergency shelter, where she tested HIV-positive. Although the baby showed no signs of apnea (transient cessation of respiration), she was placed on an apnea monitor as a precautionary measure. She was a little jittery at the time of her referral to Kaleidoscope, but otherwise was responsive, alert, and eating well.

The agency placed Joy in the home of Mrs. Smith, a newly licensed STAR professional foster parent. Mrs. Smith was well qualified for the job. She had successfully raised seven children of her own, as well as two children of a distant relative who had become addicted to cocaine. She is also the grandmother of 12. Her parenting experience is coupled with training and experience as a homemaker, a job she held at another private child welfare agency before becoming a STAR parent. Although Mrs. Smith is not involved in organized religion, she is a devout woman who would describe her interest in helping child AIDS victims as a calling. She is divorced and lives with a son and two daughters, one of whom she trained to operate the apnea monitor.

Joy is thriving in Mrs. Smith's home. She remains on the apnea monitor but continues to show no signs of apnea. Her jitters have subsided, but she remains an extremely active child for her age. She is achieving developmental motor and cognitive tasks appropriate to her age, thanks to lots of attention from Mrs. Smith and her daughter, and to her participation in an infant stimulation program at Children's Memorial Hospital. The hospital continues to monitor her health monthly. Several months ago another HIV-infected infant was placed in the Smith home; both babies benefit enormously from having a sibling, and Mrs. Smith, aided by her daughter, has found the responsibility of caring for two babies manageable.

Mrs. Smith is also well supported by Kaleidoscope in her work. At least one STAR team member visits the home twice weekly to monitor Joy's progress and offer support. Staff members also accompany her to medical appointments and are in touch by phone at least once a week. Mrs. Smith attends a support group for STAR foster parents once a month and attends monthly training. She also knows she can reach a STAR team member 24 hours a day, seven days a week, via the team's rotation on-call system.

The baby's permanency plan is still return to her biological mother. Accordingly, STAR staff members have set up a weekly visiting plan with the mother at the agency, but she has failed to come. After she last contacted the agency, the program's family development specialist went out to her home, where she gave the mother information on applying for public assistance, receiving emergency food assistance, and enrolling in a cocaine abuse treatment program, as well as information on and carfare for an AIDS treatment clinic. Her prognosis for resuming parental responsibility is questionable, but the program staff will continue with efforts to assist her in doing so. The agency is also in the process of contacting the mother's sister to see if she might be a possible permanent caregiver, and we would consider Mrs. Smith a candidate should Joy be freed for adoption.

Program

The primary goal of the program is to provide loving, nurturing, skilled foster parents for HIV-infected children and to afford them the opportunity to live in a family home as normally and as fully as they possibly can. Other permanency goals, including reunification with biological family members and freeing babies for legal adoption, are pursued when appropriate. Secondary goals include obtaining appropriate therapies, medical care, and educational resources. The care of these children is a team effort, involving a number of people inside and outside the agency; the boundaries of Kaleidoscope's responsibility are defined in staffings, but as a rule the program provides or obtains the range of resources the children need.

Currently there is room for 13 children in the program, and it operates at capacity, usually with a waiting list. All of the children currently in care are black, Hispanic, or of mixed race, typical of the population of young HIV-infected children in Chicago. They range in age from three months to 2½ years, and were usually referred to the agency within a month of birth. Eleven of the current 13 were also born addicted to cocaine. The children's mothers have contracted the HIV infection through drug injection or prostitution. In several cases, the mother has abandoned the baby; in others, the state has intervened because of the mother's illness or lack of fitness as a parent. The only intake criteria are an HIV-positive test, state responsibility for payment, and room in the program. Most children will not leave the program; in rare cases, they are able to be placed in a relative foster home or an adoptive home.

Professional foster families are recruited and trained solely for the HIV-infected children to be placed (that is, the families are not permitted to have other foster children) and are compensated for their work. Room, board, and other direct costs are provided by the agency. The foster parents' job is extremely demanding. Foster parents are expected to provide excellent parenting (nurturance, discipline, guidance in achieving age-appropriate development tasks, and so on). They are also expected to monitor the children's health, to maintain special sanitation precautions, and to obtain special medical care and other resources, such as babysitters, as indicated. They are expected to participate in treatment planning for the children, to communicate closely with the agency staff about the children's progress and problems, and to participate in ongoing training.

Foster parents are supported and supervised by a specially trained agency staff. The STAR staff team currently includes a clinical social worker/program director, two social workers, and two nurses. All have received extensive training on the special service needs of HIV-infected children, but, like the foster parents, their primary goal is to offer these children the chance to live as normally as they possibly can. STAR staff members are assisted and supported by the administrator and foster parent recruitment specialist of the Therapeutic Foster Families Program.

By and large, the STAR program has been carried out according to the program plan, but a few changes have been made. First, the original program plan called for one foster child in a foster family, but in several instances two have been placed, the agency having found that some children benefit more from having a foster sibling than they do from the special attention given only children. Second, the program has considered accepting children older than age three, in response to requests of the DCFS. And, third, the program has added a social worker trained to work with families, to provide additional support to the foster families, to identify and screen prospective adoptive parents and family day care providers, and to work with biological families.

At STAR's inception, it was not thought that any STAR clients would have the possibility of family reunification. Nevertheless, one child was in fact returned to her mother, who committed herself to drug rehabilitation. Sometimes it has also been possible to locate and persuade adult relatives of children to become their caregivers. Currently, three biological families are working toward reunification. The family development specialist searches for suitable caregivers among the children's relatives, encourages visiting between these relatives and the children, helps the foster parents to encourage and monitor involvement of biological families, and provides counseling and support to biological family members. Obviously, in the case of biological mothers, this support includes referral to and monitoring of drug abuse treatment programs.

At this writing, the STAR program is supported almost entirely by a $99.02 per diem purchase-of-service contract with the DCFS. (At contract capacity of ten children in care, this amount totals a $361,500 yearly program budget.) The program has also received small private-sector cash and in-kind donations, as well as $80,000 within the past two years from the Department of Public Health to assist in foster parent recruitment. The budget, of course, is largely earmarked for staff salaries and foster parent stipends and board payments. Despite the generous appearance of the budget, it remains glaringly deficient in certain ways. Staff salaries remain low, approximately $5,000 per position less than those of state workers. The budget did not support start-up expenses, nor does it support out-of-state training opportunities. Although the budget supports tax-free stipends for foster parents, these stipends are not at parity with salaries of child-care professionals, and insurance needs of foster parents are not covered. Finally, recruitment of foster parents has proven so difficult that the program has obtained funding support, through a grant, for a recruitment specialist.[2]

Staff

The STAR team staff was recruited from the ranks of the agency staff. It was encouraging that so many excellent staff members would want to work with this population; clearly, they were drawn by the extreme vulnerability of the children, and by their being such innocent victims of their plight. None of these staff members had had previous

[2]The STAR program has developed copyrighted policy and program materials for staff and foster parents. A list of available materials appears in the Appendix to this chapter, available for a nominal fee from the agency.

experience with HIV-infected children, although most had known something about the AIDS epidemic. Pre-service training consisted of compulsory reading of a massive amount of literature, attendance at a number of extramural seminars on AIDS, and formal training that included bringing in medical experts.[3]

Staff and foster parents work closely together in planning services, in treatment, and in monitoring progress. The caseload is divided between two staff teams; each nurse is reponsible for the health care of one group, including visiting each family at least weekly, checking the health status of each child weekly, attending medical appointments with the foster parents to make sure everyone has a common understanding of the child's medical needs, and providing brief respite care (babysitting services) when needed. One social worker and the team's supervisor share responsibility for documentation, report writing, liaison with other agencies, and foster family support. These two persons also visit one group of foster families per week, although they rotate caseloads every week so that both know each foster family well. The other social worker, the family development specialist noted earlier, develops resources for family reunification (finding biological and extended family members who might be willing to care for the children) and for day care, supports the foster families, and assists in the adoption process. (To date, six of the children currently in the program are likely to be freed for adoption, and four of the foster parents have expressed interest in adoption.)

Foster Parents

Recruitment of foster parents has been difficult enough to warrant obtaining resources for a marketing campaign and for a staff specialist. The agency first tried to recruit foster parents from the ranks of its other programs' foster parents, and from their friends. There was little interest, for misconceptions and judgments about AIDS were common in that group, largely one of working-class and middle-class black people who were extremely active in churches and fostered our children, in part, out of religious convictions. Nevertheless, a couple of veteran foster parents came forth, as did a DCFS foster parent. The agency then

[3] We are indebted to Terry Zealand of the St. Clare House in Newark, to Mary Boland of the Children's Hospital in Newark, to Ted Allen of the New Jersey Department of Youth and Family Services, and to Phyllis Gurdin of Leake and Watts in New York for their assistance in developing our staff and foster parent training programs.

turned to new possibilities—young single professionals, other minority communities, and the like. These efforts were greatly furthered by a print advertising and marketing campaign developed with private funds by a local marketing-advertising firm. The STAR program has also generated sympathetic publicity; newspaper and TV coverage has brought forth initial expressions of interest from a number of current and prospective foster parents.

The STAR program has nine foster homes at this writing. This group includes single women, single men, adult roommates who share parenting responsibility, and married couples. Four of the families have two infants in care; five have one each. The program was initially designed to place only one child per home, but the great demand for the program and the recognition that some children profited from having a foster sibling led to the practice of placing two children in some homes.

The agency requires all of its foster parents to have demonstrated excellent parenting skills and educational achievements sufficient to the tasks of reporting, working with medical and psychiatric jargon, and so forth. One foster parent per family must also give up outside employment to be available to the foster child on a 24-hour basis. Also required are attendance at pre-service and in-service training (see Figure 1), at staffings, court hearings, and the like, and weekly submission of the written logs of the daily activities of their child.

All of these duties are required of STAR foster parents, and more. STAR parents cannot have biological children under five. They must have their own washer and dryer, and they must maintain tedious sanitation practices, including wearing rubber gloves when bathing or diapering clients, washing dishes in extremely hot water, and using a chlorine bleach solution for household cleaning. They must complete a rigorous pre-service training curriculum as well as attend in-service sessions regularly. The pre-service training consists of an 18-week course that includes 20 hours of therapeutic foster parent training and an additional 14 hours of AIDS-related content. In-service training requirements include one meeting/training session per month with the entire foster parent group, one support group per month with STAR parents only, and attendance at special training events.

Relationships

Within the agency, STAR is a subprogram of the Therapeutic Foster Families Program. STAR staff members provide AIDS-related counseling

Wednesdays, 1:00–6:00 P.M.

SESSIONS ═══════════════════════════════════════

March 15, 1989   Welcome—Introductions
                        What is AIDS??
                        Presentation
                        Videotape
                        Questions

March 22, 1989   Issues in Fostering an HIV Infant

March 29, 1989   Review STAR Child Care Guidelines
                        Demonstrate use of rubber gloves
                        Review STAR documentation/paperwork
                        Practice using paperwork
                        Sign forms

April 5, 1989   No class

April 12, 1989   "Normal" early childhood development
                        Drugs and babies

April 19, 1989   Pediatric AIDS and
                            early childhood development
                        Statistics/health-medical management/
                            experiences/physical problems

April 26, 1989   Issues of death and dying

May 3, 1989   Stress—how to cope

Figure 1. STAR Foster Parent Training.

129

and expertise to the agency's Youth Development and Satellite Family Outreach programs when clients in these two programs are discovered to be at risk of AIDS. STAR, like all the other agency programs, is ultimately governed by a statewide Board of Directors, shared with the sister downstate agency. (In an expected division of the corporation, Kaleidoscope-Chicago will be governed locally.) The agency had considered convening an Advisory Board specifically for the STAR program to provide community support and to provide professional expertise, but experts have made themselves available informally, and the community has been supportive, making a formal advisory board unnecessary.

Since the goal of the program is to help children live normally in the community, STAR staff members and foster parents have relationships with many community agencies: for example, hospitals, clinics, schools, playgrounds, and babysitters. Staff members work especially closely with DCFS and with Children's Memorial Hospital, the city's most expert medical care provider in treating pediatric AIDS. Conflicts with community institutions have so far not been a problem—the young age of the children and the diligence that the foster parents have exercised to maintain confidentiality are probable reasons; this situation has also been true of the one school-aged child STAR has cared for. Problems in convincing the medical community to permit these children a normalized family life had been resolved several years ago when an adolescent in another program tested positive for the HIV virus.

The business community has also been extremely interested in the program and has had a feature article about it in the major business weekly (*Crain's Chicago Business*, November 30, 1987). A small advertising and marketing firm has developed a foster parent recruitment campaign at rock-bottom prices and has given many pro bono hours to this work as well. A business-based federated fund-raising drive for children's charities has chipped in, as have the employees of Playboy Corporation.

Senior staff members individually maintain close ties with other AIDS-related organizations, but, except for a funding group, the AIDS Foundation, and a group that focuses on AIDS education in the black community, STAR has not worked particularly closely with other AIDS-related groups because they do not deal to any great extent with pediatric AIDS.

The relationship with DCFS, the principal funding and referral source, has been relatively supportive. Differences of professional opinion about the program between our two agencies are natural products of different vested interests that occur between funder and funded agency, as well as the potential volatility of the AIDS problem. One obvious example is that DCFS has, on occasion, questioned the rate established for the program; the agency, of course, believes STAR is a bargain since DCFS would otherwise have had to spend $400 to $1,200 per day on hospital care for these babies. As of this writing, however, DCFS is using STAR more than fully. Furthermore, after two years of providing regular foster care for some HIV-infected children, DCFS has come to agree with us that specialized foster care is the program of choice for this difficult population. (Indeed, several STAR referrals have come from DCFS foster homes, when families have found themselves insufficiently paid and trained to care adequately for HIV-infected infants.) DCFS has recently obtained federal funds to develop its own specialized foster care program for HIV-infected children and youths and has already approached STAR for assistance. Both programs will no doubt be needed.

Successes, Failures, Surprises, and Plans for the Future

Success in this program is little different from success in any of the agency's other programs—the ability to help special-needs children live normally with families and in the community. Successes would also include family reunification and adoption, the completion of age-appropriate developmental tasks, and acceptance without prejudice by the foster family's extended family and by neighbors and classmates. In addition to client-centered successes, success for STAR would include the ability to recruit as many qualified foster parents as are needed and the ability to serve and to encourage others to serve every HIV-infected child who comes into state care. Our ultimate goal is that no HIV-infected child should spend even one extra night in a hospital or shelter for want of a family home to go to.

It was especially satisfying to be able to return a STAR baby to his mother with the confidence that, with continuing agency support, she would be a loving and competent parent. In this case, Satellite Family Outreach Services (the intensive family-based program) were provided to the mother at the same time that STAR services were provided to the infant. The mother received help in getting into a drug treatment program and help with parenting skills. This family remains in the Satellite program and is doing well; in a few months, the agency will likely recommend termination of its service but with continuing monitoring of the family's well-being by community agencies. Family reunification service needs of this population are multiple and complex; special staffing and funds are needed to provide these services adequately.

The agency did not anticipate in planning the program that so many of the children would be so healthy. The vast majority of the children have not yet progressed to ARC or AIDS, and their behavior is not extremely problematic. Thus, with two nurses on the team and minimal specialized medical care needs, some of the work of the nurses could be refocused (although monitoring sanitation, health, and preventive care remain, of course, critical) to more generic child welfare work. This readjustment reflects a flexibility that is critical in developing successful programs for HIV-infected children, for information on AIDS is constantly growing and changing. When STAR began, it was predicted that 60 percent of HIV-infected children would develop AIDS; now, estimates are somewhat lower.

The health of the babies has also encouraged STAR to strengthen its service support for family reunification and adoption. A social worker was added to concentrate on making and strengthening biological family ties. Many of the foster parents have expressed interest in adoption (which would come at great financial loss to them, for adoption subsidies do not approach the current foster parent payment levels), a service in which the agency was relatively inexperienced. Staff members have learned more about when they should be considering adoption and how they can support clients and foster parents in achieving this goal.

At the other extreme, the agency did not expect that children might die as young as two months of age; the baby was a dual victim of cocaine addiction and an HIV-infection, and died of sudden infant death syndrome (SIDS). Depressingly, neither the mother, who had abandoned him, or other biological family members, could be found in time for the funeral. Also depressing were the public aid-supported funeral arrangements; finding additional funds for dignified funerals has become a fund-raising necessity of the program.

Like any other child welfare agency in this country, Kaleidoscope has adjusted somewhat to the crisis-driven nature of the system. Nevertheless, the agency has been surprised at the extent to which children are referred to STAR on emergency (or a moment's) notice, particularly when the hospitals have been able to forecast the date at which hospital care will no longer be medically necessary. Since July 1987, STAR has accepted on an emergency basis 11 of the 16 children it has served; the hospital notified DCFS of its intent to discharge the children, and DCFS requested placement at a moment's notice. Some of these placements have been made with less than 24 hours notice and little referral information. The STAR staff has had to develop the ability to prepare for clients very, very quickly, including late night and weekend work, to assure that everything possible has been done to help the foster families accept the children smoothly. Private sector child welfare workers in Illinois are not protected under collective bargaining; readers with collective bargaining systems will have to cost out the implications of weekend and night staff work.

Note must also be taken of the full effects that this program can have on agency liability insurance. STAR foster parents have signed a waiver of agency liability should they contract an HIV infection (an extremely unlikely event), but even the waiver did not prevent the insurance estimates from going through the ceiling. The agency settled with the company on a plan that excludes HIV infections from our coverage.

The importance of adequate start-up funds in developing programs for HIV-infected children bears reemphasis. The agency's failure to press this issue brought about high, unremitted operating costs and an inestimable drain on staff resources. STAR staff members were doing double duty, carrying existing caseloads as well as learning their new positions. Furthermore, because no similar program existed in the state, of necessity the agency had to bear out-of-state travel and phone costs, which the state government is reluctant to reimburse.

Finally, the agency was pleasantly surprised by how sympathetic and supportive the community was of this program; the agency had been so accustomed to keeping a low profile because its children, especially the troubled adolescents, do not elicit public compassion. It is clear now, though, that in the eyes of Chicagoans, HIV-infected babies truly are seen as innocent victims, and people who work with them are viewed almost as saints.

Still more AIDS babies are coming into care than there are foster families for them, so current plans are to add a couple of family homes to our contracted capacity. Future directions for the STAR program could include three additional populations: older youths with HIV infections, children who are terminally ill from diseases other than AIDS, and infants born with cocaine in their blood. For the first two groups, STAR foster parents are trained in hospice care and in special medical care. The last group, "cocaine babies," is at present the major unmet service need in the Illinois child welfare system; foster parents with training both in treating behavior-disordered children and medically needy children are in great demand.

Other agencies have been exceptionally helpful to Kaleidoscope in developing STAR. Clearly the time is ripe to find the means to establish a nationwide network of specialized foster care agencies, to make the path of developing new programs a little smoother, to provide mutual support when clinical and political problems are encountered that one cannot solve alone, and to promote the development of practice wisdom in serving special-needs children.

Appendix

STAR Program

Copyrighted program materials available for a nominal fee from Kaleidoscope include:

STAR Program Plan
STAR Program Staff/Foster Parent Orientation and Training: Description and
    Outline
STAR Program Staff/Foster Parent Job Descriptions
Special Payment Provisions
TFFP STAR Program AIDS Fact Sheet
Guidelines for Kaleidoscope-Chicago Foster Homes: Special Health, Safety, and
Sanitary Procedures
Daily Child Care Log
Daily Child Health and Medication Report
STAR Program Intake/Referral Packet

11

Foster Care for Children with HIV Infection: Special Mission in a Loving Environment

SEMA COPPERSMITH

IN FEBRUARY OF 1987, THE STATE OF FLORIDA HAD OVER 2,000 AIDS CASES reported to the Centers for Disease Control [CDC 1987], ranking third in the country behind New York and California. Miami had 916 cases. Equally alarming, with 60 reported pediatric cases, Florida ranked third after New York and New Jersey.

A consortium of health, social service, and public service organizations had been formed, the South Florida AIDS Network (SFAN), to provide care, treatment, support, and education to persons with AIDS-related illnesses, their families, and their support systems. SFAN was deeply concerned about the growing number of HIV-positive babies at Jackson Hospital, a county-operated medical facility. The hospital, which was part of the network, was also concerned about having many boarder babies who were homeless—abandoned by their parents; these babies could not receive sufficient love, care, and nurturing in a hospital setting. In addition, the per-child cost of keeping these babies in the hospital was $800 to $1,000 a day. The hospital agreed to provide financial assistance for beginning a foster care program, far less expensive and far better suited to caring for children than unnecessary hospitalization, and SFAN asked The Children's Home Society of Florida to consider a specialized foster care program for HIV-positive children.

The Children's Home Society (CHS) was founded in 1902; it is the oldest private agency caring for children and families in the state. Committed to "promoting the health, happiness and welfare of South Florida's youth," the board of directors carefully reviewed SFAN's request and approved recruitment, home study, and licensing of foster homes to provide care for HIV-positive babies and children with AIDS. The contract for service was the result of a cooperative effort of the Florida Department of Health and Rehabilitative Services (HRS), SFAN, and CHS.

The request for services was made in February 1987, recruitment of foster homes began in late September, and the project, named Special Mission in a Loving Environment (SMILE), officially began with its first foster parents in January 1988. Within that year the number of reported AIDS cases in Florida had nearly doubled, and 29 new Florida pediatric AIDS cases had been reported to the CDC [CDC 1988].

Recruitment and Networking

The recruitment of foster parents began through extensive involvement with community groups and organizations and with publicity. Recruiting, including media coverage, remains a continual priority in preparation for increased demand for substitute care for HIV-positive children [Steinbaum 1989].

A central feature of both recruitment and the project as a whole was the establishment of a pediatric AIDS task force. Composed of representatives of community agencies, school system representatives, and community and political leaders with an interest in AIDS, this group promoted the project, guided the agency in setting priorities, and consulted with the project director on solving problems as the project developed.

Within five months, four foster homes were recruited. The home study included assessment of the foster parents' knowledge of the illness, emotional maturity and stability, child-rearing ability, ability to deal with death and dying, acceptance of their role with the agency and hospital, and ability to abide by medical obligations. Licensure was not approved until the parents had received intensive training in infection-control practices and procedures provided by the nursing staff of Jackson Hospital, where all foster parents were directly involved for regular physician care in addition to speciality services and hospitalizations.

The first four foster homes were a diverse group of caregivers: (1) a retired couple with two adult children in the home caring for two foster infants, one with considerable developmental delays; *(2)* two adult sisters, former nurses' aides, caring for four HIV-positive children (one five-year-old, two four-year-olds, and one three-year-old); *(3)* a single-parent mother with an adolescent daughter caring for two foster infants less than six months of age; and *(4)* a woman, who was a former nurses' aide, caring for one foster infant girl. They had different needs for respite care and agency support based on the strengths of their own support systems. In common, they were new foster parents, religious, extremely dedicated to their foster children, and didn't want to dwell on the children's diagnosis.

By early 1989, 15 foster parents had been licensed and over 30 children had been placed. After very brief placements, several foster children died in the hospital, and their foster parents requested and received another HIV-positive child. Many foster parents are considering adoption. One 15-year-old girl with AIDS was placed in a specialized foster home one year ago.

Almost all of the foster parents are black Americans; one foster parent is white. The children are black American, Haitian, and white. Haitian and some white children have been placed with black foster parents. The process of matching foster parents and children is designed to move children quickly from the hospital and to find a good fit between foster parent and child. No foster parents have asked for children to be removed, and no foster parents have left the program.

Services

The need for a range of services for HIV-positive children increased as the number of infected children grew or became better understood. By February 1989, the number of pediatric AIDS cases in Florida reported to the CDC had grown to 161, constituting over 11 percent of all reported children in the United States. The number of reported AIDS cases in Miami—2,209—surpassed the number of reported cases in the entire state two years earlier [CDC 1989a].

The CHS offered special foster homes for HIV-positive children abandoned in the hospital by biological parents or given up by other foster parents who discovered that their foster child was HIV-infected.

Baby Meg was placed in regular foster care at birth; her mother was in a county correctional facility. Before her first birthday, the baby began to have difficulty in breathing, and her foster mother brought her to an area hospital where she was diagnosed as having pneumonia. As the hospital stay extended and the pneumonia persisted, the diagnosis was refined and the illness was identified as pneumocystis pneumonia, an opportunistic infection symptomatic of HIV infection and a diagnosis of AIDS. Her first foster parent did not want to care for a child with AIDS, and a referral was made to the project. Repeated attempts to move Meg into foster care were thwarted by continuing and varied infections, and it was several months before she could be moved into a foster home. Medical care was transferred to Jackson Hospital. In a home with other children, she has been showing improvement and has been relatively healthy despite some difficulty in walking. In placement for one year, she has had only one brief hospitalization, due to congenital syphilis that had been dormant since birth.

Foster parents are trained by hospital personnel and visited at least twice a month by project social workers; they return to hospital clinics for follow-up visits and ongoing monitoring and treatment. Because AZT is an experimental treatment, HRS has required biological parents' permission to authorize its usage; since this consent has been difficult or impossible to obtain, the children are treated in standard ways.

Foster parents are required to participate in a monthly foster parent support group that provides practical information and advice as well as the sharing of problems, concerns, and successes. The therapeutic value of foster parents talking with each other has continued outside the support group meetings—foster parents have developed friendships with each other and an informal support network has evolved.

The project has tried to locate and work with the biological parents of HIV-positive children in foster care, but many parents are ill or not located; others have not wanted to maintain contact with their children. Particularly frustrating have been those cases in which women with HIV infection have continued to have children, producing infant sibling groups that are HIV-infected. Biological parents could benefit from the supportive services that are being created for foster parents.

As a subset of the project, a program was designed to recruit foster parents specifically with nursing experience to care for children who were more seriously ill with HIV-related illnesses and to prevent hospitalization to the extent possible. This program has been expanded to include respite care for HIV-positive biological mothers who need to be hospitalized for a limited period of time but have no one available to care for their children. Social workers provide counseling to the family members, as well as support to the biological mothers while the children are in temporary care, including discussion of AIDS-related issues. It is this program's goal to return the children to their mothers as quickly as possible if and when their condition improves.

Through working with biological parents, it became clear that there were few programs to assist single-parent mothers of HIV-positive children to continue employment. Well enough to work, and needing both the income, interaction, and increase in self-esteem that employment can provide, these mothers had nowhere to leave their children. The project is seeking funding and intends to begin a day care program for HIV-positive children as soon as possible. The day care service will also provide a respite setting for ill mothers who can maintain their children in their own homes with community supports, as well as a place for HIV-positive children who are too ill to be mainstreamed easily in community day care programs but well enough to be with other children.

The project's primary aim through its foster care programs and proposed day care center is to keep HIV-positive children out of the hospital and in home environments in order to provide a life of quality.

> In addition to a diagnosis of full-blown AIDS, at nine months of age, test results indicated that Helen was at least moderately mentally retarded. She had missed developmental milestones and was poorly coordinated physically. Doctors told the foster parents to take the child home, give her loving care, and make her as comfortable as possible for what little of her life remained. They did just that. To the doctors' surprise, she has not been rehospitalized and is in classes at a special center for the developmentally delayed. At age two she still has AIDS and emotional and physical difficulties, but with agency and school support the foster parents can cope and are proud of the progress that Helen has made.

Caregivers are encouraged to treat these children like other children and to provide a normal environment to the extent possible, including being in the community (shopping, going to church), and enjoying recreational and entertainment opportunities, such as trips to Disney World. These activities in the community require special attention to confidentiality. Foster parents are encouraged to use discretion as to whom they tell about the child's health care status. Telling others about the child's HIV may violate the child's right to privacy and subject the child and foster family to discrimination. Unfortunately, there continues to be a stigma for having an "AIDS baby" in one's home; some people continue to believe HIV is so contagious that they can be infected by toilet seats, doorknobs, and coughs and sneezes, despite all evidence against transmission by casual contact.

Project Staff

When the project began, the staff consisted of the project director and a supervisor, who was also involved in several other agency departments. They launched the recruitment effort and divided the lengthy licensing procedure necessary to open a foster home. At this writing, the project director supervises the homes, responds to foster parents' telephone calls and requests, and facilitates the foster parent support group. The project director has been assisted by graduate social work students from Barry University whose field placement has been with the project and who are instructed by the previously mentioned supervisor.

As of August 1989, there were 28 children in the project. With a limited staff, the quality of care of this project would not be possible without bright, experienced, committed foster parents. Recruiting a talented group of foster parents has been made possible, in part, by a stipend that enabled foster parents to leave other jobs and serve as full-time foster parents. The demands of the work have more than warranted the stipend, but stipend funds were cut this year by $250 a month.[1] As state funding is decreasing, the incidence of pediatric AIDS in Florida is increasing; with a cumulative number of 230 pediatric AIDS cases, Florida has surpassed New Jersey and trails only New York State in the number of children under the age of 13 who meet the CDC's narrow case definition [CDC 1989b]. The reduction of foster parent stipends may have a negative effect on recruiting further foster parents.

In addition to increasing numbers, children are coming into care at an older age, as parents who have maintained them at home become ill and unable to care for them in their own homes. The illness of older HIV-infected children has probably advanced to some definitive stage of symptomatology. They are more medically involved children, which has increased the need for recruiting foster parents with special skills in nursing care and will result in greater demands for staff assistance than

---

[1]Level II stipends for foster children who are HIV-positive, asymptomatic, were reduced from $1,700 a month to $1,450; Level III stipends for HIV-positive symptomatic children were reduced from $2,700 a month to $2,450.

in the project's initial years. The project should add at least one new staff member.

Conclusion

The project has to date successfully placed 28 HIV-infected children in foster care homes. Rehospitalizations seem clearly to have been reduced, as consistent medical follow-up and a loving environment are provided for each child. With the rise in the number of pediatric AIDS cases in Florida, with the orphaning of children as parents with AIDS die, and confronted by the continuing difficulty in preventive efforts with drug users, the primary challenge facing this project is to expand its services while working with regional networks to prevent the spread of HIV.

REFERENCES

Centers for Disease Control. AIDS Weekly Surveillance Report. Atlanta, GA: HHS, Public Health Service, February 16, 1987.

Centers for Disease Control. AIDS Weekly Surveillance Report. Atlanta, GA: HHS, Public Health Service, February 15, 1988.

Centers for Disease Control. HIV/AIDS Surveillance. Rockville, MD: HHS, Public Health Service, February 1989a.

Centers for Disease Control. HIV/AIDS Surveillance. Rockville, MD: HHS, Public Health Service, September 1989b.

Steinbaum, Ellen. "Are you going to love me? Children with AIDS." McCalls 66 (10) (July 1989): 57–59.

12

St. Clare's Home: Shelter and Transitional Care for Young Children

TERRY P. ZEALAND

THE EFFORT TO PROVIDE SHELTER AND TRANSITIONAL CARE FOR CHILDREN who are HIV-positive is a challenge that has to be addressed by an increasing number of organizations, governments, and individuals who are prepared to handle fear, sadness, hopelessness, and frustration with love and understanding. Children in transitional care have acquired HIV passively—through parents who often unknowingly contracted the HIV virus through intravenous drugs. This use of drugs was often the result of ignorance and despair, a hopelessness that permits the disregarding of one's safety and health in an effort to escape poverty and pain, most evident in inner cities where high drug use and ignorance about AIDS continue to rule the day. Given the devastation in the inner city and the spread of AIDS, both personal and professional action are required.

In New Jersey, pediatric AIDS cases accounted for 218 children under the age of 13 at the time of diagnosis, as of January 1990. Of the total number of pediatric AIDS cases in the nation, New Jersey has been second only to New York, with 13.5 percent of all children from birth to five years of age. From 1987 to 1988, the number of children under the supervision of the New Jersey Division of Youth and Family Services (DYFS) who have AIDS, AIDS-related complex (ARC), or test positive for HIV infection rose from 65 to 129. Of these 129 children, 71 are being cared for by their families or relatives, and the remaining 58 are either in foster care, hospitals, temporary housing, or in one of the two St. Clare's Homes for Children operated by the AIDS Resource Foundation for Children (ARFC).

The death of a long-time, close personal friend of the author became the stimulus to learn about AIDS and to become actively involved in helping people with HIV infection. Although the author's awareness was heightened, it is not possible simply to announce one's intentions and then hope that one's help will be enlisted in a worthy cause. St. Clare's Home began with research on AIDS and direct contact with the people and agencies who were already caring for the afflicted.

In 1985, before founding ARFC, our investigation concerning AIDS took us to Dr. James Oleske, M.D., and Mrs. Mary Boland, R.N., who had begun the Children's Hospital AIDS Program (CHAP) in Newark, New Jersey. We met children of intravenous drug abusers who were alone because caregivers had either died, disappeared, or were unable to care for them. In order to become more actively involved, the author's wife became a volunteer at the CHAP clinic as an early childhood specialist working with the children. In response to the high number of children in need and to prevent the long-term hospitalization of infants and young children, the plan for St. Clare's began to evolve.

The Organization of St. Clare's

A place was needed for HIV-infected children whose medical condition did not require their hospitalization but who had no appropriate discharge destination. Family members may have lacked the resources to care for their chronically ill child; some were homeless; others were incapacitated due to drug use and illness. The parental incapacitation could be addressed by services to the family or through family foster care for the child, but foster homes prepared for HIV-infected children were scarce. A transitional home between hospital care and return to one's family or to a foster home was needed.

After an 18-month search for a home, Sister Elizabeth Ann Maloney, S.C., the administrator of St. Elizabeth's Hospital in Elizabeth, New Jersey, offered a rent-free two-story home, owned by the hospital and located across the street from it, as the site for a transitional residence. She intervened with city goverment officials to obtain the necessary permissions.

A start-up grant ($150,000) from the New Jersey Department of

Health was instrumental in beginning the program. In addition, many building renovations and expenses were carried out or underwritten. For example, the local AFL/CIO building trades council offered its assistance. Staff members and students from the Collier School (a private school of which the author had been a former director), friends, neighbors, workers from DYFS and the Department of Health, and many others volunteered their time and skills to renovate and furnish the home and to improve its general appearance.

As renovation progressed, neighbors were informed of the purpose of the Home and were invited to tour it and to meet with staff people. Their response was uniformly positive and supportive. The goodwill of neighbors and volunteers was instrumental in launching and continuing the Home. Only one negative event occurred: on the first night the Home was open with its first resident, a nine-month-old girl, someone drove by, tossed a rock through a window, and shouted a vulgar phrase about AIDS. The rock is currently in use as a paperweight in the administrative offices.

The Home, licensed to house five children, was opened in May 1987, six months after it had been offered to ARFC. It was named St. Clare's because St. Clare was historically the companion of St. Francis of Assisi and the patroness of children in distress. A second St. Clare's Home was opened in Jersey City, New Jersey, in January 1989. As in the Newark/Elizabeth area, Jersey City has a high number of AIDS cases in general and of pediatric cases, due to intravenous drug use. A third Home, in Neptune, New Jersey, will open in the near future. Each Home will care for five children, who range in age from neonates to six years. All have been diagnosed as having AIDS or ARC, or are HIV-positive, but do not require the acute care usually provided by a hospital. In the first 18 months, St. Clare's served 29 different children. With the opening of two new residences, the number served will multiply.

Intake

ARFC has developed a formal intake process in collaboration with DYFS, CHAP, and local community hospitals. An intake committee establishes the eligibility and appropriateness of the child for St. Clare's. The formalization of an intake process has been necessary because an increasingly long waiting list for placement has developed.

Intake begins with receipt of a complete referral packet (see Figure 1), which is assigned a priority based on the day of its arrival at ARFC.

**AIDS Resource Foundation
for Children Inc.**
182 Roseville Avenue
Newark, N.J. 07107
201–483–4250

REFERRAL FORM

Name of Child _____ Age ____ DYFS KC# _____

Location of Child _____

Guardian _____ Tel. # _____

Street Address _____

City _____ State _____ Zip _____

Referral Agency _____ Tel. # _____

Street Address _____

City _____ State _____ Zip _____

Contact Person (DYFS Worker) _____ Tel. # _____

PARENTS:

Mother _____ Address _____

Father _____ Address _____

Significant Others _____

Address _____

Significant Others _____

Address _____

Medicaid # _____ Attending Physician _____

Address _____

_____

Telephone _____

MEDICAL INFORMATION	☐ Date	_____
PSYCHO/SOCIAL HISTORY	☐ Date	_____
FAMILY HISTORY	☐ Date	_____
(current periodic assessment)		
DYFS CASE PLAN	☐ Date	_____
RELEASE OF INFORMATION	☐ Date	_____

5/27/87

Figure 1. ARFC Referral Form.

1. *Medical Information*

   A. Medical History and Physical
      (Immunization, C.D.C. Classification for HIV infection
      children under 13 years old and all other pertinent
      medical information)
   B. Pertinent Lab and Test Data
   C. Current Health Status
   D. Current Medication
   E. Other Health Care Providers (consultants)
   F. Last Date Medically Seen/Next appointment date

2. *Psycho/Social History*

   A. D.O.B. __ /__ /__ Birth WHT ____ Sex ____ Race _____
      Language Spoken at Home: _____
   B. Developmental Status
      Measuring Instrument:
      Denver Development _____
      Bailey _____
      Other _____ (name) _____
      Results _____
   C. Description of Child's Behavior/Personality

3. *Family Composition*

   Mother
   Father
   Siblings
   Grandparents
   Relatives
   (information should include all medical data available,
   whereabouts, extent of current involvement with child)

4. *DYFS Case Plan/Foster Placement Plan*

   A. Case goal and plan with service agreement or court order
      attached.
   B. Legal Status with specific requirements and/or conditions.
   C. Foster Placement, documented efforts toward identifying
      placement plan within thirty days.
   D. Visitation Plan.

DYFS District Office _____ Tel. # _____
Monitoring Case Practice Specialist _____ Tel. # _____

The committee reviews the materials and contacts the referring agency or hospital regarding the child's eligibility for the Home; the child's medical history is of primary importance. St. Clare's offers non-acute medical care. If children do not require hospitalization and can receive care in a homelike setting, they are candidates for St. Clare's. To keep files current, there is a weekly review of all pending referrals.

When space becomes available, the agency or hospital that is responsible for the child is notified and prepares the child for the move to St. Clare's; DYFS provides necessary transportation. When the child is placed at St. Clare's, activity is immediately begun to locate the most appropriate long-term environment for the child (return to parents, relatives, or a foster family), a goal which is difficult to fulfill quickly. If, after 60 days, placement in a foster home does not take place, ARFC will consider, case by case, whether to keep the child for a longer period of time or return the child to the referring organization. In the first 14 months of the foundation's existence, length of stay has ranged from as long as nine months to as little as ten days. When discharge or transition to another program or hospital is considered, a pre-established program that includes DYFS advice is used while also considering the child's social and medical well-being.

Services

Children admitted to St. Clare's are tested to determine their cognitive, affective, and psychomotor abilities, and an individual education program for each child is developed. The implementation of the plan is facilitated by weekly visits from members of the CHAP program of Children's Hospital in Newark. Consultation is also provided to the child-care workers who provide daily stimulation and play activities for the children.

The following services are offered to children, their families, and foster families:

Medical

A full-time nursing staff (registered nurse 40 hours a week; on-call nurse at other hours) monitors and provides for the medical needs of the chldren. The nursing staff carries out the orders of the medical director of ARFC (Dr. James Oleske, Children's Hospital), who has admitting privileges at St. Elizabeth's and the Jersey City Medical Center in case of emergencies. The medical director coordinates the individual medical plan with the child's pediatrician or other health care personnel involved with the child. In addition, ARFC has a formal transfer agreement with United Hospitals/Children's Hospital of Newark.

Social

The home has a family-like atmosphere with round-the-clock health and child-care workers trained in procedures and techniques to provide comfort and solace for the children. A full-time housekeeper cooks nutritious meals and performs all housekeeping activities. There is a sense of shared responsibility in respect to the care of the children, together with an effort to provide extra benefits such as music lessons, trips, and special events when financially possible.

Family Involvement

Family visiting is arranged and family members are offered supportive counseling, referrals for specific services, and educational information. The visiting takes place either at the residence or at the ARFC offices. The principal goal of the social service program is maintenance of the parent-child relationship to the greatest extent possible. Parents may have died of AIDS or disappeared, but vigorous efforts are made to locate and involve family members.

Foster Parent Training

In a transitional residence, the preparation of the child and the foster family is an important consideration. Foster parents have educational sessions as well as hand-on experience in caring for HIV-infected children.

Respite Care

Temporary placement at St. Clare's, called respite care, is available to the HIV-positive child and family for medical or social reasons. If respite is needed by the parents, foster parents, or caregiver relative, a referral can be made to St. Clare's. If the potential for respite care for a particular child exists (mother may be in ill health, the foster parent may need a vacation), a respite referral form is submitted to ARFC. If a bed is available, short-term placement is made.

Emergency Placement

When it is in the best interests of children with HIV infection to be placed on an emergency basis, the Division of Youth and Family Services makes a referral and the request is considered, depending on the availability of the bed and the health of the particular child.

For example, DYFS called one evening, requesting immediate placement for two HIV-infected brothers, aged two and four, living in a motel room. Their mother was hospitalized due to AIDS, and the boys were being supervised by a relative who refused to enter the motel room without wearing a mask, gown, and gloves. These boys needed a more secure, nurturing environment and were transported to St. Clare's, whose workers reached the mother and planned family contacts, beginning with a reunion in the hospital on Mother's Day. Long-term planning for the boys' care also began.

Discharge Planning

The transition policy goal is to move children in a timely fashion to a suitable placement that will facilitate bonding of the child to a primary caregiver (a parent, relative, or foster parent). The potential foster parent or family member is encouraged to make regular visits to the Home. During these visits they are given not only an orientation in child care and procedures for handling the child's bodily fluids, but developmental training as well. This training helps the family to continue the care that the child received at St. Clare's. These sessions also help the parents to become aware of community support services.

Case Example

A two-year-old girl came to St. Clare's with severe complications from HIV infection. She had already endured a stroke and suffered aphasia as a result, which meant that she could not communicate verbally with others. Her condition was so serious that her medical instructions included an order not to resuscitate her if she experienced medical distress. She was not left to die, nor would we permit her to live in a silent world. It is our purpose to give hope where there is little or none left.

The girl began to receive AZT therapy, an experimental drug used to slow the progress of AIDS. She was constantly given oxygen, but, as therapy began to take effect, the amount of oxygen could be reduced to the point where only nebulizing her was necessary. Our health care worker decided that the best way to communicate with her was through sign language. Slowly she began to learn signs, and a simple dialogue could be achieved. Today she can sign 21 words, and that number is increasing.

The Early Intervention Program of Children's Hospital provided suggestions for caregivers so that they could interact appropriately with this girl. These instructions illustrate the consultation provided for each child.

Talk and sing to the child in the course of daily play and caregiving. Respond promptly to any attempts at vocalization, providing the word she approximates. For example, if she says "muh" and points to milk, say "milk" and give it to her.

Play games of naming body parts with her, especially at bath and dressing times. Try this technique using a mirror or a doll for variation.

Provide collections of small blocks and other safe objects and open containers to use in games of emptying, sorting, and filling.

Encourage play with toys that reinforce cause and effect, such as "Poppin' Pal" toys. Any household activity, such as turning off and turning on the light switch, is also good for this purpose.

Model and engage the child in symbolic play with baby dolls, bottles, telephones, and such objects.

Increase finger-feeding opportunities, using bits of scrambled egg, diced cooked vegetables and canned fruits, ground meat, and dry cereals.

Encourage mobility, with free access to safe living areas. Place toys out of reach, or blow bubbles and roll balls to entice the child to move toward them.

These guidelines gave direction to the various caregivers and provided the child with tasks that should help her to gain a more developmentally normal childhood.

This child's mother was very sick with AIDS. St. Clare's staff members provided many good visits for the mother and her daughter. The girl knew and loved her mother, who was deeply grateful for the opportunity to spend time with her daughter; she was also comforted to know that her daughter was receiving the best possible care.

Sadly, the mother died while her daughter was still at St. Clare's. She left her child in the hands of those who loved her and with the assurance that her child knew her and knew that she was loved by her mother. We took this girl to her mother's funeral. She was much depressed by the death of her mother, yet this story does not end on a note of tragedy. Today this beautiful child is in the care of a loving foster mother, who frequently brings her to St. Clare's, and who avails herself of the various services that St. Clare's continues to offer to her.

Haller House

To assist families and foster families, ARFC has established Haller House Family Resource Center. This building, donated by retired pediatrician Dr. Olga Haller, is the administrative center of the foundation and its operations. Haller House provides the setting for a variety of programs and services to individuals, families, and groups coping with AIDS and its effects. One program offers a monthly parent support group or social event—for example, a potluck dinner and party for 17 adults and 23 children. Other programs offered at Haller House include bereaved parent counseling, foster parent training and support groups, clothing and toy distribution, information and referral services, training for volunteers, educational programs, and a training bureau for speakers. To inform the public, Haller House produces a quarterly newsletter.

Providing Transitional Care

It is the philosophy of ARFC to maintain and promote continuity of care for resident children. The primary goal of transition policy is to move children in timely fashion to a suitable placement that will facilitate foster parent bonding with the infant or young child. This relationship is supported by familiarizing the foster parents with the individual characteristics of the infant or child and by increasing the foster parents' knowledge of HIV infection and existing supportive services.

Potential foster parents are required to make regular visits for two weeks to one month before the child's designated date of transfer. Regular visiting is minimally defined as two or three two-hour visits each week. The administrative review committee may choose to shorten or extend these visits, based on individual case considerations. Visiting should include instruction in providing for physical needs of the child, including feeding, diapering, and bathing, and instruction in providing for social/emotional and developmental needs, through playing, holding, and early intervention exercises.

Potential foster parents should spend one two-hour session with the head nurse and social worker to discuss the special needs of HIV-positive children, to review the guidelines adhered to at St. Clare's, and to discuss the adaptation of children to a new home environment. These sessions should help the parent to become knowledgeable about supportive services that are available in the community, such as WIC, Medicaid, respite care, home health care, support groups, babysitter and day care services, emergency medical care, medical clinics, and early intervention programs.

This commitment to serving a transitional function and to empowering the foster parent or, in some cases, the biological parent to take the child to a home and there provide loving, appropriate care is the central mission of St. Clare's. It is grounded in the conviction that children, particularly young children, need a family and a home environment for their well-being, but they also need a loving place to live while a more permanent place is located and prepared. Although this aim is designed for the child's best interests, it poses some significant challenges in its implementation. The two main challenges have been those of relationship demands and financial support.

Relationships

A transitional residence requires its staff members to love the young children but then to let them go. For the staff at St. Clare's, this brief time with the child is not only a consequence of the child's life-endangering illness but a deliberate goal of the Home: to move the child to another setting with foster parents or relatives. The staff members quickly bond to children and watching them leave the residence is difficult, not only because the workers have become attached to the children, but the children have also become attached to the workers. One worker noted how a nine-month-old baby responded to him in a special fashion as soon as they met: she would cheer up and move toward him when he entered the room. He felt that she had chosen him as someone special, and to plan for and assist her transition to another home was a challenge. There is a general tendency to judge potential foster parents with some severity, as if to consider them not good enough to care for the child or unable to care for the child as well as the present worker. Loving and letting go is never easy.

To assist each other in this transition process, supervision, both individually and in groups, is intensive and frequent. St. Clare's purpose is repeated over and over again, and particularly strong attachments are recognized and explored. When it is time for a child to leave, a party is always given to honor the child. Children who were former residents, along with their caregivers, are invited to return to St. Clare's for these parties. This ritual eases the transition and allows continuing positive contact with children who have been discharged from the residence. The opportunity to meet with children who have left the home provides great encouragement to the staff members who cared for those children when they were residents, because they can then see how the children are progressing.

The transition difficulty is also met by the Home's continuing involvement with the child and the foster parents or relatives after the child has been moved. The Home maintains contact with the family by providing follow-up services and inviting children and their families to return for parties and other such events. Workers' continued involvement with families after transition is not as rivals for the children's affection but as supporters and helpers (even as extended family members) to the children and caregivers. Loving the child means preparing the child and potential parents for life together and then letting the child go while maintaining realistic ties to the family.

Financial Support

Despite the support of public agencies and private charities, transitional care presents a funding challenge. The medical and care needs of the children and their families require more intensive services than traditional residential care. In addition, moving children to foster homes or to homes of relatives loses the assurance of funding that comes from long-term Medicaid-eligible care. Many times, children in need are not Medicaid-eligible, yet there is nowhere else for the child to live. St. Clare's has chosen to accept children based on need, not on funding eligibility, with financial distress for the program as a result.

St. Clare's work with biological families, with its continuity during the children's stay at the Home and after their discharge to families and relatives, enriches the care given children and their families but expands the mission and scope of the agency. This expansion is not adequately noted or funded. St. Clare's has become a multi-service community agency rather than simply an institutional residence with limited discharge planning.

Staffing

A range of trained, professional persons is necessary to carry out ﹅ residential and family service program such as St. Clare's. The program has a medical director from the Children's Hospital, and children are also attended by a physician from the New Jersey Division of Youth and Family Services. In addition to a full-time registered nurse, a nurse is on call 24 hours a day. A social worker deals primarily with family members and foster parents. Each residence has a house manager, housekeeper, and child-care staff (two staff members on eight-hour shifts, round the clock; none sleep in the residence). Currently, there is an initiative to increase the medical competence of the child-care staff, creating a medical child-care worker position requiring 100 hours of instruction and a 200-hour internship under nurse supervision. This high level of medical training for child-care staff members, in addition to nurse and physician involvement, allows St. Clare's to serve children with a range of medical treatment needs, including nasogastric feeding, monitors, and antibiotic treatments.

All staff members are trained in universal health precautions (refer to Table 1). They receive periodic HIV-antibody testing. No instances of transmission of HIV from children in care to family members, other children, or staff members have occured.

The house staff members meet regularly once every two weeks to reassess the children's needs. Evening staff members are required to attend and are paid overtime. House managers, nurses, and administrative staff members also meet once every two weeks.

St. Clare's has depended upon volunteers to provide a number of

Table 1

Guidelines for Basic Hygiene and Infection Control

Handwashing is the single most important way to prevent the transmission of infection:

1. Before washing your hands, remove the rings from your fingers to facilitate thorough cleansing and drying. If your watch has an expansion band, slide it above your wrist. Adjust the water to a warm temperature, and rinse your hands.

2. Lather your hands thoroughly. Remember that it is the friction from rubbing your hands together that removes potentially infectious organisms from your skin. A ten-second vigorous handwashing will adequately remove most transient flora.

3. Wash each wrist by vigorously sliding the opposite hand around its surface area.

4. Interlace your fingers and thumbs, and slide them back and forth. Clean under your nails and around the nail beds with the fingertips and nails of the opposite hand.

5. Thoroughly rinse each hand from the wrist down. If your hands were grossly soiled, repeat steps 2, 3, 4, and 5.

6. Dry your hands with disposable towels.

7. To protect your hands from the contaminated surface of the faucet handle, turn off the faucet by placing a dry section of your used towel over the handle.

Gloves are indicated in the following situations:

1. When providing care when there is a potential for contact with blood or body fluids, such as when changing diapers, or in cleansing and dressing the wound after a child gets a cut or abrasion

2. When handling materials, cleansing surfaces, or objects that have been contaminated with blood or body fluids

3. When cleaning with bleach solution, to avoid irritation to your skin and prevent cracking and chafing

4. If you have abrasions or wounds on hands or arms and are unable to cover them properly with protective bandage

5. When caring for a vascular access such as a broviac catheter

Masks should be worn:

1. When the health worker has an upper respiratory infection

2. When infant or child has a productive cough and is coughing sputum into the air

Smocks should be worn:

1. When there is a potential for contact with blood or body fluids (e.g., if infant or child has diarrhea)
2. When child health care workers wish to protect street clothes

Care of environment and household:

1. Cleaning solution for disinfection is 1:10—

   1 part bleach to 10 parts water
   or
   1 cup bleach to 1 gallon water

2. When spills of blood or body fluids (urine/stool) occur, wear gloves, remove soil, and then clean with bleach solution, rubbing vigorously.
3. Rugs and upholstery should be cleaned once a month. When cleaning up spills on these surfaces, use Lysol and warm water.
4. Floors should be cleaned once a day with hot, soapy water. Bathroom floor should be disinfected once a week with bleach solution.
5. When possible, dishes should be done in the dishwater, after rinsing them. When there are only a few dishes, wash them in hot water and soap. (Dishwasher is preferred for proper and thorough cleaning.)

Laundry:

1. Dirty linen should be double-bagged before bringing it to the laundry room.
2. If linens or clothes are soiled with blood, feces, or urine, wash them separately.
3. One cup of bleach with *hot* water should be used for laundry. If material is not color-fast, use non-chlorine bleach (Clorox 2).
4. Cleanse washing machine with bleach solution and rinse thoroughly after completing laundry.

Disposal of garbage:

1. Garbage should be double-bagged.
2. Garbage should be disposed of at St. Elizabeth's after the day shift and 11 P.M. to 7 A.M. shift. On late evening and night shift, if linen or clothing is soiled with blood, urine, or stool, place in hot water and soap in the basin in the basement sink.

valued services. As mentioned earlier, volunteer labor and skill were instrumental in preparing the residence. In addition, seven volunteers are involved in direct child care, having completed formal and on-the-job training requirements, and seven volunteers assist with various administrative tasks.

Statistics on pediatric AIDS demonstrate that almost nine of ten children with AIDS are black or Hispanic. This finding has several implications for staffing. First, it is crucial that an agency such as St. Clare's have a significant number of black and Hispanic staff members. Second, all staff members need to be sensitive to cultural diversity and issues in child care. For example, actions that may seem relatively unimportant to the staff, such as clothing or hair care and styling, may have great significance to family members who have very distinct preferences and want an active role in caring for their child's appearance.

Conclusion

There is a great danger that HIV-infected children will be overlooked. As a relatively small percentage of the total population of AIDS sufferers, their needs may not be paramount or adequately presented. Without outward signs of sickness, many will suffer stigma but will not receive services. In need of homes and, in some cases, families, many were abandoned in large city hospitals, and some continue to suffer unnecessarily long hospitalizations, awaiting a stable home with reliable, nurturing caregivers. A transitional residence can provide this care for such a child while working to establish a permanent home for him or her. It is difficult to love a child and then let the child go, but the child's needs are primary. Despite obstacles and a world that often does not seem to care, individuals, agencies, and governments need to recognize suffering children and their families and respond.

13

Reaching Out to High-Risk Adolescents

OLGA C. HERNANDEZ

STEPHEN E. TORKELSEN

> In the fall of 1987, a Covenant House counselor finally persuaded Robert to drop into our medical clinic for a checkup. He looked awful. He had lost about 40 pounds and a lot of his teeth due to infections. To complicate matters, he was addicted to crack. A blood test mercilessly confirmed that Robert had AIDS. That was the first tragedy. The second was that there wasn't much we could do for him except help him die with a little dignity.
>
> —Covenant House Staff Member

THE NEWEST PROGRAM AT COVENANT HOUSE FOR HOMELESS BOYS AND girls under 21 opened officially on December 30, 1988, but, in a certain sense, its 26-bed residential treatment program for runaway and homeless adolescents suffering from AIDS really began that day in October 1987, when 20-year-old Robert walked into its medical clinic. He complained of an abscessed tooth, but the result of several tests quickly confirmed that he was sick and getting sicker, not from an infected tooth but from AIDS. Within just a few weeks he was dead. The official diagnosis was pneumocytis carinii pneumonia (PCP), but Robert really died from AIDS.

In the days and weeks following the young man's death, a steady stream of homeless young males and females began walking into the

159

clinic near New York's Times Square with a variety of HIV-related symptoms—sudden weight loss, tooth abscesses, enlarged lymph nodes, night sweats, and high fevers—that pointed to the devastating verdict: AIDS was beginning to have a disproportionate effect on homeless youth whose high-risk behavior on the street put them at great risk of getting this deadly disease.

High-Risk Behavior: Against the Odds

At 20 years of age, Robert was addicted to street life, trapped in a vicious cycle of drugs, sex, and petty crime that offered him little relief or escape; the news that he had AIDS was only the latest and most tragic consequence of the high-risk behavior that had characterized much of his life.

From the moment he was born in a prison cell, Robert almost seemed destined to a short and bitter life. Abandoned at an early age, taken in by relatives who didn't really care for him, and finally, sexually abused by an uncle when he was ten years old, Robert ran away to the streets where he could learn to live on his own. The only problem was that he didn't know how to do so. He never learned to read or write. His only real skill at communication was "getting over" on the adults he came in contact with by manipulating them, a practice that finally landed him in jail for petty theft before he was barely out of his teens.

In many ways, Robert was typical of the homeless and high-risk male and female youths between the ages of 17 and 21 whom Covenant House sees at its shelters (located in New York, Toronto, Houston, Ft. Lauderdale, New Orleans, Anchorage, and Los Angeles). Fewer than a third of these youths have homes to which they can return; the rest have less and less chance to enter or remain in a child welfare foster or group home because of their age, funding ineligibility, or aggressive behavior.

When they are rejected or discharged from these settings, they see their home as a series of couches in "squats" or "crash pads," temporary beds in temporary shelters, or a hotel room at night with days and evenings spent entirely on the street. As the founder of Covenant House has said, "The street is a brutal parent," teaching them values that slowly but gradually destroy their lives.

Having already suffered early, chronic, sexual and/or physical abuse and neglect at home, these youths, if they cannot find meaningful work, begin a deteriorating spiral of abuse and neglect of themselves and of others, by begging, stealing, and using alcohol and/or drugs daily. After a short time on the street, most are chronically undernourished and suffer from colds and upper respiratory infections. When panhandling brings too little to pay for their room, board, and drugs, most homeless youths use sex to survive—with a boyfriend, a pimp, or as part of the lifestyle of a squat or crash-pad apartment.

If they do not quickly leave these precarious living arrangements, they rapidly lose more and more of whatever self-esteem they have and turn increasingly to hustling as their main occupation, selling themselves in arcades, train and bus depots, in front of pornographic bookstores or movie houses in entertainment zones, or, in some cities, at bus stops and corners of known male and female prostitution zones, commonly called "strolls."

Underneath the denials, the rationalizations about alternative lifestyles, and a growing malaise about changing their behavior, they gradually embrace a unique hopelessness. At 19 or 20 years old, when the rest of their peers are beginning their adult lives and looking forward to the future, these youths feel that theirs are already over.

With no home, no work, and no family support, they can survive only by forced choices. These high-risk choices can result in a recurring cycle of illnesses and diseases such as gonorrhea, syphilis, herpes, and chlamydia that, unpleasant as they are, can be treated and even avoided if intervention is successful. For a growing number of street youths, however, a diagnosis of AIDS is final and fatal. It also can come too late.

That, perhaps, is one of the greatest tragedies of the AIDS crisis, especially among street youths: If the disease is already in its advanced stages, it does not give these youths, who are at risk to begin with, or the service providers who try to help them, time enough to change their behavior.

There was little we could do any more for Robert. Even with the minimal structure imposed on residents (regular meals, daily appointments with a counselor, and a 9 P.M. curfew), he refused to stay at our shelter; he had become too used to living on the street with its totally unregulated lifestyle. As an alternative, he was housed in a nearby hotel. He was willing, however, to come to the clinic every day for checkups. As he became weaker, a member of the nursing staff visited him every day to make sure he was safe and to maintain contact with him.

At first the staff hoped that somehow matters would improve if Robert accepted medical attention and proper food and rest. It was hard not to believe that somehow he would get better, but it was a false hope.

One day we knocked and knocked on his door, but no one answered. The nauseating smells in his room told us what had happened. The youngster had been suffering from severe diarrhea and vomiting. After a frantic search, he was found wandering in the lobby, in shock and suffering from an abnormally high temperature. It was clear that Robert needed to be hospitalized immediately.

We checked him out of the hotel and brought him back to the shelter with us. We knew that Robert would probably have to wait for hours before being admitted to the hospital because of the bed shortage that the AIDS crisis was causing in city hospitals, and we wanted to make sure someone would be able to wait with him and make him as comfortable as possible. On that particular day, however, we had already used all of the staff members we could spare to help Robert, so we called on the Hetrick Martin Institute, an agency in New York City that had also worked with the youngster, and asked if a volunteer might be able to take him to the hospital. From the very beginning of our response to this crisis, we had learned that no one agency can provide all the needed services all the time for a youngster infected with HIV, particularly when the youngster becomes sick; in fact, collegiality and cooperation among agencies is vital to helping these youngsters.

That was the beginning of an uncomfortable two-day hospital wait for the sick youngster until a bed became available. Like many others needing medical attention, Robert had to wait in the hall of the hospital until there was room for him. During his wait, however, Covenant House staff members visited him daily to keep up his spirits and even provided such services as emptying his bedpan or making sure he ate, when the harried hospital staff did not have the time. The extra services such patients require were taking their toll on all of us. Most of the visiting had to be confined to after work. Covenant House staff members felt frustrated that they could not give Robert more attention.

The end came swiftly. A week later, attached to a life-support machine after suffering his first heart attack, Robert suffered a second massive coronary and died. The memory of him hooked up to a life-support machine waving a silent goodbye to the staff etched itself deeply into the hearts and minds of the staff members who surrounded him in his final days.

The shock of Robert's death galvanized the staff into action. Something more had to be done than simply helping youngsters like him to "die with dignity." A way had to be found to help them live, regardless of what their future held, and that meant reaching them *before* the disease reached its final stages. In view of the many homeless youths whose very existence increases the likelihood of contracting AIDS, that was a daunting challenge. Just a month before, in October of 1987, the agency had begun conducting a blind study with the New York State Department of Health to assess the prevalence of HIV among homeless youths; the results, released in November 1988, were alarming: Of the first 1,096 specimens, 74, or approximately 6.75 percent, tested positive for the virus, a rate hundreds of times higher for this group than normal [from an unpublished study, by Dr. James Kennedy and others, "HIV seroprevalence of adolescents at Covenant House/under 21 New York City," presented at the American Public Health Association Conference, Boston, Massachusetts, November 1988]. Clearly Robert was only the first of many potential teenage casualties who would occur at Covenant House if we did not act quickly.

That realization set several policy and procedural changes in motion over the next few months, remarkable even for an agency whose response to crisis in behalf of homeless adolescents has been its hallmark. In the words of Dr. James Kennedy, head of the agency's medical clinic, "AIDS was like a train out of control bearing down at full speed and headed straight through the middle of Covenant House."

Responding to a Crisis

What was needed as quickly as possible was a specialized residential unit to serve adolescent males and females infected with HIV-related illnesses. Several weeks after Robert died, an AIDS Planning Committee consisting of the Director of the Health Services Department at Covenant House, along with staff members from the clinic and residential program of Covenant House/New York, was formed and began meeting regularly.

The rising statistics among young adults in their twenties, whose disease had obviously begun when they were teenagers, made it clear that AIDS would be a threat to the youths at Covenant House when they reached their twenties. It was also clear that, by acting now to reach these youngsters early enough, we could perhaps stop the train or at least soften its effect.

Questions emerged. First, how complex were the medical and other needs of adolescents infected with HIV? There was a general lack of knowledge about AIDS at Covenant House at the time and nothing definitive about how to help adolescents who were affected.

Second, by responding to these massive medical needs, would Covenant House in effect become a hospital, or a hospice, thereby moving outside its formal mission, which is to provide 24-hour emergency shelter and programs as well as long-term residential services for homeless adolescents?

Third, to respond properly to the needs of these youths, should a separate facility be set up for this new program, or should it be integrated into the existing residential structure? The agency had already developed several programs to meet the special needs of the young residents, including programs for adolescent mothers (the Mother-Child Program); drug and alcohol-addicted adolescents (the Covenant House Addictions Management or CHAMP program, developed at the Ft. Lauderdale center); older unemployed teenagers (Rights of Passage, which started in New York); and young hustlers and prostitutes who are gathered through various street outreach programs at Covenant House centers in North and Central America. All of these programs are integrated into the structure of the larger residential program.

It was also clear from the beginning of the discussion about the shape of the so-called "Special-Needs Unit," however, that the special medical needs of homeless, HIV-infected adolescents would demand a radically different approach in its staffing and structure.

What was needed was a holistic program that addressed their social, psychological, spiritual, and medical concerns as well as met their complex medical requirements. To accomplish that purpose, the staff would have to be expanded and the facilities enlarged, to include, for instance, a larger laboratory and an x-ray machine. The clinic could not continue serving both a general and a special population. AIDS patients would need continuing medical attention, for example, while the majority of Covenant House residents are treated on an outpatient basis. The predominant medical needs of these special residents made it necessary for the Health Services Department, not the regular residential crisis-care staff, to direct the program.

Responding to these complex medical needs obviously demanded extraordinary financial resources which the agency did not have. As with other programs at Covenant House, which raises over 90 percent of its funds from private contributions, a special group of donors provided the funds necessary to finance construction. Cost of operating the floor was estimated at $617,000 (or $70 per bed per day) for the first full year of operation.

At the end of 1988, the new 26-bed facility was dedicated and received its first three residents, all of whom had been residents at Covenant House in the past and were known to the health services staff. Like the rest of the Covenant House program, this new floor looks more like a home than an institution. Comfortable sofas and armchairs dominate the living room of the common area where residents gather to talk and watch television. At one end is a separate dining area with small round tables and chairs next to a built-in kitchen. At the other end is a large table, where residents can read and play board games. Bedrooms with private bathrooms are located down the hall from the lounge and are decorated with simple but tasteful furnishings. Creating a homelike environment is one way to show the youths that we care.

Despite the best efforts, though, the future remains unknown for these youths. In five years, perhaps, this program will shut down—or perhaps the numbers will escalate and demand more and more space and services from us and other organizations. What matters is that the agency is going forward now to meet the needs of desperate youngsters whose homelessness gives them few options and fewer places to turn for help.

Putting a Plan into Action

Only two of the staff members required for the special-needs unit were in place when planning began: the medical director and the director of health services. During this early stage, however, it became clear that an effective residential program would include several key components. An adequate and well-qualified staff was essential to providing the individualized, nurturing, and holistic care needed. A multidisciplinary staff of professionals, paraprofessionals, and volunteers with a ratio of 1:5 was the goal, to ensure that each resident would have the full range of services (medical, social, psychological, cultural, nutritional, spiritual, educational, and vocational) to improve the quality of their lives.

Through newspaper advertisements in general circulation publications like the *New York Times,* word of mouth, and professional associations, the search for new staff members began. Previous experience with adolescents, the homeless, and HIV infection was given as the ideal qualification for these openings, in addition to technical and professional qualifications. We also looked for professionals who could respond to this special population with the type of personal care and commitment that marks the best of a Covenant House program—professionals who were competent but who also felt drawn by the challenge of meeting homelessness in ways that would exemplify the Covenant House principles of unconditional love and support of homeless youths.

The Specifics

A director with a master's degree in nursing or a related field (such as a psychiatric nurse with drug experience and knowledge of adolescent behavior), experience in program development, and knowledge of adolescent behavior and AIDS heads the program and manages and supports the senior team, which consists of a casework supervisor to provide supportive services to staff members and residents and coordinate all casework and counseling services; a chemical drug specialist to provide treatment approaches that modify, alter, or stop the chemical abuse process; a life management specialist to help adolescents develop the skills necessary to succeed in their individual plans; and a nurse coordinator to give special attention to the physical, environmental, and medical needs of the adolescents and to obtain the best possible liaison with any medical services available both in-house and from outside agencies.

The core staff currently consists of residential advisors who are available on a 24-hour basis. Shifts are scheduled from 8 A.M. to 4 P.M.; 3 P.M. to 11 P.M.; and from 10 P.M. to 8 A.M.

Additional staff members include a dietitian to provide nutritional assessments and individual help and to monitor dietary standards for the special-needs unit, and a pastoral counselor to address the spiritual needs of each adolescent, on a voluntary basis. The pastoral counselor visits residents regularly to offer support and guidance. In addition, announcements are broadcast concerning religious services and other opportunities for spiritual support.

Volunteers are also regarded as a vital part of any successful staff. Their presence alone sends a clear message to sick adolescents that the community at large does indeed care about them and gives them the additional support and guidance they need at a critical time in their lives. Finding these volunteers was not a problem for us once the call went out. Volunteers can apply for the program only after they complete regular volunteer training (three evenings of seminars and observation) and have worked 50 hours in the regular Covenant House program. Upon acceptance as a volunteer on the special-needs unit, they are required to attend an additional week-long training on the needs of these special residents.

The general shortage of available licensed practical nurses, however, was, and still is, a major staffing concern. In the early stages of planning we visited nursing schools and placed newspaper advertisements in general circulation newspapers and professional journals to attract these urgently needed staff members, with little success. Currently the agency is considering hiring part-time nurses and using the visiting nurses program.

The agency also has an AIDS prevention program staffed by a coordinator, a nurse-educator, a health educator, and a clerical person. This team offers groups and seminars for residents and staff members and one-to-one counseling and referrals. Counseling attracts young people who are worried about infection, who have family members with HIV/AIDS, who have children born with HIV/AIDS, and those interested in taking the HIV antibody test.

Ongoing training would have to be part of any program serving HIV-infected individuals and be available to the entire staff, from administration to housekeeping. It is conducted by both in-house staff members and outside consultants. Considering the nature of and knowledge available about AIDS, it was clear from the beginning that intensive and ongoing staff training would be essential to the program. In addition to providing information, training also offers support, which helps avoid staff burnout.

Information-sharing and cooperation with outside agencies responding to the AIDS crisis were vital to the agency's own efforts. Wide-ranging and growing contacts and relationships with those professionals in the field responding to the AIDS crisis provide us with an invaluable network of referral services for our clients, as well as access to a wider body of information and resources as the program continues. For instance, Covenant House/New York has been a member of the AIDS Services Delivery Consortium/NYC since its inception. Approximately 28 state, local, and community-based agencies and hospitals that deliver AIDS-related services belong to the consortium, which is funded by the Robert Wood Johnson Foundation and the United States Public Health Service. Agency members serve on several subcommittees and also host meetings, among other activities, while the coordinator of the agency's AIDS prevention program actively participates on the adolescents and AIDS working group that developed from the consortium.

In addition, the staff has worked with other agencies and individuals fighting the AIDS crisis, such as the Hetrick Martin Institute; the Streetworks Projects associated with the New York Victim Services Agency; and the AIDS and Adolescent Clinic at Montefiore Hospital in New York City. The agency is also a member of the Child Welfare League of America, which provides standards and practices for residential programs involved in the care of AIDS patients. Information-sharing and collegiality will be essential links in continuing to find solutions to problems.

Bridge to Hope: The Design of the Special-Needs Program

The special-needs program for HIV-symptomatic youths provides not only emergency and short-term residential services, but also longer-term and transitional care—hospitalization, hospice care, or even independent living, as the needs of the residents change during their stay at Covenant House.

The aim of the special-needs unit is to provide a supportive, trusting, and nurturing environment to help HIV-infected adolescents to gain control of their own lives, by providing three types of services:

1. Specialized medical care to arrest or slow down the disease process, with particular attention to known preventive and therapeutic medical regimens, including pharmacological treatments such as AZT, pentamidine, and antibiotics; dietary treatments; and substance abuse rehabilitation;

2. Psychosocial support and life management skills to encourage residents to seek a healthier lifestyle;

3. Spiritual support, to help residents seeking to come to grips with meaning, usefulness, death, and other life issues.

To be admitted to the unit, an adolescent must be HIV-symptomatic and display emotional, psychological, or physical symptoms. Particular emphasis is also placed on educating and involving all direct care staff members, especially intake and outreach staff members who come in contact with high-risk adolescents and are able to recommend them for entry into the program. Youngsters also learn about the program via word of mouth and through other child-care agencies.

Upon admission, the adolescent is oriented to the unit, and a primary counselor is assigned who helps the resident during the initial adjustment phase, and serves as both advocate and service coordinator for the resident's individual health plan, developed with the resident during the first 48 hours of admission. Through individual and group activities, the primary counselor supports the resident's health plan, which serves as the main instrument for assessing the adolescent's needs and potential growth.

The health plan involves all aspects of the resident's life, including short- and long-term goals as regards physical, social, mental, cultural, educational, spiritual, and vocational needs. The plan is reviewed and modified weekly by the senior team.

Overall organization of the unit is comprehensive and oriented toward the personal growth of each resident. Activities include the reestablishment of daily living routines for the individual and the group; educational programs, both in-house and outside (currently the unit offers yoga lessons, meditation, support groups, and physical fitness groups); and referrals to outside educational services such as vocational training programs. Residents are also required to do regular chores, keep their rooms clean, and follow curfew.

One problem common to the adolescents currently being served is intensive drug abuse, with crack use the most serious. Drug programs that meet the needs of crack addicts are hard to find, and, when they are, waiting lists are long. At present, the program uses outside day programs as an alternative.

Currently, family members and close friends can visit residents in a supervised setting. A visitor's policy for this unit, which is located on the third floor, is being studied in order to balance residents' concerns for confidentiality and security. Many of these residents have been exposed to violence from their life on the street, and need to be protected from people seeking retaliation.

If the behaviors of any residents are negatively affecting the unit and they are unable to modify their behavior (e.g., drug abuse, violence, sexual activity), discharge will take place. Every effort will be made to discharge residents to positive living situations where supportive resources are in place. An aftercare program is also provided for the adolescents, who will still be able to obtain health, counseling, and support services. In addition, protocols for reentry will be developed should an adolescent warrant further residential services.

Making the Difference

The definition of success will vary depending on the extent to which the residents can accept help and are willing to change their behavior, especially if they are now using drugs and engaging in other high-risk behaviors. For those residents, the agency will do as much as it can to help them understand that they can take control of their own lives and begin living healthier and more productive lives. For those adolescents too sick to reach that goal, however, success will be defined as improving the quality of their lives in the time they have left.

There is, however, always hope, even in the bleakest of circumstances. Eighteen-year-old Angel (not his real name) first came to Covenant House when he was 14. For the next two years, he was heavily involved in drugs and prostitution on the street. When he was 16, a counselor with the agency's street outreach program talked to him about how he could change his life and the teenager stopped using drugs, went back to school, and began living in a group home.

After being clean for about a year, Angel took the AIDS test—and tested positive. Friends and staff members at the group home where he lived withdrew from him. He had to clean the bathroom every time he used it, wash his clothes separately, and eat his meals from paper plates. Desperate and depressed, he went back to the streets. For the next year, we saw him on and off in the medical clinic, where he came for outpatient care. He listened politely whenever we talked about the new program that was starting, but he said he just wasn't interested. He claimed that he liked street life and felt accepted there for what he was. Then, one day, about a week after we opened the unit, Angel changed his mind. He has stopped using drugs, is still in the program, and is thinking of completing his general equivalency diploma.

The turning point? In his own words, "I remembered how I had been treated when I came to Covenant House, and that made me come back and give things one more shot. Now I wouldn't think of leaving. The people here treat me like I belong to a family."

14

Training for HIV Infection Prevention in Child Welfare Services

J. BURT ANNIN

THIS CHAPTER IS NOT ABOUT CURRICULUM DEVELOPMENT, SEQUENCING, adult learning theory, or learning curves. It is about the challenges encountered in training on HIV-related topics—societal dilemmas that confound training efforts and how the training technique that works best resembles, perhaps is, clinical social work.

Let us begin by asking you, the reader, to indicate your thoughts, feelings or beliefs concerning the following statements by placing yourself on a continuum. As you evaluate each statement, think about a colleague who would respond differently.

I am worried that I, or someone I love, will get AIDS.

| Strongly agree | Agree | No opinion | Disagree | Strongly disagree |

Homosexuals are responsible for the AIDS epidemic in the United States.

| Strongly agree | Agree | No opinion | Disagree | Strongly disagree |

I would be uncomfortable sharing an office with a person with AIDS.

| Strongly agree | Agree | No opinion | Disagree | Strongly disagree |

Distribution of explicit sexual information that eroticizes and thus promotes safer sexual practices is a legitimate approach to changing sexual behaviors.

Strongly agree   Agree   No opinion   Disagree   Strongly disagree

Teenagers who are already sexually active should be educated about safer alternatives to intercourse (for example, mutual masturbation).

Strongly agree   Agree   No opinion   Disagree   Strongly disagree

All children eligible for adoption should be tested for the presence of HIV antibodies.

Strongly agree   Agree   No opinion   Disagree   Strongly disagree

Youth in residential care who are known to be or suspected of engaging in behaviors likely to transmit HIV should be tested with or without their permission.

Strongly agree   Agree   No opinion   Disagree   Strongly disagree

The government would be doing more if so many of the people infected weren't black or Hispanic.

Strongly agree   Agree   No opinion   Disagree   Strongly disagree

It would be surprising if you had difficulty imagining a wide range of responses to these questions, taken from a Child Welfare League of America Training Institute Values Clarification Exercise. (See Appendix.)

Consider how disparate the beliefs and opinions in a roomful of 20 individuals might be. How would one go about advising a workshop leader where and how to begin such a difficult task? That is why this discussion about AIDS training may not be what you expect.

The Child Welfare League of America Task Force on Children and HIV Infection recognized that developing its *Initial Guidelines* required a great deal of debate, negotiation, learning, stretching, and catharsis. As highly motivated and informed as its members were, each meeting required a re-covering of ground once gained but lost in the regression inevitably associated with the isolation, loneliness, frustration, and discomfort of being a leader in a cause not fully embraced by the public or its elected leadership. A passionate advocacy—not an intellectual one—

would be needed to forge a responsible, responsive course for the child welfare community.

The Task Force shaped the concept of training institutes that would help the field transform its recommendations into practice. Ideally, the sequence of the institutes would begin with "Emotional Support for People with AIDS, Their Families and Caregivers." To progress effectively, however, practitioners must assume some leadership responsibilities and commit themselves emotionally. The passionate advocacy that is needed would not come from knowledge and existing levels of commitment.

Practically speaking, the first question raised must be the first question addressed. What should the child welfare response be and how should its policies reflect it? Hence, the institute most subscribed to was "Responsible Policies/Responsive Practice." Child welfare agencies demonstrated a remarkable willingness to apply resources toward developing programs and policies to serve the already infected child or family member. Discussions took many turns, raising a surprising range and depth of issues. Any solutions arrived at through this process inevitably brought participants back to two issues: discrimination and prevention. It became clear that we had to end one and begin the other. This chapter encompasses both.

Commitment to Prevention

Child welfare agencies' willingness to serve children who are already HIV-infected and their families and the agencies' accompanying commitment to prepare to do so can be used to redirect some of that energy toward prevention activities. In a sense, it is paradoxical that HIV is preventable even while many of us have already had to learn about medical needs, assumed the leading role in case management, developed capacities to respond to psychosocial issues, and led advocacy and resource development efforts. Practitioners create comfort zones by demonstrating professionally responsible individual and agency behavior toward the already infected children and their families, but, for us to be truly responsible, our policies and activities must encompass prevention. HIV infection prevention must be incorporated into every case plan for every child.

When effective prevention is genuinely included in our casework, many questions of policy regarding the already infected child would not be so difficult to answer—especially questions related to such areas as testing, confidentiality, the need to know, the duty to warn, whether to serve or not, or the type of setting in which to serve.

Consider the following hypothetical case study used to prompt discussion on the issue of duty to warn:

> G.G. is a 16-year-old girl who turned to prostitution to survive after running away from home. She has entered your residential program under court order. Her HIV status is unknown. She reports to her counselor that she intends to maintain a sexual relationship with B.B., her boyfriend, who is also 16. He has spent time in a juvenile detention facility for use and possession of illegal intravenous drugs and was tested at his request. He claims that he is HIV-negative. The juvenile authorities will not even confirm whether B.B. was tested nor tell you his status. Despite close supervision, you are not convinced that will won't find a way for G.G. and B.B. to find the time and the space to have sex.

Points for Discussion

Testing

Should B.B. be required to be tested? Should G.G.?
If so, by what authority?
How should the authority be obtained?

Need to Know

Who needs to know B.B's HIV status? G.G's HIV status?
Why?

Duty to Warn

Assume G.G. is HIV-positive. Is there a duty to warn anyone?
Who?
Why?
How?

The extent to which the decision makers in the foregoing situation had undertaken aggressive prevention efforts with B.B. and G.G. would have directly affected and simplified the social work and legal decisions. General and individualized HIV infection prevention education avoids dropping a "startle bomb" on anyone and minimizes the issues involved. This approach reverts to the recommendation: Use the issue of AIDS-response training to advance a prevention agenda.

The Prevention Agenda

The welfare of children in their own homes, in out-of-home care, involved in any way with the public or volunteer service delivery system, and in our own homes today requires that we caregivers, parents, counselors, and advocates provide age- and developmentally appropriate prevention education for all children. Prevention education must describe HIV and how it is transmitted in explicit terms that children use and understand. We cannot, for example, expect children or adolescents to hear the words "high-risk sexual behavior" and inventory those behaviors. We can't even expect them to hear the more explicit words "unprotected anal or vaginal intercourse" and universally understand them. What does unprotected mean? What is anal intercourse? What is vaginal intercourse? These terms derive from our need to communicate comfortably with each other. Until we know how youths understand those terms in their own words, we cannot begin to communicate effectively with them. Prevention education and counseling must connect sexual information to self-esteem development and decision-making processes; it must deal with the sexual nature and development of human beings at all ages. Our capacity to do this is limited by our share in our society's inability to deal with human sexuality and sexual development.

The intervention system that brings child welfare practitioners into contact with children and adolescents requires us to apply appropriately skills associated with enhancing physical, intellectual, emotional, and spiritual development. It has not historically or generally included sexual development. It is an evasion to say that four out of five isn't so bad, or that sexual education and development are exclusively within the province of parental functions and family privacy. The first four areas of responsibility are equally parental functions. The time is past for us to recognize that we have the responsibility, that we must learn what to do, and that we must do it.

Child welfare practitioners are expert in assessing and enhancing self-esteem at all developmental levels; it is an issue for every child and adolescent on our caseloads. We are less highly skilled in enhancing decision-making skills at all developmental levels. In our casework with younger children, we haven't interpreted as well as we might the appropriate analogues to what we do in our work with youths and with decision making as part of interdependent-living skills. Younger children make decisions and choices, just as adolescents do; they must have the self-esteem to know and exercise the power and responsibility to make or to participate in making decisions in their own behalf. Social work's challenge for the prevention agenda is to connect self-esteem, decision making, and development of sexuality—a task made difficult by our lack of personal ability and by public obstacles.

Do we lack the personal ability? In parenting, modeling is our primary informer. Whom do we model for the sexual development component of parenting, and how skilled were they? Who were their models? Is our parenting model sexually naive or even repressed? At some point in every training session we ask the question: If you use your own parents as your model for the sexual education and development of your children or of children in your care, would those children be able to remain HIV-negative? At least one person in attendance could answer yes, but never more than two. Let us then assume that this task is going to be extremely difficult and that we are starting with a deficiency. To do less would be to overestimate our capacity and to fail our children in the process.

As soon as we accept the challenge of becoming informed about how best to guide sexual development and all its attendant behaviors, we will have to accept the challenge of battling constraining public policies and laws such as federal legislation that forbids the expenditure of federal dollars to develop any material for AIDS prevention that promotes homosexuality or depicts it positively. Any money misused would be reappropriated. AIDS prevention education, therefore, faces a dilemma: How do we speak directly and with developmental appropriateness about high-risk behaviors engaged in by homosexuals and heterosexuals alike? Do we refuse to acknowledge and address homosexual youths or youths engaging in sexual experimenting with members of their own sex? We know, or should know, that aside from sharing intravenous needles, engaging in anal intercourse without using a condum and a water-soluble lubricant containing HIV-inhibiting spermacide presents the greatest risk of transmitting the virus, and that anal intercourse is engaged in by the sexually active—heterosexuals, homosexuals, and bisexuals. We do know that information abut negative consequences of behavior alone won't change the behavior of many people. In my own search to find out what we must do and how to do it, I met with Rodger McFarlane, the education director at Sloane-Kettering, who was originally with the Gay Men's Health Crisis in New York. He offered this example:

> If information alone changed behavior, would anyone smoke? Twenty years after placing warnings on cartons and restricting advertising, kids still take up smoking. Adults—including pregnant women—continue to smoke. This despite the multimedia, prime-time exposure of the Great Smoke Out Campaign? Can you envision AIDS prevention getting the same exposure? No! Even if it should, it wouldn't be enough. "Don't do this; don't do that" won't work. For sexual behavior to change, desirable behaviors have to be substituted. That means safer sexual practices must be made desirable—eroticized.

The federal legislation, which passed the Senate almost unanimously, hampers us because it intends to eliminate an essential part of the prevention message. For example, eroticizing safer forms of sexual activity is subject to challenge as promoting unacceptable forms of sexual activity. It also hampers prevention efforts because it supports a natural tendency to retreat into comfort zones that tend to exclude all that prevention must encompass. How comfortable are we when promoting, for example, erotic and safe forms of mutual masturbation?

The debate on the federal legislation did not fully consider the consequences of the proposed limitations. Lawmakers did not necessarily know how far prevention efforts must go to be effective. Lawmakers at the national and local levels must be educated; the consequences of the legislation they propose must be considered by the people to whom it applies, if lawmakers are to support effectively the battle against HIV transmission and infection.

Religious teachings that forbid Catholics, for instance, from promoting or practicing birth control also limit the prevention activities of some practitioners and a number of agencies. More general is the religious teaching that young people (all people) should reserve sex for marriage. Until then, we should abstain from—say no to—sex. This belief informs much public and voluntary agency policy and reflects the thinking of a great many practitioners. The same practitioners and agencies acknowledge that youths in their care are sexually active, and the personal and professional moral dilemma of the agency staff member is painful. Someone has to resume the efforts at the place where theirs fall short.

Joyce Hunter of the Hetrick Martin Institute in New York City works with street youth and has helped practitioners throughout the country who are working with hard-to-reach youth in order to develop prevention agendas. She offers this advice to those who would limit their prevention efforts to teaching abstinence.

> Since people admit that many youths are already sexually active, just saying no to doing it again is very different from just saying no to doing it the first time. To illustrate the point I ask all in the room who have ever had an orgasm to raise their hand. Now, everyone willing to just say no to having one again, leave your hand up!

Following Hunter's recommendation, we repeat this exercise. The debriefing has always resulted in admissions by participants that they must broaden their message.

Just as universal administration of the smallpox vaccine was required to eradicate smallpox, it will take universal, individualized, comprehensive, age-appropriate prevention education with everyone to halt the spread of HIV. So far, too little has been done, judging from our experience.

During each of the CWLA Attention to AIDS Institutes following an explicit safer sex training demonstration, practitioners were asked this question: "How many of you have been doing effective prevention since 1986? 1987?" No one was. No one indicated that he or she had incorporated effective HIV infection prevention into case practice until 1988. But the number of reported cases of AIDS is growing most rapidly among the 20- to 29-year-olds. The fact that the latency period (the time between infection and the onset of symptoms) can be eight years or more forces the recognition that a significant number of these individuals with AIDS became infected during their adolescence.

We have a choice to make. Either we must begin prevention efforts now, accepting that we will have to confront and overcome intense, passionate, personal, institutional, political, and societal challenges, or accept the consequences of knowing that children once in our care or in our agency's custody are HIV-positive, have AIDS, or have died.

If the risks of lost funding, censure, excommunication, lost community support, bad publicity, isolation, and burnout seem so great that we choose to let someone else do the hard part of prevention, or we choose to limit our activities to the ineffective type or to do nothing, we are, in effect, doing nothing.

The Challenge for Staff Training

Training for the community-based organizations that formed in response to the HIV crisis was made easier in that those who came forward, who volunteered and applied for jobs, were personally highly motivated. The people infected with AIDS were their friends, family, lovers, colleagues, co-workers—but they are getting used up. During the Child Welfare League of America "Attention to AIDS: Commitment to Prevention" forum in Miami, in April 1989, Sally Dodd, former executive director of the Miami Health Crisis Network, described a future challenge. She pointed out that few human services practitioners realized the challenges found in an AIDS caseload of one, let alone many—but the human services delivery system will become more and more involved, and, given high turnover, increasing caseloads, and the burnout factor, trainers will face either a demoralized, exhausted group or a group who are not present willingly but who have been forced to take on the challenge.

As with training on any subject, learning about HIV stops and starts again as the content touches participants' experiences, values, and beliefs, or recalls their personal histories, or challenges their assumptions. In child welfare, the personal life history of everyone in the room is always a consideration, so we must think about who will be trained.

Today's work force is young. Many staff members are single or just entering marriage or remarriage. When we talk about high-risk behaviors in terms of adolescent behavior to a group of new child welfare staff members, we must be aware that we are encompassing the sexual behavior of the people in the room. And we must not assume that it is only the youngest of the work force who may be sexually active outside a long-term monogamous relationship. What we refer to as an adolescent's practicing serial monogamy (one's only girlfriend or only boyfriend or only sexual partner over a given period of time) may be practiced by many, regardless of age. When seemingly remote information strikes close to home, hearing stops; learning stops. The presumed objective response is actually a subjective response. For the trainee, it is tantamount to trying to watch a movie through a strobe light. Words and images are missing. The picture is confusing, the plot lost.

The trainer/social worker must perform unceasing assessments of the group to learn where the trainees are and to deal with their issues as training begins and continues. Otherwise, the training will be ineffectual, just as are case plans based on incomplete, inaccurate assessments.

Many child welfare agencies have made HIV training mandatory or universally available. But what may well not be clear is what actual social work is required to get what appears to be a training job done. It is the responsibility of the training specialist and the AIDS educator/advocate (in tandem, if they are not the same person) to spell out for administration what is required to achieve the objectives of HIV training. They must demonstrate how HIV training provides an opportunity to assess and respond to staff members' personal issues individually and agency morale collectively.

How many cases of sexual abuse were revealed before we learned how many people had been sexually abused and never treated? How much more time elapsed before we realized that we were asking child welfare workers to take on sexual abuse cases without knowing that, in having to confront their personal sexual abuse issues, they not only agonized personally but possibly did harm to clients? Let us not ask ourselves to overcome our personal HIV issues on the job. Let us make proper counseling available. Let us make ongoing clinical assessment part of the training, not just for the practitioners but also for the administrators.

The Complexity of Multiple Perspectives

We are asking people to understand extremely complex issues. These complexities were fully revealed to the CWLA Task Force by its inability to address completely an HIV-related child welfare practice matter without putting it through three filters: medical, legal, and psychosocial. The three filters are equally important. Until all three aspects are considered in answer to a question, a recommended course of action is not comprehensive and is potentially dangerous. Unfortunately, the three professions involved in the filtering process are not perceived as having equal power and stature, as they should.

Practice implications include psychosocial considerations which may be as significant to clients as medical or legal considerations or even more so. Social workers represent the psychosocial aspects of every decision and must not permit them to be subordinated to the medical and legal aspects, if clients are to be treated more kindly, gently, and comprehensively.

Training then must answer this question: How do we represent the strength of the social work profession in decision making on an issue that has so many people so badly frightened that they defer to someone else or to some other authority? In designing workshops, therefore, we must be certain to assess our ability and skill in case management, our belief that the psychosocial aspects must be aggressively considered in decision-making forums, and our belief in social work's equal stature with law and medicine on the decision-making team.

Catharsis

Elisabeth Kubler-Ross gave me a woods creature named Trusty that wears a backpack—used with children to tell stories or thoughts to or to ask questions:

> Meet Trusty. This little creature comes from the blueberry patch. Trusty listens to the secrets of children and grown-ups who have stories or questions they must share with someone. But, these are the kinds of questions and stories that sometimes are not safe to tell out loud. Therapists working with children who have been sexually assaulted have introduced them to Trusty as a way of helping them to tell their secrets. We will use Trusty the same way.

Training participants are given the following instructions:

> In front of you are several index cards. If a question occurs to you but the tenor or the timing does not feel right for asking it aloud, write it on the card and slip it into Trusty's backpack. You may be making a statement—having a catharsis and getting something private off your mind—and don't want to have the issue brought up. In that case, write *Private* across the back of the card. Or you may need to have the question answered or the group ponder the challenge. In that case, write *Discuss* across the back of the card. Following each break we will check Trusty's backpack and respond.

Comments solicited by this technique have included the following:

Discuss: What should you do as an agency employee if you disagree on liability or ethical issues in the management of a specific case?

Private: I've never considered myself homophobic—live and let live. But I can't help being angry at gays for unleashing this epidemic.

Private: My brother has died of AIDS.

Private: A favorite counselor from our center died. It was probably AIDS, but we don't know for sure. The children need to process it, but what about his right to privacy and respect, even after death?

Private: I am married. I have four children. Twice I have had sex with men. I am scared.

Private: I don't think it is fair to place for adoption children who are going to die. Foster care, of course. Adoption? It seems unethical.

Confronting Racism and Sexism

Racism and sexism, including institutionalized racism and sexism, must be dealt with in training or the training will miss a vital component. Child welfare admits to racism and sexism, but group discussions are usually limited to demographic imbalances. The issues must become more real than statistics, or they will persist insidiously.

AIDS is a riveting subject, and AIDS training affords the opportunity to confront these issues. Separate workshops on sexism, racism, and AIDS do not bring everyone together. The issues should be incorporated into every topic.

As an example, we hear almost everywhere how cultural (as contrasted to societal) homophobia in black and Hispanic communities makes prevention a different issue for them. In training we accept a basic premise, often set forth by black and Hispanic trainers, that black and Hispanic men have male identity pressures on them that in turn exert pressures on women to avoid insisting on use of condoms, which puts both the men and the women at higher risk of HIV infection. Problems with generalities aside, perhaps the premise does not seem racist on the face of it. But to ascribe homophobia to black and Hispanic men without including white men is racist. White men are homophobic, too, often extremely so. Consider these two examples:

> The social work profession is dominated in numbers by women; social work administration is dominated in numbers by (white) men. CWLA held an administrative retreat on HIV so administrators could become more informed, share personal and professional experience and anxiety, ask questions and debate issues safely—without being scrutinized or held to expectations of knowing what to do. Thirty-one public child welfare administrators originally registered. Of those, 12 were men. Nineteen women ultimately attended. No men did.

> In the Attention to AIDS Institutes, half of which were designed specifically for administrators and executives, fewer than 10 percent of the participants all across the country were men. On some occasions, there would be no men.

Why no men? Participants discussed this question. Our shared perception: Men (regardless of ethnicity, culture, or race) seem to believe that if they express open concern about HIV they will be perceived to be homosexual, bisexual, or suspected of leading a double life. If this perception is accurate, homophobia, racism, and sexism come to the fore in AIDS training.

People with knowledge and resources will join with others who have analogous knowledge and resources to solve common problems. When problems are viewed as somehow uniquely *their* problem, solutions are left to *them*. If white male decision makers in child welfare or anywhere else are excused because they are not perceived as homophobic, not perceived as part of the problem, we will not have their full support in solving problems, advocating for resources, or shaping responsible policies. We will further institutionalize racism, homophobia, and sexism. AIDS is not a homosexual problem; it is not a black problem; it is not a Hispanic problem; it is not a drug addict's problem. AIDS is truly a societal problem.

Strategies for AIDS Training

A number of steps can be taken to increase the effectiveness of AIDS training:

Link HIV education to teenage pregnancy prevention education and initiatives that reinforce common themes of self-esteem, effective decision making, and healthy sexual development.

Acknowledge the fear that accompanies addressing AIDS. The American culture places high value on recreation and leisure; youth, beauty, and sex appeal; mental competency; and mobility; the culture fears death, disfigurement, age (physical infirmity), mental illness, and homosexuality. AIDS involves every one of these fears. HIV/AIDS education will need to discuss a range of fears beyond sexuality. Listen for and assess the fear that is stated or implied in group members' questions.

Provide a safe environment for learning so that questions can be asked and risks taken by participants. Ground rules for feedback need to be established; do not respond cavalierly or disrespectfully to questions.

Assume that someone in the group knows someone with AIDS; assume that someone in the group is HIV-positive. Acknowledge that people learn to keep some secrets.

Expect that people are influenced by what they read and hear in the media, but this knowledge is often based on headlines rather than thoughtful exploration of news sources.

Involve an interdisciplinary group of presenters to address complex issues.

To accomplish these tasks, training and educational initiatives might (1) include persons with HIV infection to answer questions and to change statistics into hopes, dreams, and changes in real people's lives; (2) use effective videos to enliven, vary, and make more realistic the issues discussed in training; or (3) involve community experts on HIV from a range of local organizations. When training or consultation on medical aspects of HIV infection are sought, it is important to recognize that this study is a specialized area of medical practice. On the one hand, an agency's favorite pediatrician may never have seen an AIDS patient; on the other, the doctors most experienced in treating AIDS patients might have an adult-only perspective that does not correlate with children.

Most important, a medical professional should be able to communicate with non-medical caregivers. Some terms that are comforting to medical researchers, such as "theoretical transmission risk," may sound extremely frightening to non-medical personnel, who hear "it is possible" rather than "it is highly unlikely, existing only in theory."

CWLA's Task Force recommends that organizations include an AIDS expert or coordinator on staff to keep abreast of developments and inform ongoing in-service training.

Conclusion

There may be a temptation to complacency because many people with HIV have been quite well cared for, and reports of treatments and cures are always imminent. In the absence of national leadership on AIDS, however, it is up to each individual to become informed and to accept some measure of leadership for AIDS education, prevention, and service. With information, dedication, and skill, we must not only reach our colleagues and the children in our care but also communities. Each one of us has a leadership responsibility. So part of what training must do is to provide the time and the opportunity for this discussion—people personally asking, "What am I going to do with this information?"

Appendix
Facing AIDS: Values Clarification Exercise

Indicate your thoughts, feelings, or beliefs about these statements by "placing yourself" on the continuum.

1. The AIDS epidemic has changed my life.

   strongly agree   agree   no opinion   disagree   strongly disagree

2. Sexual activity should be reserved for marriage.

   strongly agree   agree   no opinion   disagree   strongly disagree

3. I am worried that I, or someone I love, will get AIDS.

   strongly agree   agree   no opinion   disagree   strongly disagree

4. Information about AIDS changes so rapidly that I won't accept that it's not spread by casual contact.

   strongly agree   agree   no opinion   disagree   strongly disagree

5. Homosexuals are responsible for bringing the AIDS epidemic to the United States.

   strongly agree   agree   no opinion   disagree   strongly disagree

6. It should be a crime for people with AIDS to have sex without telling their partners.

   strongly agree   agree   no opinion   disagree   strongly disagree

7. It should be a crime for people who are HIV+ to have sex without telling their partners.

strongly agree   agree   no opinion   disagree   strongly disagree

8. All people who are sexually active and not monogamous should be required to be tested.

strongly agree   agree   no opinion   disagree   strongly disagree

9. All known IV drug users, homosexuals and bisexuals should be tested.

strongly agree   agree   no opinion   disagree   strongly disagree

10. Quarantine is an option to control the spread of AIDS until a cure or vaccine is found.

strongly agree   agree   no opinion   disagree   strongly disagree

11. I would be uncomfortable sharing food with a person who has AIDS.

strongly agree   agree   no opinion   disagree   strongly disagree

12. I would be uncomfortable sharing an office with a person who has AIDS.

strongly agree   agree   no opinion   disagree   strongly disagree

13. I would be uncomfortable using the same bathroom as a person who has AIDS.

strongly agree   agree   no opinion   disagree   strongly disagree

14. Teenagers should be educated about alternatives to intercourse (including, e.g., mutual masterbation).

   strongly agree   agree   no opinion   disagree   strongly disagree

15. Encouraging proper condom use to prevent HIV infection gives people a false sense of security.

   strongly agree   agree   no opinion   disagree   strongly disagree

16. IV drug users should be given clean needles to prevent infection with HIV.

   strongly agree   agree   no opinion   disagree   strongly disagree

17. Distribution of explicit sexual information which promotes and eroticizes safer sexual practices is a legitimate approach to changing sexual behaviors.

   strongly agree   agree   no opinion   disagree   strongly disagree

18. All children eligible for adoption should be tested for the presence of HIV antibodies.

   strongly agree   agree   no opinion   disagree   strongly disagree

19. Government would be doing more if so many of the victims hadn't infected themselves by breaking laws against drug use and homosexual behavior.

   strongly agree   agree   no opinion   disagree   strongly disagree

20. Government would be doing more if so many of the people infected weren't gay.

strongly agree   agree   no opinion   disagree   strongly disagree

21. I would date someone who would not get tested.

strongly agree   agree   no opinion   disagree   strongly disagree

22. I would not let my child, brother, or sister attend school with an HIV+ child.

strongly agree   agree   no opinion   disagree   strongly disagree

23. I would be afraid to receive a blood transfusion if I needed emergency surgery.

strongly agree   agree   no opinion   disagree   strongly disagree

24. I would not use the spa facilities in a health club if I knew gay men used them.

strongly agree   agree   no opinion   disagree   strongly disagree

25. Youth in juvenile detention centers who are known to be or suspected of engaging in high-risk behaviors should be tested with or without their permission.

strongly agree   agree   no opinion   disagree   strongly disagree

26. I never have and never will participate in "high-risk" behaviors.

strongly agree   agree   no opinion   disagree   strongly disagree

27. Government efforts to prevent further spread of HIV infection are sufficient.

strongly agree   agree   no opinion   disagree   strongly disagree

28. All students entering college at any level should be tested.

strongly agree   agree   no opinion   disagree   strongly disagree

29. Government would be doing more if so many of the people infected weren't Black or Hispanic.

strongly agree   agree   no opinion   disagree   strongly disagree

30. All high school students participating in contact sports should be tested.

strongly agree   agree   no opinion   disagree   strongly disagree

15

Working with Drug-Dependent Parents and Children at Risk for HIV Infection: A Community-Based Model of Service Delivery

GENEVA WOODRUFF

ELAINE DURKOT STERZIN

FAMILIES WITH A HISTORY OF INTRAVENOUS DRUG USE REQUIRE THE SERvices of a variety of providers and agencies. Delivering home-based clinical intervention, parenting education, and case-management services to this population requires an understanding of the behaviors of addicts and the ability to work with multi-problem families. It requires the service provider to be knowledgeable as well as willing and able to work as a team with other service providers and community agencies.

In an effort to increase the effectiveness and streamline the delivery of services to this population, Project WIN, a model demonstration program operating in Boston, has developed the transagency model of service delivery. Service providers from a variety of community agencies plan services together with the families, assign roles and responsibilities for delivery of services, and regularly monitor their service implementation. The transagency model has proven to be effective with people who receive services from a number of agencies. This chapter describes the model and two of the families WIN has served, and discusses skills necessary for effective intervention.

The Model

Project WIN is a Boston-based model demonstration project funded by the Handicapped Children's Early Education Programs and the Boston Foundation. It grew out of a previous demonstration project, PACT (Parents and Children Together), which was the first project to employ the transagency service delivery model with multi-problem, intravenous drug-dependent, alcoholic, or incarcerated women and their children.

WIN is a direct service program for children from birth to six years of age who are at risk for or diagnosed as having HIV infection because they come from families in which a parent has a history of intravenous drug use. Direct services support the parents' recovery from addiction, identify and provide home-based early intervention for the children's developmental needs, and help the family members find and use the services they need. WIN's principal goals are providing and mobilizing community-based services for families at risk for or diagnosed as having HIV infection so that they can stay together in their homes and community, making hospitalization for custodial purposes unnecessary.

The WIN team consists of a director, coordinator, clinical supervisor experienced in family systems and addiction, three case managers from different disciplines, and a consulting speech and physical therapist. Staff members function as a transdisciplinary team, assessing children and planning family-focused interventions together. Each case manager carries a caseload of ten families. Case managers provide recovery support, parenting education, case-management services, and developmental intervention with the children. Small caseloads allow the WIN case managers to provide families with the intensive attention they often require. The children and their families are seen in their homes, motels, or shelters. The family is defined as the client, and all members of the family are eligible for services.

Case-management efforts coordinate the implementation of community services to ensure that families receive all necessary supports in a cohesive and manageable service plan. The service providers involved with the family are in frequent contact with one another through informal discussions and regular case conferences. Together, the service providers and the family design and work from one service plan that addresses all the family's service needs, review the service plan and interventions, define roles and responsibilities, and decide the timing of service delivery.

All activities of the project are guided by a transagency board composed of representatives from 31 health, education, addiction treatment, and child and social service agencies who meet monthly to plan and monitor services to families. Board members refer children and families for WIN services, recommend interventions, develop a community service plan that is appropriate and manageable, review and evaluate service plans, and monitor delivery of services.

Delivery of services is governed by the philosophy and principles of the transdisciplinary (TD) and transagency (TA) models. The TD model requires team members from different professional disciplines to plan services with the family. These interventions are then carried out by one team member, called the primary service provider, and the family. Transagency service delivery expands the TD model in that providers from a variety of community agencies meet to develop a coordinated service plan across agencies that is then managed by one of the service providers. Both models have proven effective with multi-problem families requiring the services of many agencies and providers.

The TD model reduces service duplication, overlap, and fragmentation for the child and family by encouraging communication and planning among professionals serving the families. Similarly, the TA model reduces duplication of services among multiple community agencies. The model bridges service gaps by establishing a process for defining providers' roles and responsibilities and by assigning one provider to act as the family's case manager.

The Families

WIN has worked with people in all stages of drug addiction—from continued active use of intravenous drugs to active recovery. All of the client families are at risk for HIV infection because of sharing needles or prostitution, or because of sexual relationships with other drug users. Some of the clients experience pervasive anxiety about HIV infection, but do not change high-risk behaviors, including needle sharing and unprotected intercourse. In some of the families, the parents and child are HIV-infected.

Two families are described below, after which the direct and case-management services are discussed.

The M. Family

Ms. M. was referred to WIN for parenting support by a hospital social worker after she delivered a five-pound baby boy six weeks prematurely. She is a 23-year-old divorced black woman who has a four-year history of intravenous heroin and cocaine use. She said that she last used drugs two weeks before Mark was born, and he had negative drug screens at birth. Ms. M. conceived Mark when she was working as a prostitute. She is involved with Mr. P., who is not the baby's father. Mr. P. works as a laborer with a construction firm. Ms. M. has worked as a nurse's aide and would like employment training that would lead to a degree in nursing. At the time of referral, she was not employed and was supported by public assistance.

Ms. M. also has a seven-year-old child, Tiffany, whom she has not seen for over a year. Although Tiffany is in the father's custody, she lives in the Virgin Islands with Ms. M.'s mother, who also has a long history of drug and alcohol use, as does her father. When Ms. M. was a young child, her mother divorced her father. She told the children that she had divorced him because she did not want the children brought up by an addict. Her mother's latest partner is in jail for drug-related crimes.

Ms. M. said that she wanted WIN's help with her recovery. She also wanted Mark's development watched because she felt very guilty about the effects her drug use might have on his learning. She said that she would soon want help finding day care for him so that she could enroll in employment training.

After her discharge from the hospital after Mark's birth, she was followed by a visiting nurse to monitor Mark's growth and health. No primary drug treatment agency was involved.

Mother and child lived in a rooming house in a Boston neighborhood. Although she had no baby furniture, she explained that soon she would be moving to an apartment with Mr. P., where there would be a room and furniture for the baby. Within a week after Mark was born, the mother began bleeding profusely and was readmitted to the hospital. The baby stayed with Mr. P. and his family.

The WIN case manager did not know that Ms. M. had been readmitted to the hospital, and no one was home when she arrived for their first home visit. Because Ms. M. did not have a telephone, the case manager left a note on the door informing her when she would come again. On the second visit, the case manager met the landlady, who told her about Ms. M.'s hospitalization.

Ms. M. called the case manager from the hospital to arrange a home visit, telling her that Mr. P had found them an apartment, but that they could not afford to have a telephone installed. She reported that she was feeling much better and that the baby was healthy and growing.

At the next home visit, Ms. M. talked with the WIN case manager about her wish to be clean and to get her life together so that she could provide a good family life for Mark. She wanted to enter drug-free counseling, saying that she realized how important it was to all her goals to be able to work on her recovery. She also said that she would not give up smoking pot, but that she did not view this as a problem. She admitted to having strong cravings and dreams about using cocaine again. She felt that she could not go for inpatient treatment because it would take her away from Mark and Mr. P. She needed to be with them to build their family.

Ms. M. and the WIN case manager generated a list of treatment agencies, options, and the steps that she would have to take to obtain treatment. Before Mark's birth she had been involved with two drug treatment facilities in the Boston area, but she had not completed treatment. She included these programs on her list. She and Mr. P. also made an agreement that they would attend NA and AA meetings together.

Soon after, Ms. M. made and kept an intake appointment with a women's drug treatment agency with a reputation for toughness and a high success rate. She did not return for the second appointment, however, because Mr. P. did not want her traveling to the clinic, which was in a dangerous neighborhood. The following month she made an intake appointment at another treatment program. Again she kept the first appointment, but did not continue because she and the baby were leaving for three months to visit with her mother and daughter in the Virgin Islands.

When Ms. M. returned from her trip, she contacted her WIN case manager and joined a recovery support group at a treatment facility. After attending the group twice, she did not return because she said that she could not find a babysitter. She expressed strong yearnings to have Tiffany back with her, but realized that she had to prove that she was in drug treatment and to clear up outstanding arrest warrants for grand larceny and prostitution before she could regain legal custody. She was sure that the father would contest any attempt she made to get Tiffany back.

Ms. M. repeated the pattern of starting and not following through on drug treatment with three more agencies. One intake worker told the WIN case manager that Ms. M. appeared high at her appointment. She frequently talked with the case manager about craving drugs and continually asserted that she was resisting temptation. She also said that too much was going on in her life to fit in drug treatment. She was feeling increasingly stressed by Mark's demands, by her guilt over Tiffany, by her perception that her mother was pressuring her to take Tiffany back, and by her deteriorating relationship with Mr. P.

The relationship was volatile, and they fought frequently. He criticized how she cared for Mark. They disagreed about how to handle Mark's crying, night-waking, and discipline. When the baby was teething, he cried through the night. Ms. M. tried to comfort him, but he was often inconsolable. Mr. P. could not stand listening to the baby's crying, so he wanted Ms. M. to bring him into bed with them. She disagreed and asked the case manager for help. During his first year, Mark also had times when he cried whenever his mother left the room. She worried that if he didn't learn to separate from her, he would never be able to go to day care.

The disagreements between Ms. M. and Mr. P. frequently led to loud arguments, with him leaving the apartment for hours or nights at a time. After three months of intensifying arguments, their fights turned physical. Once he grabbed her roughly around the neck in the heat of an argument. Another time, he locked her out of the apartment.

Discussing their relationship with the case manager, Ms. M. said that she would not consider leaving Mr. P. or going to a shelter, because she was "just not the kind of woman who could be without a man." She felt that she was trapped and had no choice but to stay. Her resentment of Mr. P.'s freedom and independence escalated; she felt increasingly isolated. She wanted to make it in a straight world but did not think she could. She said that Mr. P. was continuing to use cocaine and alcohol, making it more difficult for her to stay clean. Mr. P. repeatedly told the case manager that he did not have a problem with drugs or alcohol and did not need drug treatment. Ms. M. admitted that her craving for drugs was becoming increasingly difficult to resist. She wanted them to go to couples counseling and asked the case manager to help them find a counselor who could see them in the evenings.

In addition to discussions in support of Ms. M. entering recovery treatment, the WIN case manager—along with the visiting nurse— monitored Mark's development and health. The case manager also helped the mother with parenting skills, counseled her regarding HIV testing, and helped her and Mr. P. focus on their relationship.

When the case manager discussed the case with the WIN trans-agency board, the members representing drug treatment agencies confirmed the case manager's suspicions that the couple were not ready to deal with their recovery and offered suggestions for confronting them about these suspicions. Board members also recommended a couples counselor with a strong background in addiction who was accepting new clients and who also accepted Medicaid.

A continuing focus of the case manager's work was Mark's development and ways that the two adults could help him to learn and grow. Developmental assessments performed by the WIN team and the visiting nurse when Mark was four months and 12 months old showed that he was a sociable, curious child, with age-appropriate skills. Unfortunately, he had frequent illnesses during his first year that required repeated trips to the hospital. He had asthma, recurring ear infections, a rash, and severe diarrhea and vomiting that caused dehydration and required his hospitalization.

When the mother and the case manager discussed with his pediatrician what they perceived as Mark's chronic illnesses, the doctor said that the baby's illnesses were perfectly normal. The mother and the case manager were distressed with this dismissal of Mark's health problems and their concern about the possibility that Mark was HIV-infected. Despite the pediatrician's assurances, Ms. M. continued to worry that both she and Mark might have AIDS.

The case manager discussed with the pediatrician the correlation between the baby's illnesses and early symptoms of HIV infection. He responded that, if the mother wanted to, she could have Mark tested, but he was certain that there was no reason to believe that Mark was infected. The case manager talked with Ms. M. about her options and, at her request, helped her locate anonymous testing sites. The case manager then accompanied them for their test, but Ms. M. was too afraid to enter the building for the test. She scheduled tests a second time, but again did not follow through "because it was just too scary." The case manager and the visiting nurse continued to monitor Mark's health and development closely and let the mother know that they would support her if she decided to pursue testing.

During the seventh month of involvement with WIN, the case manager helped Ms. M. locate and enroll Mark in a day care program. Ms. M. then found a full-time job in a nursing home. She continued to meet with the case manager to talk about drug treatment, improving her parenting skills, and trying to resolve her anxiety and fears about the possibility that she and Mark were infected with the AIDS virus.

Ms. M. has continued to work full-time at her job, trying to pay off the debts she accumulated before Mark's birth. She succeeded in paying off her outstanding telephone bills so that they could have a phone installed. She also saved enough money to pay for Tiffany to fly to Boston to spend the summer with her. Mark's health stabilized and his development was within normal limits.

Toward the end of the first year of involvement with WIN, Ms. M. admitted to the case manager that she had been using cocaine since Mark was born, although she had been restricting herself to using it only at night. She acknowledged her resistence to entering a drug program, but said that she was now so tired of it all that she felt she could no longer resist drug treatment.

She and Mr. P. have expressed their commitment to making their family work and to continuing couples counseling with their therapist. The therapist is counseling them about their substance abuse and supporting their attendance at NA meetings. Mark is walking, saying a few words, and seems well settled in his day care program. The case manager meets with the family in the evening and continues to work with them on improving their parenting skills, supporting their recovery treatment, and coordinating services. Although the mother continues to worry about their HIV status, she has not arranged testing for herself or for Mark.

In the past year Ms. M. has kept 35 of 47 appointments, cancelled two, and not appeared for ten. Keeping 74 percent of her appointments is high, considering that she was using drugs for most of the time; however, a high proportion of the case manager's efforts were spent in working with her and her partner to enter drug treatment. Because the case manager was involved in so many of the family's day-to-day issues—finding day care, dealing with Ms. M.'s outstanding warrants, finding medical treatment for Mark's frequent illnesses, discussing parenting and relationship issues, and her fears about HIV infection—it took several months to recognize her pattern of initiating but not following through with drug treatment. Assisted by consultation from addiction experts on the transagency board, the case manager was able to confront Ms. M. and help her to overcome her denial and resistance sufficiently so that she could enter and stay in treatment with the couples counselor, who is dealing with their substance use, as well as regularly attend NA meetings.

The R. Family

Ms. R. was referred to WIN a year ago by a Department of Social Services (DSS) worker. She was a homeless, 26-year-old Caucasian woman, four months pregnant and living in a shelter, where she worked in the clothing distribution office. She had a history of heroin and cocaine use, but said she had not used drugs for the past ten months. At her first meeting with the case manager she said that she was HIV-positive and was concerned about the health of the baby she was carrying. Ms. R. had met another shelter resident, Mr. O., and they have been partners for the past month. Mr. O. was a recovering alcoholic who had just completed a detox program. They attend AA meetings together. Although he was not the father of the baby, Mr. O. said he planned to care for the baby as his own.

Ms. R. has a family history of loss and abandonment. When she was four years old, her mother left the family. After a year of trying to raise four children on his own, her father placed them in foster care. For a short time, she was in a home with one of her sisters. From the age of four to 16, she was placed with eight different foster families; the longest placement lasted four years. At 16 she went on her own and lived on the streets.

When she was 18, Ms. R. married "Pete," whom she had known for five years. In their seven years together, they had four children before separating one year ago. Ms. R. said that she had occasionally used drugs when she was a young teenager, but didn't become hooked until she was 22, after her second child was born. As her addiction progressed, she neglected her children, leaving them alone for hours at a time. Her marriage also fell apart. The children, ages eight, six, five, and two, were removed to foster care by the Department of Social Services because of neglect. Ms. R. said that losing custody of her children made her come to her senses, and she stopped using drugs without treatment.

Discussions with the Department of Social Services worker handling the children's placement revealed that, despite many opportunities to visit the children, the mother had seen them only once in the past year. The father was also present at this visit. They argued loudly in the children's presence, and the DSS worker asked them to leave. Since then Ms. R. has not seen her children. The children are placed with two foster families who live in the same neighborhood. Each foster family has expressed its wish to adopt the children in their care. The two-year old is HIV-positive.

After the parents separated, Ms. R. met "Bob," whose baby she is now carrying. "Bob" was abusive, and their relationship ended after four months. She then met Mr. O, who said he wanted to be the baby's father and create a family with Ms. R. and her baby.

At the first meeting with the case manager, Ms. R talked about her goals. She wanted to stay clean, wanted to find a place where she, Mr. O., and the baby could live, and wanted to regain custody of her other four children. She openly discussed her HIV status with the worker and her concern about staying healthy.

After the first intake contact, Ms. R. disappeared for three months. One month before giving birth, she enrolled in a drug treatment program that is represented on the WIN board. Through this representative, she was once again referred for WIN services. The case manager resumed contact immediately. Ms. R. then entered the hospital and delivered a son, whom she named Miguel, Jr. At birth, the baby had a positive screen to cocaine, which the mother had used just before going into labor. When both were released from the hospital, they went to live with Mr. O. at his sister's apartment.

Ms. R. said she was pleased to be in contact with WIN again and told the case manager that she could visit her at her sister-in-law's place any time after noon when they usually awakened. She also asked that the case manager say nothing about drugs or HIV infection in front of her sister-in-law.

When the mother and the baby came home, Mr. O. quit his job so that he could help with child care. At the time of the case manager's first visit, they were both reading the infant care pamphlets they had been given at the hospital and talking about their hopes and plans for the baby.

Ms. R. said the baby had been up most of the night crying. She felt that she could not let him cry because she was afraid that the family would be evicted from the apartment. She asked the case manager for the Parents' Anonymous number, saying that as the baby got bigger, she would need it.

After a month of living with Mr. O.'s sister, they moved out with no advance warning and without telling the case manager where they were going. Ms. R. called the case manager from the hotel where social service workers had found emergency shelter for them after they had spent over two weeks living in abandoned trains and buildings. Ms. R. reported that they had no food, clothes, or supplies for the baby. They had only the clothes they were wearing. The case manager arranged for an emergency food voucher, so that they could eat over the weekend, and arranged a joint visit with the DSS worker to plan more permanent housing and basic arrangements.

When the case manager and DSS worker arrived at the hotel, Ms. R.

was not there. The case manager left a message at the hotel desk and called the desk for two days, before finally reaching Ms. R. She was upset and cried frequently during their conversation. She said she had missed all her appointments because she was sitting in the welfare waiting room for two days trying to get benefits. While at welfare, she saw her previous DSS worker who told her that the visiting nurse reported that she had missed Miguel's well-baby checkup. The worker told Ms. R. that she would risk losing custody of the baby if she did not take him promptly to the hospital for his checkup. She did as she was told and reported that the pediatrician said that the baby was in "perfect" health. She was furious that the DSS worker thought she was not caring for Miguel responsibly and vehemently repeated that no one was going to take him away from her.

The case manager discussed the need for all the workers to meet and obtained the mother's permission to arrange a case conference with the DSS worker, the visiting nurse, Miguel, Jr.'s medical team, and the welfare housing advocate. Within two weeks a case conference was convened and agreements were made about responsibilities, priorities for finding housing, and facilitating the mother's use of health and social services. The transagency board provided support and consultation about working with the hospital staff to coordinate the mother's and Miguel, Jr.'s health care in one location.

The family occupied a room at the hotel for three months. For the first month, until the case manager was able to find them a crib, the baby slept with them in their double bed. Mr. O. cleaned the hotel room and painted it himself. Initially he was employed by the hotel management as a custodian, but he lost this job. Ms. R. said that he was fired after the visiting nurse made trouble by complaining to the management that their room had inadequate heat. Mr. O. wanted to look for other employment but did not have suitable shoes or clothes to wear to job interviews.

During this time, the case worker helped them look for and prepare the documents necessary to be eligible for emergency housing. She also arranged for them to go to charitable groups and service agencies that provided them with emergency food, vouchers for baby formula, clothing, diapers, and supplies for the baby, and clothes for both adults. The visiting nurse continued to visit weekly, and the mother kept Miguel, Jr.'s monthly appointments at the hospital infectious disease clinic.

Ms. R. had a deep and persistent cough during this time, for which she refused to seek treatment. A discussion with the family about their safe sex practices to prevent transmission of the virus revealed that Mr.

O. had been tested for the virus when they first got involved and was negative. They were not practicing safer sex because "he was not that kind of man," when it came to using condoms, and besides, he would love only Ms. R. Continued discussion about the need for everyone to stay healthy resulted in both agreeing to go for counseling at a confidential HIV testing program, and consent on his part to consider using condoms. When Miguel, Jr., was four months old, they proudly informed the case manager that Ms. R. was pregnant.

Through the coordinated efforts of the transagency team, the family found housing in a city outside Boston. Finding housing in Boston near the hospital where they received treatment was impossible. When the case manager visited them at their new apartment the day after they moved, she found them both intoxicated. They said that they had been celebrating their good fortune.

Miguel, Jr., has had repeated illnesses. He has weeping eczema over his entire body, which cracks and bleeds in his skin folds. He has had thrush and enlarged lymph nodes. He has been treated for flu symptoms, including diarrhea and vomiting. When he was a newborn he cried frequently, appeared to have increased tone in his arms and legs, and frantically sucked on his bottles and pacifiers. He would cry when a face came into view, and he did not make eye contact with adults. His growth is within normal limits, in spite of high caloric intake that would usually cause a child his age to be overweight. Developmental assessments performed at five months indicated that his skills were age-appropriate, but the team had reservations about the quality of his responses.

Ms. R. and Mr. O. are involved with a number of practitioners and agencies. They are followed by a caseworker from the Department of Social Services, have regular home visits from a nurse, and are followed by the infectious disease team at a hospital. The mother is receiving prenatal care and drug treatment at this hospital as well. In addition, she is involved with a housing advocate and welfare worker. The team meets at least every three months to coordinate services, keep up-to-date on the family's evolving needs, and monitor their health status.

As of this writing, the family is settled in their new apartment. Mr. O. did not follow through with HIV testing or counseling, and he says that he is still thinking about using the condoms the case manager gave them. The mother is fairly regular in keeping appointments with WIN, drug treatment, and the hospital. She is highly motivated to work with the service providers because she is extremely lonely and isolated. The service providers are her only connection to the outside world.

She is now telling the case manager about her feelings about being HIV-infected and asking her questions about who should be informed. She is concerned about keeping it a secret from friends and family members and from practitioners who do not need to know. She is also talking about her concerns about Miguel, Jr., her four children in foster care, and the baby she is carrying, with the result that she has decided that she will have a tubal ligation when the new baby is born. She has also decided to discuss permanency planning for her other four children with the Department of Social Services. Discussions with Mr. O. and Ms. R. about safer sex practices are continuing. These discussions take place within a framework of understanding and respect for Mr. O.'s culture and beliefs.

The mother's goals in working with WIN are to help her keep connected to the many individuals and agencies involved with her family. To attend appointments at the hospital where Miguel, Jr., is seen each month, the family must travel 15 miles through intense city traffic, either by cab or by public transportation. As her pregnancy progresses, it is becoming increasingly difficult for her to make the trip. She wants to do whatever she can to stay healthy and to take good care of Miguel, Jr. The transagency team is working closely together to arrange convenient transportation for her and to coordinate medical services so that they take place in one location and at one time.

Discussion

As these cases illustrate, working with families affected by drug addiction and HIV infection and assisting them to acquire and use the services necessary to help them survive, demands an extraordinary amount of time and effort. Many more hours than a once-weekly, 50-minute office session are required to help the families identify their needs, find the necessary services, and then aid them to acquire the skills to use the services available. Services must be family-centered, reality- and present-focused, multifaceted, and flexible enough to respond to many and repeated crises. Practitioners serving the families must function as a team, assign roles, streamline and coordinate their services and the timing of interventions [Johnson et al. 1989; Woodruff et al. 1989]. No one agency or practitioner could possibly provide all the services these families need.

Providers must be knowledgeable about the lifestyle, habits, and behaviors of drug addicts (refer to Figure 1). They must be experienced in recognizing and confronting drug-related behaviors and activities. They must also be sensitive to the cultures and ethnicity of these families and deliver services in the primary language of the family and in ways that demonstrate respect for their clients' values, beliefs, roles, and expectations. The stage of recovery from addiction is an important determinant of how well families respond to intervention (see Figure 2). Those working at their recovery and committed to sobriety were better able to set priorities, follow through on service plans, and deal effectively with the problems as they occurred. When the family members were still using drugs, they were not free to expend energy to accomplish other goals. Drug use was such a central force in their lives that other aims, obligations, and dreams were secondary. Continued drug use correlated with a high failure rate for appointments, limited perseverance on planned interventions, and frequent interpersonal and parenting difficulties, including misjudgments in parenting and fights with partners and providers.

Service plans developed with the families focus on their strengths, resources, needs, and priorities. Drug treatment, however, is a nonnegotiable goal written into every service plan. Talking about the recovery process is always part of the work, but it is not the sole focus. Discussing the addiction and the effect it has on behaviors is not done in isolation, but in conjunction with helping families to deal with their needs, parenting behaviors, and health issues. Improvement in these areas reinforces the recovery process and builds the parents' self-esteem [Black and Mayer 1980].

To work effectively with this population, practitioners must know how to recognize the behaviors that indicate drug use as well as techniques to confront suspected drug use and to support recovery. An alliance with the family is necessary, however, before confrontation techniques will be effective [Jacobs 1981]. As Ms. M. illustrates, it can take months of regular intervention and building trust before the confrontation results in positive behaviors.

Consultation from the drug treatment specialists on the WIN board has been invaluable in understanding the addiction-related behaviors of clients and successful intervention strategies. Similarly, consultation with the various minority agencies on the board assisted the team to

- Change in personality
- Loss of interest in other activities
- Changing companions
- Disappearance of money or valuable possessions
- Vague illnesses, frequent accidents
- Physical signs: slurred speech, giddiness, reddened eyes, "nodding out", tremors
- Legal problems
- Bizarre behavior: asocial, aggressive, hostile, infantile
- Impulsive behaviors, demonstrating poor control over emotions
- Self-defeating behaviors—appear to be own worst enemy
- Poor tolerance for anxiety—activity wards off anxiety
- Poor self-image, poor self-esteem, much guilt over behaviors
- Perpetual state of crisis
- Demanding of attention/repeated testing of worker
- Difficulty with problem solving, planning, and decision-making
- Unrealistic view of the future
- Low tolerance for frustration
- Inconsistency in behaviors between straight and high times
- Obsession with drugs makes all other goals secondary/creates conflict and tension that can only be relieved by using drugs
- Poor quality of relationships and use of appropriate supports
- Isolation from mainstream of society, but high involvement in drug culture
- Inappropriate expectations for children to behave like adults
- Undependable—frequently misses scheduled appointments, is late, unavailable, does not follow through with planned interventions

Figure 1. Drug-Related Behaviors.

Figure 2. Progression Of Substance Dependence Recovery

Adapted from a handout by Roger Weiss, M.D., McLean Hospital, Institute for Addiction, Belmont, Massachusetts, 1987©

SOCIAL

First Introduction
Use At Social Events for Stimulation

Obsession with Substance

Sex Heightened by Substance

Only When Others Have and Offer

Increasing Tolerance

Morning After Financial Regrets

User Starts Buying Substance

Using Until Sunup

Missing Work and Commitments

Begins to Deal/Criminal Activity

Loss of Other Interests

Buys More Quantity and Hoards

Changing Companions

Loss of Normal Will Power

Paranoia Begins

Can't Stop Until Substance Is Finished

Grandiose Behavior

Promises and Resolutions Fail

Using Substance Alone

Inability to Perform Sex When High

Missing Social Events Because of Substance

Work and Money Problems

Searching for More Drugs After Original Purchase is Finished

Onset of Substance Binges
• Overdose
• Physical Deterioration

Efforts to Quit Substance Fail

Persistent Remorse

Using Substance with Inferiors

Family and Friends Avoided/Neglected

Frequency and Length of Binges Increase

Intense Paranoia and Hallucinations

Impared Thinking at All Times

Loss of Family

Moral Degradation

Bizarre Behavior

Financial Ruin

Stops Taking Primary Substance

Total Defeat Admitted

PROBLEM

CRUCIAL

CHRONIC

Assisted in Making Personal Stocktaking

Spiritual Needs Examined

Onset of New Hope

Appreciation of Possibilities of New Way of Life

Regular Nourishment Taken

Realistic Thinking

Natural Rest and Sleep

Family and Friends Appreciate Efforts

New Circle of Stable Friends

Facts Faced with Courage

Increase of Emotional Control

First Step Toward Economic Stability

Care of Personal Appearance

Rationalizations Recognized

Group Therapy and Mutual Help Continue

RECOVERY

Honest Desire for Help

Learns Addiction Is an Illness

Told Addiction Can Be Arrested

Meets Former Addicts Normal and Happy

Right Thinking Begins

Physical Overhaul By Doctor

Start of Group Therapy

Diminishing Fears of the Unknown Future

Return of Self-Esteem

Desire to Escape Goes

Adjustment to Family Needs

New Interests Develop

Rebirth of Ideals

Application of Real Values

Confidence of Employers

Contentment In Sobriety

Increasing Tolerance

Enlightened and Interesting Way of Life Opens Up with Road Ahead to Higher Levels Than Ever Before

May Change Drug of Choice to One Less "Serious" Alcohol, Marijuana, Pills, or Mode of Ingestion

Obsessive Substance Use Continues in Vicious Circles

Three Options:

1. Recovery   2. Insanity   3. Death

206

locate services that the families would be most likely to use and to deliver them in a way that respected their cultures. Focusing on addiction treatment, however, did not exclude attending to other family needs and parenting skills. Treating the behaviors related to addiction and providing parenting education and support for basic needs occurred at the same time. Feeling good about their ability to care for their children often provided necessary incentives for working on recovery [Black and Mayer 1980].

It is especially challenging to build a relationship and work with people who are resistant and frightened of changing the only lifestyle in which they have ever felt able to get along. Breaking down barriers of mistrust and surviving the lengthy testing process and the lying and concealment of drug use, as well as the cravings, take time, patience, and fortitude. Initially, clients miss more scheduled appointments than they keep and do not follow through on planned activities [Colten 1980; Gomberg 1976]. Consistency and perseverance are required of the worker to get beyond this stage in the therapeutic process.

A trusting relationship is a prerequisite for helping people to change destructive behaviors, especially people with limited problem-solving ability and limited capacity to form mature and lasting relationships [Kaplan 1986]. In many instances, the case managers gave concrete assistance—rides to appointments, food vouchers, clothing, bleach bottles, condoms, and so on—not only because the families needed immediate assistance, but also because it was a tangible way of demonstrating concern and trustworthiness.

It is as important for workers to be able to set realistic goals for helping families as it is for the families to set realistic goals for their progress. Rescue fantasies have no place in effective intervention with this population. Maintaining attention to the needs of the family when organizing and delivering services often alters what services are offered and how they are introduced. For example, an intervention that may be in one family member's best interests may be harmful to other family members. Service providers must recognize that the family defines itself; members do not have to be blood-related to be a family. The family must also be viewed as the client. Workers must learn about family members' strengths, priorities, and needs. They must also maintain a non-judgmental approach sensitive to the values, culture, ethnicity, and traditions of the family. This perspective results in interventions that are meaningful and manageable [Shelton et al. 1987].

Working with families in their homes conveys to them a belief in their own value and worth: "I am important enough for them to come to me." It also gives the case manager a clear view of the family's environment, needs, and interactions. An intimate knowledge of family resources and factors that impede their ability to function affects how and what services are delivered. For example, after witnessing firsthand the difficulty that Ms. R. and Mr. O. had in living with a newborn in a hotel room with no cooking facilities and no crib, the case manager had strong evidence to support advocacy efforts to find more suitable housing. The urgency of the situation convinced the case manager not to wait for an apartment closer to the hospital.

When families are coping with HIV infection, their existence is further complicated. Already isolated and stigmatized by being members of the drug culture, infected adults and their children experience additional stigma and ostracism [Lewer 1988]. In some cases, these attitudes were shown by practitioners in the very systems that are supposed to provide service and support. The case managers have had to educate service providers about risk factors and what can and cannot happen to them if they provide services to families. It has been the case manager's task to stimulate (i.e., to hound or nag) social agencies to provide services to families. The case managers also have acted to protect clients' civil rights, especially as to breaches of confidentiality and disclosure of HIV status.

Having one or more HIV-infected and symptomatic family members requires workers to spend a great deal of time on indirect services, repeatedly calling a number of agencies to arrange services, checking to ensure that services are given, and then starting all over again when services fall apart. Strong management and negotiation skills are required of case managers working with large numbers of service providers, agencies, and institutions, some of whom feel that it is not their job to deal with the HIV-infected, and some of whom believe that they should be the sole service providers. Although employing the trans-agency model has streamlined service delivery, at times working with inflexible and narrow agency policies has resulted in frustration for the case managers.

Work with these families has required that staff members be culturally sensitive and possess stamina, fortitude, strong self-esteem, and creativity. WIN case managers visit people in their homes in dangerous neighborhoods, where violence occurs daily. They work with people whose lives are continually in crisis, who are not home at appointed hours, especially when they are still using drugs. Even with daily team support, weekly supervision, and monthly consultation from the transagency board, staff members have often felt overwhelmed, overburdened, and powerless. Despite the dangers and difficulties in providing home-based services, however, it is absolutely necessary to work with these families in their homes and communities.

The efforts of the WIN staff and the transagency model have resulted in improved delivery of services for the families, but there are still gaps in services. The need for a flexible, family-focused continuum of services that anticipates and responds to families' increasing or diminishing needs is glaringly apparent. Agencies must allow for periodic hospitalization of clients and must restore services without major delay or paperwork. These services include home health support, home-based nursing care, and round-the-clock home support. Other required services include transportation on request to and from hospitals and health centers; parent and sibling counseling; day care for children; support for meal preparation, shopping, and errands; and buddy or volunteer services for families.

The healthy children of infected parents are carrying an inordinate burden of responsibility, yet they are in the unenviable position of possessing no identified support system. Often they feel compelled to maintain secrecy about the nature of their parent's or sibling's illness. Sometimes they are not told directly what is happening and what to expect, which compounds their fear, guilt, sense of responsibility, and sadness. Yet many of these children seem to be holding their families together, assuming an adult burden of care for their sick parents and their younger siblings.

Families with HIV infection can be served in their homes and communities. With support and services, families can continue caring for their HIV-infected children at home. The community can respond to the needs of families and deliver coordinated services, making it possible for families to stay together.

REFERENCES

Black, R., and Mayer, J. "Parents with special problems: alcoholism and opiate addiction." Child Abuse and Neglect 4 (1980): 45–54.

Colten, M. E. "A comparison of heroin addicted and non-addicted mothers: Their attitudes, beliefs, and parenting experiences. In Heroin Addicted Parents and Their Children." DHHS Pub. No. (ADM) 81-1028. Rockville, MD: NIDA, 1980.

Gomberg, E. "Alcoholism in women." In Kissen, B., and Begleiter, H. (editors), Social Aspects of Alcoholism. New York: Plenum Press, 1976.

Jacobs, M. Problems Presented by Alcoholic Clients: A Handbook of Counseling Strategies. Toronto: Alcoholism and Drug Addiction Research Foundation, 1981.

Johnson, B., McGonigel, M., and Kaufman, R. Guidelines and Recommended Practices for the Individualized Family Service Plan. Washington, DC: National Early Childhood Technical Assistance System and Association for the Care of Children's Health, 1989.

Kaplan, L. Working With Multi-Problem Families. Lexington, MA: D.C. Heath, 1986: 40.

Lewert, G. "Children and AIDS." Social Casework: The Journal of Contemporary Social Work 69 (June 1988): 348–354.

Shelton, T., Jeppson, E., and Johnson, B. Family-Centered Care for Children with Special Health Care Needs. Washington, DC: Association for the Care of Children's Health, 1987.

Woodruff, G., Durkot Sterzin, E., and Hanson, C. "Serving families with HIV infection: A case study." Zero to Three IX (5) (June 1989): 12–17.

ADDITIONAL RECOMMENDED READINGS

Kosten, T., Hogan, I., Jalali, B., Steidl, J., and Kleber, H. "The effect of multiple family therapy on addict family functioning: A pilot study." In Stimmel, B. (editor), Alcohol and Substance Abuse in Women and Children. New York: The Hawthorne Press, 1986: 51–62.

Lief, N. "Parenting and child services for drug dependent women." In Beschner, G., Reed, B., and Mondanaro, J. (editors), Treatment Services for Drug Dependent Women. DHHS Pub. No. (ADM) 81–1177. Rockville, MD: NIDA, 1981: 455–498.

Lief, N. "Some measures of parenting behavior for addicted and non-addicted mothers." In Beschner, G., and Brotman, R., (editors), Addicted Families and Their Children. 480. Rockville, MD: NIDA, 1976: 38–47.

Reed, B., Beschner, G., and Mondanaro, J. (editors). Treatment Services for Drug Dependent Women VII. DHHS No. (ADM) 82-1219. Washington, DC: NIDA, 1982.

16

Foster Parent Education: Preparing for Informed and Compassionate Caregiving

GARY R. ANDERSON[1]

To DEVELOP IN A HEALTHY MANNER, CHILDREN NEED A HOME ENVIRON-ment with the consistent attention of a loving caregiver. When parents are unable to provide such attention adequately, children are cared for by relatives who are familiar to them and have a tie, commitment, or duty to provide it. When relatives are unavailable or unable, families called foster parents have volunteered or have been recruited to provide a home for the children. The word "foster" means to keep affectionately, to cherish, giving and sharing shelter, affection, and care. AIDS has overwhelmed ill parents, overburdened their extended families, and severely challenged those persons who might cherish unrelated children who desperately need nurturing homes.

[1] The author wishes to acknowledge the helpful comments and advice given by Susan Bear, Coordinator for Foster Home Services and Director of Project Hope, New York Foundling Hospital; Nicki McNeil, Intake and Homefinding Coordinator, and Helen Oakun, Director of Foster Care and Adoption, Lutheran Community Services, New York, New York; Sister Elizabeth Mullane, Director of Specialized HIV Foster Care Program, St. Vincent's Children's Services, Brooklyn, New York; and Joe Pietrangelo, Director, Children with AIDS Training Project, Center for the Development of Human Services, Buffalo State College, New York.

The Need for Foster Parent Education

The demand for foster homes will rise as the number of women with HIV dramatically increases, and parents become unable to care for their children. A cohort of foster parents is needed to provide for HIV-positive children, and for those young children who will seroconvert to negative status but who will be stigmatized by the earlier presence of their mother's antibodies and her illness, or who will suffer medical complications due to neonatal drug addiction.

Preparing specialized parents for the challenges posed by the medical, psychological, and social circumstances of HIV is an immediate child welfare priority. In addition, all foster parents need information about HIV and AIDS. A number of foster parents will discover that the foster child in their home has HIV or that a family member of the child has HIV.

> Last June the foster parents of a three-year-old girl suffering from respiratory distress took her to Lincoln Hospital in New York. Her condition deteriorated and she lost weight. After extensive tests, doctors found that the girl had AIDS . . . soon after, the foster parents told hospital officials they were giving Tracy up [New York Times 1984].

> The foster mother had taken the two-year-old boy as an infant. He had always seemed a little sickly and underweight. Now he was hospitalized with a form of pneumonia that was associated with AIDS. With some nervousness, the hospital physician and social worker asked her if she would continue to provide care for the boy, who would soon be ready for discharge. She replied that she had not bargained for a child with AIDS but she loved him and was committed to him and would not leave him now even though she was uncertain and fearful about the future.

All foster parents need to be educated concerning AIDS so that, if confronted with an HIV-infected child, or a child who has a family member with AIDS, they can respond with informed compassion. Many will also be concerned and will know of friends and others with AIDS. In fact, foster parent educators should be prepared for foster parents' questions concerning the foster parents' personal behaviors or those of other family members or friends of the foster parents. Ideally, education can prepare foster parents for unexpected crises; reduce anxiety, fear, and prejudice; and increase openness, understanding, and empathy for

HIV-infected children and their families while correcting misconceptions and stereotypes.

In regular foster parent education, it is important to clarify the fact that the primary goal is not to recruit foster parents for HIV-infected children but to provide information so they can develop a personal degree of comfort and accurate knowledge about AIDS that they can convey to others [Pietrangelo 1989]. A subset of the general foster parent population has been recruited to acquire specific skills and knowledge about caring for HIV-infected children. This group of foster parents requires additional, intensive education and training to provide quality care for potentially ill children.

The Content of Foster Parent Education

The Child Welfare League of America's Task Force on Children and HIV Infection [1987] recommended a range of subjects for foster parent education. These subjects include:

Medical Issues

Basic information on infectious disease

Medical specifics about HIV infections, including transmission, risk behaviors, testing, symptoms, treatment, and HIV prevention

Infection control procedures

Psychosocial Issues

Death, dying, and grief

Alteration in the quality of life, loss of self-esteem, intensity of emotion, anger, and denial

Cultural and ethnic concerns and viewpoints

Addictions and their role in HIV risk and coping

Types of medical and emotional crisis situations that may be encountered with HIV-infected individuals, families, and significant others, and how to access services in these situations

Practice Issues

Confidentiality and disclosure of information

Display of affection and appropriate, caring physical contact

An outline that can be adapted to a two-hour, half-day, or full-day educational session could address *(1)* foster parent attitudes and values, including negative judgments associated with AIDS and positive impressions about children with HIV; *(2)* medical information, highlighting transmission of HIV; *(3)* the effects of AIDS on children, exploring the social and psychological aspects as well as medical and developmental conditions; *(4)* care of HIV-infected children, including fluid and blood precautions and the protection of the child; and *(5)* self-care to prevent burnout [Pietrangelo 1989].

Foster parents need to be sensitized to their own emotional responses to AIDS and to those infected with AIDS as well as to the feelings and perceptions of HIV-infected children and family members. These responses might include strong negative attitudes toward biological parents or viewing the child as an oddity and overlooking the child's normal needs and abilities.

Enhancing foster parents' cultural sensitivity enables them to recognize and appreciate diverse traditions and viewpoints. Some generalizations about racial and ethnic groups have been made to provide a guide to beliefs and actions [Medina 1987; Ell et al. 1988; Schilling et al. 1989]. Some statements might, unfortunately, risk negative stereotyping [De La Cancela 1989]. Encouraging learning about an individual's rituals, traditions, values, and views (for example, on illness and health) would increase understanding and reduce excessive generalizations.

In addition to broad AIDS educational content, foster parents who are preparing to care for HIV-infected children require training sessions on caregiving skills. Detailed training should cover *(1)* the general backgrounds of children coming into care and the placement process; *(2)* the medical, developmental, and psychosocial conditions that children with HIV can display, and the assessment of symptoms and appropriate responses; *(3)* the medical treatments required for infections and ailments and the identification of medical resources; *(4)* the range of agency services—what to expect and how to access social work, nursing, educational, and spiritual resources; *(5)* the physical care of children, including instructions on cleaning and glove use; *(6)* the agency expectations, including visiting with biological families, participation in foster parent support groups, and medical appointments; and *(7)* the laws that govern confidentiality and the determination of need-to-know and informing others.

Strategies for Foster Parent Education

The methods of introducing information about AIDS to foster parents include *(1)* integration of AIDS content into the agency's foster parent curriculum, *(2)* presentation of educational sessions devoted solely to AIDS education, *(3)* introduction of AIDS tutorials, or *(4)* utilization of formal and informal foster parent support networks.

Integration

An integrative strategy results in all foster parents learning something about AIDS at the time of initial foster parent orientation and throughout mandated and voluntary educational sessions. This content can be naturally integrated, for example, into discussions on medical care, child development, and permanency planning.

This approach to education has several advantages. Everyone is exposed to the information, whereas, in specialized sessions, foster parents may choose not to attend, or be unable to attend because of a schedule conflict, and therefore miss the content. Integration not only ensures at least a minimum of information to all foster parents, it also normalizes the content and does not stigmatize it as a special, mysterious matter that is talked about only at certain times by certain people. When an agency unknowingly places an HIV child or seeks to place a child with known HIV, that occurrence might present a challenge but should not precipitate an agency crisis. Continually hearing about AIDS may help foster parents to absorb the content over time; it often requires multiple hearings of the same information to develop a genuine comfort with regard to such an issue as transmission.

Integration of information can offer several disadvantages. The AIDS content may be dealt with quickly and superficially because it competes with other required topics that must be discussed. The trainer would not ordinarily be an expert on AIDS. The presentation format may not allow sufficient time to consider the issues raised and may omit the sensitizing experiences that are important for motivation beyond a simple grasp of minimal medical facts. Limited time and attention can affect the educational techniques used. Some foster parents may need or desire more detailed information and guidance because they are caring for HIV-infected children or children with high-risk backgrounds who may eventually test positive for HIV.

Specialized Sessions

Offering a number of sessions devoted only to HIV infection and children and their families is a second strategy (refer to Table 1). It could include a half-day or a full-day session, multiple sessions over a series of weeks, or some other allocation of time. The key element is sufficient time for presenting content and also for the thinking and talking together that facilitate understanding and attitude transformation based on the knowledge gained. After this period of specialized education, a plan for follow-up and updating is useful at some future time, given the increase in AIDS knowledge and the potential reactions and changes experienced by foster parents.

On the one hand, this specialized strategy offers several advantages. In addition to sufficient time for thorough presentation and discussion, it also allows some creativity in presentation because use of audiovisuals or guest experts may be easier. Consequently, foster parents may be better informed, more sensitive, and better prepared to care for an HIV-positive child.

On the other hand, there are several disadvantages. A foster parent may miss an all-day or half-day session or series of sessions. The time demands may be difficult to negotiate, given the other demands on a foster parent's time. Considerable planning time and some expense may be necessary to prepare and carry out specialized education and training. Some foster parents may feel that the time spent on AIDS is not justified, given other competing content areas of greater relevance to them, particularly in geographic areas of low incidence.

It may be possible to provide this specialized knowledge for foster parents without overtaxing agency resources by networking with other agencies for joint sessions on AIDS. It may also be possible to send foster parents and staff members to educational sessions provided by other organizations within the geographic area or to pertinent programs or conferences rather than mounting an agency effort. Despite losing the tailoring of information to one's agency and setting, this method may satisfy the need to inform a cohort of foster parents.

Table 1

Outline and HIV/AIDS Presentation

1. *Medical/Epidemiological Information*
   a. Definitions
   b. Syndrome process and clinical symptoms
   c. Modes of transmission and risk behaviors

2. *HIV/AIDS and Cofactors in Geographic Area*
   a. Number of reported cases
   b. Incidence of sexually transmitted disease
   c. Drug-related mortality

3. *HIV Antibody Test*
   a. What is it? How is it done? Is it accurate?
   b. Counseling issues
   c. Where can one be tested?

4. *Sociocultural Issues*
   a. Incidence among Hispanics and blacks
   b. Issues in effective preventive education

5. *Psychosocial Issues*

6. *Prevention of HIV Infection*

7. *Wrap-up/Questions and Answers*

   Adapted from Project Hope, New York Foundling Hospital

Tutorials: One-to-One Training

A number of agencies have found that small group and individual educationally focused interviews can impart information, respond to foster parents' questions and concerns, and prepare foster parents to care for children with HIV or AIDS. This combination of home study issues and orientation can be conducted in the office, agency, or, quite frequently, in the foster parents' home. The latter facilitates involving the foster parents' children as well as the foster parents in the discussions of HIV and to solicit and respond to their questions and concerns.[2]

---

[2]For example, one such discussion elicited one boy's concern that so much attention was directed to the foster child that he felt neglected by his parents.

This small group setting may also increase the participants' willingness to voice their fears and prejudices because the potential intimidation of a large group is absent and a heightened contact with the worker is present. This educational approach encourages a close relationship between staff members and families and facilitates the trusting, supportive ties that sustain both foster parents and workers.

The tutorial process also educates the worker. After placement, workers learn about HIV in general and about a particular child from foster parents who are involved in the child's daily care. This mutuality of learning characterizes each strategy but may be enhanced by the intensity of ongoing individual interviews.

The tutorial strategy requires a high staff member-foster parent ratio because it involves considerable time and mobility on the part of the worker. A number of workers must be quite knowledgeable about HIV issues and possess strong interviewing and teaching skills. This ongoing, less formal approach to education and training is therefore most easily employed for HIV children by specialized programs with expert knowledge, experience, and small caseloads. In addition, there are times when foster parents may need information from specialists that can only be delivered through a larger group format, and bringing a larger group of foster parents together for training may provide encouragement and a sense of cohesion.

Foster Parent Support Groups

Educational issues and training in caregiving skills can be incorporated into the groups comprising foster parents caring for children with HIV. These groups are usually set up to encourage and support foster parents by sharing experiences and by feeling that one is part of a group of people who understand the challenges each is contending with. They have proven vital for foster parents caring for children with HIV because of confidentiality laws and the foster parent's justifiable caution in sharing their concerns with others. Incorporating an information and referral exchange as well as medical, legal, and psychosocial updates as part of the group time seems natural, efficient, and effective.

The development of foster parent support groups is relatively easy when there are high concentrations of foster parents. Child welfare agencies with specialized HIV programs and medical centers serving a number of families through outpatient clinics can compose groups without too much difficulty—particularly so with the help of babysitting and transportation reimbursement. Many foster parents caring for HIV-infected children, however, are not in specialized programs and may feel isolated, particularly in geographic areas with a lower incidence of pediatric AIDS. Forming a consortium of agencies to bring together foster parents for support and education is one way to solve this problem [Leake and Watts Children's Services 1989].

Case Example: St. Vincent's Children's Services

When a person expresses an interest in becoming a foster parent for an HIV-infected child, the program director or program social worker of St. Vincent's, Brooklyn, New York, meets with the person to begin a series of discussions about AIDS and foster care. One session may take place in the program office, but most are conducted in the applicant's home, with immediate family members present. The program's goal is to create a team—foster parents and workers—who can offer feedback and support to each other in order to provide the best possible care for children.

Although a number of applicants have considerable knowledge about AIDS, each is given a booklet, *The Child with AIDS (Human Immunodeficiency Virus): A Guide for the Family* [Boland and Rizzi 1986], to discuss with the worker. At least three sessions are planned with the family, and a general outline is flexibly followed (refer to Table 2). One-to-one discussion permits an accelerated educational experience.

In these sessions, several subjects are emphasized. It is imperative that foster parents understand how HIV is transmitted. If an applicant expresses some concern about getting AIDS, the program director might ask, "Are you going to have sex with the children?" There are also scenarios related to blood transmissions; techniques of drawing blood and sharing needles are briefly presented to illustrate the conditions for transmission of HIV. Another topic for careful exploration is the person's image of what an HIV-infected child will look like and be like. The program director chooses to paint a difficult scenario—a child with physical and emotional complications due to maternal drug and alcohol use, frequent hospitalizations, the possibility of death, and an older child versus an idealized infant girl—and then end with a verbal depiction that reflects the positive aspects of caring for these children.

The director points out that she has seen children thrive in foster

Table 2

Sample Specialized Training Outline

Session One: To develop an understanding of HIV, its transmission, effects, precautions, and prevention
  Overview and definitions
  Transmission
  Physical effects of HIV infection
  Opportunistic infections
  Precautions
  Current treatments
  Statistical data

Session Two: To develop a positive attitude and skill in caring for HIV-infected children
  Children and HIV
  Hygiene, diet, and physical exercises
  Household chores
  Dealing with illness and accidents
  Medications
  Immunizations
  Medical coverage

Session Three: To develop an understanding of the psychosocial aspects of HIV
  Confidentiality
  Coping with HIV
  Reactions to HIV
  School issues
  Special needs and special services
  Growth and development
  Safety

Adapted from St. Vincent's Program, Brooklyn, New York

care due to regular meals and consistent, loving care. Child development is discussed; children with HIV have the same needs as other children—play and socializing, love and attention, and food. The director notes that many foster parents "forget" the HIV and realize that they are caring for a child, not a disease. During office interviews, the director may point to a collage of children's photographs on her bulletin board and ask the person to pick out the children with HIV and the children without HIV—it is impossible to distinguish among them.

In the in-home sessions, prospective foster parents are told that the child may return to a parent or relative; even though this experience is rare, foster parents should be informed of the possibility. Foster parents are told the exceptional board rate, but staff members recognize that compassion is the primary motive in caring for HIV-infected children, not financial gain. Also addressed is confidentiality, with some foster parents so well sensitized that they were later hesitant to tell the child's pediatrician that the child was HIV-infected.

In addition to this series of introductory and orienting tutorials, education-focused sessions in the foster parents' home continue after placement of the child. First, a session describes the incoming child and discusses his or her background and medical needs. Weekly follow-up visits and educational discussions become an integral part of the care of the child.

Some foster parents express anger at what they assume were the biological mother's past actions and the consequences of risky drug and sexual behaviors. The worker will try to help the foster parent understand what biological parents endure—a composite description of biological parents' backgrounds and stresses intended to develop empathy for the parent: "The mother did not get pregnant to give a child AIDS." Educational discussions thus address attitudes and beliefs, as well as providing information.

Discussions of death and dying require a balanced handling. There are times when foster parent denial of dying is allowed and supported. At other times, the worker will press a foster parent to prepare herself for a child's death. This process can become quite complicated. For example, one foster mother was despairing because she believed that a young child's eternal destiny was based on the mother's behavior. The foster mother concluded that, based on the biological mother's behavior, this infant girl was doomed to an eternity in hell and could not talk about it or prepare for the child's impending death. The director pointed out that in the eyes of the state she, the foster mother, was the girl's mother; she was the only mother that the child had known, and therefore it was the foster mother's loving behavior that influenced the child's destiny. This viewpoint comforted the foster mother and freed her to prepare for the girl's death.

Staff members and foster parents have noted the powerful effect on everyone of children dying of AIDS. The director noted that a 13-month-old who died "touched many lives, invoked a response of love, and created more love in her short life than some people who live to be 90 years old."

In addition to tutorials, foster parent education and training are accomplished through biweekly support groups where information and ideas are exchanged together with encouragement and sympathetic listening, and through formal AIDS educational seminars sponsored by New York State. Despite this multifaceted preparation of foster parents for response to whatever needs a child might present, circumstances arise that seem to defy response.

> An eight-year-old girl and her seven-year-old brother were both sexually abused by their mother's live-in boyfriend. He had a violent nature and in one of his rages he brutally murdered the mother. The children were then placed with a series of relatives where they were physically and emotionally abused. They were placed in foster care and were moved from foster home to foster home. When it was learned that the man who sexually abused the children was HIV-infected, they were tested and found positive. The foster parent then asked for removal. They were transferred to St. Vincent's where they were placed in neighboring foster homes, giving the children individual attention but proximity, and providing a respite exchange for the foster parents. Staff members wondered how to help foster parents deal with such a traumatic life experience.

> The young infant had quickly responded to the foster mother and she loved the child. A case of chicken pox that would not have disturbed a child with a healthy immune system resulted in five hospitalizations for this HIV-infected girl. The foster mother remained with her constantly during hospitalizations. The physicians regretfully informed her that they were not making progress against mounting medical complications and the girl was going to die soon. The mother and the staff members could barely face this outcome. How do you prepare foster parents for these moments, made even more difficult by the denial and grief of staff members who are closely involved with parent and child? Thankfully, the girl survived and recovered to return to the foster mother's home [Mullane 1989].

Other Educational Issues

In addition to content and strategies, foster parent educators should consider other issues: trainee resistance to the content, conflicting demands on the foster parents and educator, and the personality and style of the educator [Freeman et al. 1987].

Resistance

Foster parents may attend sessions "ready to not believe the presenter." In addition to having accurate, up-to-date facts, educators must be able to convince participants by their own calmness, experience, genuineness, and patient response to repeated questions. Transmission of HIV is a universal point of concern. Medical information on transmission may have to be repeated on several occasions. Engaging in detailed debates with participants may be counterproductive. Searching beneath questions and objections to address parents' fears is more likely to produce desired goals [Pietrangelo 1989]. It is also important to avoid unwittingly fueling resistance by trying to shock or offend participants—some foster parents may not want to blow up condoms and punch them like balloons! Similarly, overwhelming them with information or dwelling on death and dying may make a general audience of foster parents feel incompetent for what seems to be an impossible task. AIDS education should concentrate on *living with HIV*, because such children live longer and longer lives.

Conflicting Demands

Foster parents may have difficulty hearing information about AIDS because they are preoccupied with caring for children with multiple problems. This reaction parallels AIDS education for the community:

> Any AIDS program should be done as one component of a large program that does some of the other things this community needs, that provides some concrete services. Strict AIDS education isn't going to go anywhere. For these people, your ceiling is falling down, you've got four kids, you have no money, your husband is a substance abuser, your kids are depressed and violent—AIDS is just one more thing, another stress [Freudenberg et al. 1989].

Particularly in regular foster parent education, HIV should be related to other foster parent issues and take place in the context of a training program that addresses a range of foster parent concerns.

Educator Characteristics

Quality content and careful strategies can be quickly undone by incompetent presenters. The educator's value base and experience are important considerations, as well as his or her group leadership skills. The presenter must be informed and up-to-date but also able to talk comfortably about HIV and empathic to an audience's knowledge and mood. To promote listeners' competence and comfort and to lessen fear and feelings of inadequacy, the educator must communicate a sense of respect for foster parents. Respect is demonstrated by acknowledging the difficulty of the topic, providing a safe environment for asking any question, and listening to the participants and encouraging them to listen to each other. Foster parent educators have to project trustworthiness based on honest communication. The educator's curiosity, patience, genuineness, and openness provide an environment for learning as well as a modeling of traits for others.

Teaching Methods

Educational content can be offered by staff members, community experts, or foster parents. Using staff members is sensible because they have experience and expert knowledge in caregiving and are readily available; having them interact with foster parents builds positive communication patterns. Community experts are particularly helpful in communicating specialized content such as medical information, legal issues, or insurance questions. They may include persons with AIDS who can tell their experiences to an audience in such a manner that the listeners' stereotypes are challenged and the disease is personalized to increase understanding and empathy for family members of children with HIV [Gerbert et al. 1989].

Foster parents are not only the most effective recruiters of other foster parents, they are also very effective educators of other foster parents and agency staff members. As formal presenters or as active audience members, they can communicate not only information but also a perspective and attitude about caring for HIV-infected children and their families.

The 40 foster parents at the agencywide seminar on AIDS had expressed a range of views about AIDS. At times the presenter's agenda was swallowed up or pushed around by the foster parents' recurring expressions of transmission fears—including fear of mosquito bites, reluctance to ride on a subway car with a person with AIDS, and fear of using public restrooms. When discussing the stigma of AIDS, a foster parent raised her hand and told the audience that she had an HIV-positive foster child who was relatively healthy and had any child's normal needs. She described the cruel treatment the child had received at school. The other foster parents began to nod and shake their heads sympathetically and then to speak up in defense of this foster mother and her child. The mood of the session changed.

After the meeting, a foster parent told the speaker she would like to have an HIV-positive child placed in her home.

Regardless of the presenter, however, some curriculum or content plan is necessary. It should encompass how to introduce participants and begin the session; an agenda of the topics for discussion; and a variety of formats such as brief lectures, large group and small group discussion questions, case studies [Beckler 1989], foster parent or PWA testimonials, drama, readings, handouts, or audiovisuals [Land 1987].

Audiovisuals can supplement or, at times, replace live presentations for educational purposes. For example, although primarily designed as a recruitment vehicle, the video "With Loving Arms" followed by discussion can also be used effectively in regular foster parent education on AIDS or orientation programs for families caring for HIV-positive children. A number of videos are available for use in educational programs as well as for training in specific skills [see Appendix C]. Since it is often difficult to find a video with which one is completely comfortable in regard to currency, accuracy of content, tone, and point of view, all videos should be previewed for purposeful use in educational sessions.

Written materials can also be used in conjunction with educational programs as preparation for the session, for reading at the session, or for follow-up. With these materials, as with education and training in general, it is necessary to stay up to date on the expanding information about HIV. This goal may require assigning a staff member as an AIDS coordinator or establishing and maintaining an agency library devoted to AIDS information [Child Welfare League of America 1989].

Special Issues for Specialized
Foster Parents

Certain issues stand out in educating foster parents caring for HIV-positive children:

Discussing confidentiality guidelines and risks—working on whom to talk to and what to say with regard to HIV

Recognizing defense mechanisms, particularly denial and magical thinking, and respecting their role in coping

Encouraging the exchange of information with each other and affirming the experienced foster parent as an educator and expert

Concentrating on developmental and psychosocial needs, in addition to medical care (Medical care is manageable, but sacrificing for a child who rejects adults creates anger, and a child's losing hard-won developmental milestones after a brief hospitalization can devastate foster parents.)

Encouraging foster parents to find personal meaning in life beyond their relationship with their foster children, and personal relationships beyond their ties to doctors, nurses, social workers, and other caregivers

Educators may want to offer separate sessions for foster parents in general and foster parents with HIV-positive children. There are advantages and risks to mixed group sessions that should be weighed by the educator [Pietrangelo 1989].

Conclusion

Foster parent HIV education may raise some objections that it is too time-consuming; irrelevant, particularly in geographic areas with low incidence rates; beyond the resources of the agency; ineffective; or even alarmist. Foster parents and other caregivers are already provided with education and training on a range of issues, and AIDS education may have to compete with this existing crowded agenda. Nevertheless, giving time to learning about this illness and preparing for its effect is time well spent. Many foster parents will believe the topic is important. The caregiving issues related to HIV will also be germane to many other children in care. Some foster parents have reported sharing AIDS education with their adolescent children and friends; AIDS education is prevention education.

The availability of community resources may vary greatly, and this circumstance may pose an obstacle to offering a thorough AIDS educational program. To learn of and gain access to resources may require involvement in existing broader initiatives on AIDS in all age groups. Some persons have taken the initiative to begin or strengthen pediatric AIDS networks. Others have found it necessary to travel to other parts of the country for conferences and consultations—preparing some staff members to be agency specialists. Audiovisual and written material may yield valuable assistance in geographic areas with underdeveloped or nonexistent community resources.

Is AIDS education effective? This question has not been adequately studied. With regard to AIDS education programs for foster parents and other caregivers, effectiveness in part depends on the desired goals and expected outcomes. A goal of total comfort with AIDS and HIV-positive children for all caregivers is unrealistic [Gerbert et al. 1989]. In part, outcomes will depend on the length, content, format, and presenter of the educational program, as well as on factors beyond agency control, such as foster parent exposure to persons with AIDS in their personal lives, the influence of religious values, foster parent history with life-threatening illness, and medical issues [Gurdin and Anderson 1987].

AIDS education programs should offer accurate information about the illness, particularly with regard to its transmission, to reduce ignorance and harmful myths. Reducing fear, particularly irrational fear, and increasing appropriate caution and compassion seem to be reasonable goals. An educational program should explain the distinctions between HIV infection, AIDS-related illnesses, and AIDS, to ensure an accurate understanding of the illness and related levels of care. Education can sensitize participants to confidentiality and stigmatization, so that they are respectful of privacy and more tolerant, if not sympathetic, toward those who have HIV. Substantial and lasting changes in attitudes and comfort may come only with repeated exposure to accurate information. Ongoing, even repetitive sessions, may generate positive changes in feelings as well as knowledge. This process will find foster parents at different stages of knowledge and comfort; many will have investigated and learned about AIDS from a variety of sources independent of the agency's program.

Learning about AIDS and discussing care for HIV-infected children is prudent preparation rather than fear-mongering. Centers for Disease Control (CDC) data indicate that AIDS prevalence is widespread and growing, and their data do not include the number of children who are HIV-positive or who have a family member who is HIV-positive or has AIDS [CDC 1989]. As the number of such children and families increases, child-caring agencies will be called on more and more to provide services, and many may be surprised to discover HIV children and families already among those they are serving. Ignorance of or ignoring the educational challenge will create or maintain fear and prejudice.

All agency staff members and caregivers need basic content on AIDS. Some will require concentrated training as they prepare for and provide care for HIV-infected children and their families. The need for this education is imperative, and the time for it is now.

REFERENCES

Beckler, Patricia. "A Case Example for HIV Training for Work with Children and Families." Appendix B of this volume.

Boland, Mary, and Rizzi, Deborah. The Child with AIDS (Human Immunodeficiency Virus): A Guide for the Family. Newark, NJ: Children's Hospital, 1986.

Centers for Disease Control. HIV/AIDS Surveillance. Washington, DC: U.S. Department of Health and Human Services, Public Health Service, Centers for Disease Control, Center for Infectious Diseases, Division of HIV/AIDS, July 1989.

Child Welfare League of America. Report of the CWLA Task Force on Children and HIV Infection. Initial Guidelines. Washington, DC: CWLA, 1987.

Child Welfare League of America. A Guide for Residential Group Care Providers: Serving HIV-Infected Children, Youths, and Their Families. Washington, DC: 1989.

De La Cancela, Victor. "Minority AIDS prevention: Moving beyond cultural perspectives towards sociopolitical empowerment." AIDS Education and Prevention 1(2) (Summer 1989): 141–153.

Ell, Kathleen, Mantell, Joanne, and Hamovitch, Maurice. "Ethnocultural factors in health care delivery: Implications for curriculum in health concentrations." Journal of Teaching in Social Work 2(1) (1988): 33–47.

Freeman, Edith, McRoy, Ruth, and Logan, Sadye. "Strategies for teaching the differential use of alcoholism treatment approaches." Journal of Social Work Education 23(2) (Fall 1987): 29–36.

Freudenberg, Nicholas, Lee, Jacalyn, and Silver, Diana. "How black and Latino community organizations respond to the AIDS epidemic: A case study in one New York City neighborhood." AIDS Education and Prevention 1(1) (Spring 1989): 12–21.

Gerbert, Barbara, Maguire, Bryan, Badner, Victor, Altman, David, and Stone, George. "Fear of AIDS: Issues for health professional education." AIDS Education and Prevention 1(1) (Spring 1989): 39–52.

Gurdin, Phyllis, and Anderson, Gary. "Quality care for ill children: AIDS-specialized foster family homes." Child Welfare 66 (July–August 1987): 291–302.

Land, Helen. "Pathways to learning: Using experiential exercises in teaching practice with special populations." Journal of Teaching in Social Work 1(2) (Fall/Winter 1987): 87–96.

Leake and Watts Children's Service. "HIV training and technical assistance available." Pediatric AIDS Foster Care Network Bulletin 1(1) (June 1989): 1.

Medina, C. "Latino culture and sex education." SIECUS Report 15(3) (1987): 1–4.

Mullane, Sister Elizabeth. Personal interview. June 1989.

New York Times. "Young victims of AIDS suffer its harsh stigma." June 17, 1984: I: 22.

Pietrangelo, Joe. Personal interview. August 1989.

Schilling, Robert, Schinke, Steven, Nichols, Stuart, Zayas, Luis, Miller, Samuel, Orlandi, Mario, and Botvin, Gilbert. "Developing strategies for AIDS prevention research with black and Hispanic drug users." Public Health Reports 104(1) (Jan–Feb 1989).

17

Caregiver Support Groups for Foster and Adoptive Parents

JOE PIETRANGELO

THE RESPONSIBILITIES OF PERMANENCY PLANNING HAVE BEEN SIGNIFI-
cantly challenged by the demands for child welfare services presented
by children with AIDS and their biological, foster, and adoptive families,
including services to help children with AIDS remain with their families
as long as possible, and, where necessary, the provision of foster care
that supports permanence. As with all other children served by the child
welfare system, the permanence of children with AIDS in foster care
must be met through adoption if reunification with their families is not a
possible alternative.

Support groups for biological families and for foster and adoptive
parents caring for children with AIDS where caregivers can network,
exchange information and experiences informally, and meet others who
are sharing a common experience significantly facilitate permanency
planning. It is essential that child welfare providers maintain sound
practice principles grounded in permanence for children with AIDS and
the family systems to which they are connected. Clearly, the way in
which child welfare manages this issue will directly reflect on child
welfare services for all children. Fundamentally, permanency planning
for children with AIDS must remain a definite possibility in the minds of
child welfare professionals. The permanency planning options for these
children cannot be less than they are for other children; neglecting
permanency planning for children with AIDS may result in the retrac-

tion and abrogation of permanency planning services for other challenged and challenging children.

Although support groups for biological families of children with AIDS are of paramount importance for these families, the focus of this chapter is on the establishment and maintenance of support groups for foster and adoptive parents caring for such children. The material presented here may also be useful to practitioners interested in the function of support groups for a variety of caregivers (biological families, childcare workers, child welfare staff members), who are not foster or adoptive parents.

History

At the beginning of the pediatric AIDS epidemic, the energy of human services and health care professionals was directed toward providing support to hospitalized infants. HIV-infected infants were identified as a subset of infants boarding in hospitals due to a variety of social problems and health issues that affect families. Efforts to place these infants in foster homes resulted in the development of specialized AIDS foster care resources. As it became clear that AIDS affected children differently than it did adults, and that some children were, in fact, living with AIDS, concern arose regarding support for foster parents, reunification of infants with their families, and adoption services.

Historically, training as a supplement to casework services has been the principal means of support extended to foster and adoptive parents by child welfare agencies. When training was provided to foster and adoptive parents of children with AIDS, certain unanticipated phenomena emerged. These caregivers said they were reasonably comfortable in their understanding of pediatric AIDS and well supported by medical providers, that child welfare staff members were generally responsive, and that they felt generally able to deal with the needs of the children with AIDS in their homes, but isolation and the inability to share their experiences with the usual informal supports on which they previously relied were creating great difficulty for them.

Almost universally they reported ill-informed, negative, and sometimes hostile reactions on the part of others when they sought support from informal networks of foster parents who were not caring for a child with AIDS, or from friends and family. Health care providers and child welfare social workers did not fill this gap. According to foster and adoptive parents, professional supports were either proscribed, not always available, or occasionally psychologically distant, and generally did not offer an insider's perspective. Particularly at times of crisis, when concrete and emotional supports are most necessary, effective and nurturing professional relationships were not available in ways that met the needs of these caregivers; it was on these occasions when they sought support from their informal networks and met with reactions based in stigma, blame, judgment, and hostility.

These caregivers were left feeling abjectly alone, and thinking recurrently, "I am the only person doing this." The consequence was a particular form of burnout syndrome: diffuse and undirected anger, stress, frustration, anxiety, helplessness, hopelessness, a sense of impending crisis, and a diminishing sense of competence and self-worth.

The main focus of the program for which the author is responsible is the training of child welfare staff members and foster and adoptive parents. In the early stage of the pediatric AIDS epidemic, the training process was primarily directed toward the recruitment of foster homes for infants with AIDS or with HIV infection. As specialized AIDS placements and homes developed, it quickly became clear that the traditional structured training was second on the agenda for them; they demanded opportunities to talk to each other informally about what they faced in caring for children with AIDS.

Although the need for formalized, relevant foster and adoptive parent training remains and is accepted, it cannot take the place of empowerment, competence, and strength obtained through involvement with others in a support group.

Definition

The nature of support groups for these caregivers derives from their function: any group of foster and adoptive parents that promotes and grants permission for informal sharing of information and experiences grounded in the issues confronting the members fulfills a support group function. The subjective experience of support group members dictates the support experienced as a result of group participation. Structurally, support groups for caregivers of children with AIDS can range along the continua of sponsorship, permeability, longevity, focus, membership, schedule, or organization. They can be ad hoc, open to informal support persons or to the members of the child's biological family, or include members who are interested in caring for children with AIDS but have not, as yet, committed themselves to the decision. It is advisable to permit support group structure to be dictated by group member needs and group member decisions while carefully attending to furtherance of the group functions inclusive of sharing, receiving information, and connecting with others of common experience.

Enhancing and supporting the competence, self-worth, and connections of members are the overall goals of the group process regardless of the issues under discussion. Attention to these goals is critical for the effectiveness of the group. Participants will be committed to the process and to the group if these goals are met in a caring, supportive environment.

Leadership

Critical to the maintenance of a viable support group is an individual committed to fulfilling an anchor role within the group. This individual must be willing and able consistently to provide an organizing presence for the group, to schedule meetings, and to serve as group facilitator. It is not essential that the anchor be an agency staff member, but it *is* essential to recognize that an anchor who is also a foster or adoptive parent caring for a child with AIDS has support needs independent of responsibilities to the group. Support group responsibilities cannot be permitted to supersede support group needs. To do so could jeopardize the ability of the caregiver to continue in the caregiving role or deleteriously affect the functioning of the support group.

The facilitation of a support group for AIDS caregivers requires time, basic knowledge of group process and the effects of AIDS on children and their families, and comfort with the facilitator role. It also requires the ability to create a safe, trusting, non-judgmental environment, as well as skills in the management of numerous consecutively occurring issues among members experiencing a vast range of sometimes difficult, painful, and tragic experiences.

Support Group Issues

The discussion presented here is not exhaustive; what emerges in the context of a support group meeting is as unique as the individuals who participate in the support group process. Each support group meeting, however, seems to capture a particular theme, based either on the needs of a group member or members or introduced as a topic by the facilitator. Since these themes are generally both important and common to all members, discussion tends toward a particular focus.

It is useful for a facilitator to present a topic for discussion. Individual needs may result in a change in topic direction, but facilitator-generated topics may make possible discussions that members find difficult to initiate. Many feelings and opinions are expressed by group members when talking about what affects them, and raising one point tends to result in the introduction of another. Sometimes it seems that issues are bubbling up from each group member, especially when the group has collectively shared one member's crisis, such as the death or serious illness of a child. Although it is critically important for the facilitator to follow the energy of the group, it is equally important for the facilitator to maintain focus and direction, to allow full discussion of each issue and permit participation from each group member.

As with other areas of child welfare practice, there is no judgment that good or bad feelings or opinions are being expressed by members in support group meetings; it is important to relate and direct one's facilitation to the feelings and ideas that lie below the words. The emotional nature of caring for a child with AIDS, coupled with the difficulties of providing this care due to the stigma and uncertainty of AIDS, results in a complex caregiving situation. Disagreements, judgments, and lectures with regard to what members bring to the group should be avoided; the motivating feelings of group members, rather than the facts presented in the words, should guide the facilitation of the group process. It helps for the facilitator to frame the process in curiosity rather than definitiveness and to ask open-ended, clarifying questions. Information thus gathered makes it easier to reach underlying feelings.

Parenting in the Closet

Foster and adoptive parents caring for children with AIDS react to everything that arises in daily living with a significant degree of independence whose antecedents are rooted in the difficulty they experience in functioning without the usual support systems on which they formerly relied. Although the reluctance to share concerns is realistically appropriate, the resultant isolation is akin to closet parenting; that is, fulfilling parenting responsibilities on one's own. The support group meeting is designed to counteract this effect.

The Illness-Wellness Roller Coaster

Caregivers for children with AIDS live with considerable uncertainty, which directly contributes to a feeling of helplessness, impending danger, and anxiety typical of situations over which individuals can exert little control. Support group members know from personal experience and the experience of others that an asymptomatic child can manifest symptoms at any time. Since many children with AIDS are not ill all of the time, the degree of anxiety experienced by caregivers is directly related to the duration of the period of wellness. Group members may openly express the feeling that with each day of the child's wellness they become more fearful and anxious.

It is difficult to order one's life while feeling that the future is not predictable. Although members are well aware that this state is the human condition, the thought brings little comfort when dealing with a critically ill child. Acknowledgment of this reality and discussion of what facets of life are within their control help group members to maintain a sense of empowerment.

Degree of Illness

The degree of a child's illness during symptomatic periods has little to do with the caregiver's ability to manage the child's care. Group members sometimes minimize another member's concern if their perception is that the child being discussed "isn't all that sick" or "isn't as sick as my child is or was." It is the subjective perception of the caregiver and not the degree of the child's illness that dictates the caregiver's reality.

The illnesses and conditions that affect children with AIDS range along two main continua—chronic-episodic and degree of seriousness in physical, developmental, social, and psychological spheres—and are felt differently by each support group member. Minimizing competition among members regarding individual competencies and validation of subjective experience and fostering a cooperative effort in developing competencies is imperative to the cohesiveness and effectiveness of the support group.

Anger

It is not unusual for foster and adoptive parents to express anger about some aspect of the care of a child with AIDS. In fact, anger may be an overriding feeling that relates to many other support group issues. Anger is often expressed toward a helping system or individual that is seen as "not doing enough" for the child. This feeling seems to be contagious in support groups and elicits similar feelings and examples from most members.

Anger can also be directed at oneself or a member of one's own family, at another child in the home, at a fellow group member, or at the child with AIDS. Group members may show anger with themselves at their frustration in "not doing enough" for their child when the child is undergoing a bout with illness.

Anger directed at systems or self is more easily expressed than anger at others, particularly when it is anger at the ill child for not getting well. Caregivers feel that they are not supposed to feel angry, especially at the child with AIDS. Permission to experience this feeling frequently elicits a sharing of angry feelings among members, who are relieved to find that anger is common and that they aren't alone. Knowledge that sometimes feeling angry toward the ill child or other person with whom the caregiver frequently interacts does not make a caregiver "bad" promotes management of these feelings and enables caregivers to continue with a feeling of competence.

Guilt

Guilt is felt by group members as a result of a variety of feelings and actions with regard to the AIDS-infected child. Examples include forgetting to give the child a scheduled medication, not staying with the child round the clock while the child is hospitalized, inadvertently exposing the child to someone with a contagious illness, or not being able to answer the child's questions about his or her illness.

Guilt disables caregivers. It saps strength and ability to manage the stresses inherent in the provision of day-to-day care of the ill child. Relieving guilt through open discussion alleviates a significant burden and enables group members to manage these guilt-producing situations as they occur.

The Child's HIV Status

The nature of seroconversion of children infected with HIV perinatally and the fact that some children seroconvert from HIV-antibody-positive to HIV-antibody-negative are of significant interest among group members. Although members whose children have seroconverted to HIV-antibody-negative initially share this with the group as a cause for celebration, in reality, they appear to experience greater stress than caregivers of children whose serological status is constant.

Caregivers of children who have seroconverted live with the fear that the next HIV antibody test may be positive. Furthermore, support group members whose children have not seroconverted may be angry or resentful toward those whose children have done so. They may also interpret announcements of seroconversion as bragging or as implying that the caregiver whose child has seroconverted feels superior in caregiving abilities to those whose child did not seroconvert. Seroconversion to positive or the appearance of HIV-related symptoms in children who previously seroconverted to negative further complicates the implications of this issue for group members.

Denial

Caregivers frequently show varying degrees of denial in their minimizing the child's developmental delays, the effects of symptoms, or the demands that the child's condition make on the caregiver. It is not unusual for group members to enter into a collective denial regarding a particular situation common to the group. All group members share the hope that their children will live with AIDS with a minimum of disability. The members quickly learn the condition of each other's child. When a group member describes the serious and life-threatening illness of a hospitalized child and voices the opinion that the child will recover from the current illness, as the child has in the past, most fellow members will support and encourage this belief. This kind of reaction occurs in the support group when confronted with most manifestations of denial.

Denial is a critical ingredient in the care of children with AIDS and has its uses. It is essential to the maintenance of hope and enables the caregiver to continue. Sometimes denial is what enables a caregiver to face another day in the care of a critically or chronically ill child, and it can then be viewed as the adrenalin of the psyche. Denial is not a completely effective defense, however; a part of the caregiver is cognizant of the current reality, but the fact remains that caregivers cannot deal with the totality of the sometimes overwhelming situations they confront until they are ready. Enabling this readiness and being prepared to provide support without disassembling the denial unless it presents a danger, such as not providing needed medical treatment for the child, is one of the functions of the support group.

Mourning and Grief

Sadness associated with the care of a child with AIDS is a frequently expressed feeling in the group. When confronted with a critically ill child, some members begin to grieve in a preparatory mourning before the child's death. To varying degrees, this preparatory mourning is common to most support group members. When the child actually dies, the preparatory grieving does not minimize the acute effects of the loss.

Discussion of the sadness that can accompany the day-to-day care of a child with AIDS tends to generate the acute identification of these feelings for most members. It is also common for it to trigger the discussion of other losses members have experienced that are unrelated to the child with AIDS. It is imperative for the group to remain with this topic and not to minimize its effect. They need the opportunity to ventilate, to share experiences and perceptions, and to arrive at a degree of peace with the uncertainties and potential loss that they confront.

Magical Thinking

Magical thinking is observed in support groups as related to, but separate from, denial. It is a consequence, as is denial, of uncertainty and helplessness and frequently relates to something the caregiver does, thinks, says, or believes that will prevent the child from becoming ill. Religious practices; special foods or nutritional practices; ritualized behaviors; degree of affection, involvement, or stimulation; and other aspects of child care are examples of such thinking.

This attitude can become a serious issue for the support group when the actions based on magical thinking are not effective, and, in spite of a member's best efforts, the child becomes ill. Invariably, the member feels a significant sense of responsibility, self-blame, and of "not being good enough," that can have a ripple effect on the group. Other members begin to doubt the efforts that have, as they believe, sustained their own child, and their sense of vulnerability increases. Conversely, individuals can also decide to "do it harder/better/more" to make sure it works.

Open discussion of this "super-parent" response is necessary at some point in the course of most support groups. It is important to help members gain perspectives on their sphere of limits and control in maintaining the child's health and to alleviate the sense of personal responsibility and failure that often accompanies the onset of illness.

The Child's Biological Family

The foster parent's effect on permanency planning for children is well documented in the child welfare literature. Moreover, the attitude of adoptive parents toward the child's biological family has a significant effect on the adopted child's developing self-concept. Foster and adoptive parents of children with AIDS regard themselves as the only caregiving resource for an unwanted child and, in some cases, as rescuing the child from parents who have placed the child at risk by transmitting AIDS. Given this viewpoint, it is not unusual for such caregivers to be reluctant to engage in a partnership with the agency in permanency planning if the plan is based on returning the child to the family.

Support group members frequently question the wisdom of planning to return an ill child to a family caregiver who might also be infected with AIDS; they blame the parents for the child's illness and suffering, and insist that "those people don't deserve my child." Some members say that they could manage the child's death better than they could manage the child's return to his or her family.

Enhancing the connection between the biological family, the child with AIDS, and the foster or adoptive parent support group member through discussion of caregiver concerns can assist in the development of empathy for biological families. A level of familiarity with the child's family can also serve to mitigate the blame group members experience.

The Effects of Stigma

Caregivers daily confront fears of disclosure of their children's AIDS status. Most group members have experienced the AIDS stigma in rejection from important others, criticism, threats of the risk they are presenting to other family members and friends, and negative judgments. Some caregivers have been assaulted, forced to move to a different neighborhood or to relocate where they can remain anonymous, or actively discouraged from patronizing local businesses. All group members will have heard of at least one example of the effects of AIDS stigma; many will have experienced it personally.

The support group provides an important forum for discussing the effect of AIDS stigma on members, the child with AIDS, and the caregiver's family. The effects of the stigma can be acutely painful for some members, particularly when it involves rejection by loved ones. It also makes them unsure of the rightness of caring for a child with AIDS: "If I'm doing something good for me and this child, why do so many people think it's wrong?" Airing these issues helps members to feel less isolated and outside the mainstream, shares the burden of the stigma with others who will be supportive, and helps them to develop strategies for managing the effects of the stigma.

Spouse/Family/Friend Management

The demands of caring for the child with AIDS can become a consuming experience for the caregiver. There may be periods when the needs of the ill child are so critical that the needs of other family members and significant others are ignored or minimally attended to. This behavior further contributes to the caregiver's sense of isolation. Other difficulties, such as spousal discord, acting out on the part of well children, and distancing by significant others, can be common reactions.

Distancing may also occur as a result of the magnitude of the child's illness. Although AIDS is not contagious, the stresses of caring for a child with AIDS can be. These significant others may not know how to support the caregiver or to share the caregiver's sense of helplessness and may be unable to find the right words to provide comfort. Caregivers may interpret these relationship difficulties solely as relating to the AIDS stigma. It is important to help members to look closely at themselves. They are sometimes so consumed by day-to-day demands that it becomes impossible for them to be objective about their own contribution to the situation. When caregivers project blame outward with no sense of their own responsibility or role, relationship problem solving becomes difficult to negotiate.

Experiencing Hope and Joy

When caregivers find it hard to keep up hope for the future and joy in daily life, depression frequently results. Hope and joy are critical ingredients in sustaining caregivers. A sense of hopelessness is frequently discussed by members in the meeting. They sometimes feel that experiencing joy and a rewarding personal life other than that involved in the care of the child is disloyalty to the ill child. Comments such as "How can I have fun with a sick child" or "I can't give time to myself because I don't know how long we have left together" are common.

The support group process, however, reinforces a sense of hopefulness. It is sometimes the only forum on which members can rely in the struggle to maintain hope. It is noteworthy that the simple discussion of group member issues is frequently enough to restore a sense of future. The group can also be useful to promote joy and opportunities to have fun and to become involved in some group activity not related to the care of the child, such as a social activity for group members and their significant other adults, a camping trip, or a group family picnic. Group members are frequently able to see this need in other group members and encourage an independent personal life even when they do not recognize it in themselves.

It also helps to focus participants on the joyful events they have experienced in the course of day-to-day parenting of the child. Members come to the group prepared to unburden their difficulties. Introducing the sharing of corresponding successes, pleasurable situations, and joyful events, such as the child achieving a developmental milestone, can be extremely heartening.

Setting Limits for the Child

Caregivers of children with AIDS commonly feel reluctant to set limits for their children. They may interpret all child behaviors, regardless of effect, as "cute" and "adorable" and refuse to exercise appropriate discipline; they want to provide the child with as full a life as possible. Sometimes, a caregiver will try to fill the child's life with a variety of experiences to give the ill child a lifetime of experiences in an indeterminate but, in the caregiver's perspective, limited life span.

Caregivers are sometimes confronted with children with whom they are unable to exercise appropriate parental control. The child may be unwelcome in child-centered activities and in the homes of relatives and friends, increasing the caregiver's isolation. As the child becomes older, the difficulties resulting from the lack of appropriate control become more acute, and the caregiver may begin to feel anger toward the child and feel that the child is "ungrateful" and doesn't appreciate the attention, care, and commitment.

Sharing of parenting experiences is an important support group function. Members gauge the behaviors of their child against the descriptions of the behaviors of other children, enabling them to commiserate about common experiences, compare discipline and parenting methods, and improve their own methods.

Accurate Pediatric AIDS Information

Caregivers have an acute need for current, accurate pediatric AIDS information. Even though support group members are generally well informed about AIDS, receiving information from various means (the media, lectures and workshops, family and friends, and so on), often results in misunderstanding due to the confusing and contradictory nature of these sources.

Caregivers rely on accurate and timely AIDS information as their best weapon in combating the natural doubts and questions posed by misinformation, stigmatizing, and judgmental responses to AIDS, and in educating others about the effects of AIDS on children. A sound understanding of HIV transmission and a level of comfort with this information is essential to retaining foster and adoptive families for children with AIDS.

The support group is a primary vehicle for disseminating pediatric AIDS information and an arena for members to ask questions about the information they have been getting. The group should institutionalize a mechanism for providing current, accurate AIDS information, with a particular focus on children, both as a response to member concerns and as a proactive means of supplying accurate information and reinforcing the correctness of some of the information they have received.

Accessing Services and Supports

The ability of caregivers to access services and supports with regard to their child is unpredictable; some are assertive; others struggle with the problem. Accessing of services and supports may also be related to a caregiver's sense of self-worth. When caregivers are for any reason feeling unsuccessful in the care of the child, obtaining services and supports becomes that much more difficult. Since the degree of isolation a caregiver feels is directly related to the availability of supports and services, denial of, or significant roadblocks to, these resources results in a profound sense of inability to care adequately for the child.

Discussion of these difficulties and the sharing of experiences among group members is a beginning in the management of this problem. Caregivers are invaluable resources in developing strategies as to the methods for obtaining services and supports. Assertiveness training on the support group agenda also helps to empower members.

Getting Started

Caregivers of children with AIDS are generally anxious to engage in any form of support offered to them. Ambivalence about group participation frequently stems from concern about confidentiality, the motivation of the agency, and time constraints. A positive, realistic, and encouraging description of the support group to potential group members is critical to the willingness of foster and adoptive parents to become involved. It helps if this presentation is made by a foster or adoptive parent or agency staff member who is known to, and trusted by, the potential group member. Participation should be voluntary; mandatory attendance will compromise the group process.

The initial meeting with potental group members introduces them to the support group, ascertains willingness to participate, and elicits a "participation contract" covering commitment to the group, attendance at support group meetings, confidentiality, and participation if the individual is willing to become a part of the group. The meeting should include a review of the purpose of the support group, the meeting time and location, the frequency of meetings, confidentiality, the structure of the group, description of the group facilitator, general discussion of other potential group members, and a brief review of the benefits of group participation to the foster or adoptive parent.

During the recruitment and study process, the support group service can be introduced as an option to potential foster and adoptive parents of children with AIDS. For those currently caring for children with AIDS, the opportunity to participate in a support group may require agency energy and advocacy. They may, based on previous experience, be initially suspicious of an agency-sponsored program.

As with the establishment of any group, adequate attention to housekeeping details is critical to the initial participation and involvement of support group members. Constant and reliable housekeeping details are an inanimate support group anchor, second only to the anchor function of the facilitator. The support group should convene at the same time and at the same place on a predictable schedule (such as monthly) for each meeting. Providing refreshments and child care encourages attendance and participation.

The availability of child care during the support group meeting has an added, and extremely significant, function: it provides support group members with the opportunity to bring their foster, adoptive, and biological children with them to support group meetings. Since the focus of the support group is the care of children with AIDS, it is natural for group members to be curious about the children other group members discuss. Furthermore, foster and adoptive parents of children with AIDS, like any parents, take great pleasure in any opportunity to show off their children. Given the reaction to children with AIDS and the closet parenting frequently experienced by group members, caregivers rarely experience this reinforcing opportunity that is a given for other parents.

Support Group Structure

Two matters are critical to the operation of the support group: the frequency and duration of meetings and the size of the group. These meetings can be emotional, and sometimes painful, experiences for both group members and the facilitator. There is a limit to the energy demanded by participation; once this threshold has been reached, group members begin to withdraw and distance themselves from the meeting. Three hours seems to be the maximum time that can be sustained by group members and a facilitator. It should be stipulated and adhered to.

The frequency of meetings should not create an additional concrete or emotional demand on group members. The interval between meetings should be long enough that group members do not have to distance themselves from a sometimes painful process by missing a meeting. Meeting monthly seems to provide enough time between meetings to provide this distance without sacrificing cohesiveness. Meeting monthly also does not create an additional burden on group members; they do not have to feel that it has become simply another appointment to keep.

Since each member requires both the group's attention at each meeting and adequate time to be heard, group size should be limited, although it should be large enough to promote group process and allow for group members who are unable to attend a particular meeting. In practice, a maximum group size of 12 seems right.

Support Group Maintenance

It is advisable for the facilitator to prepare a topic for discussion at each meeting by selecting from issues that have arisen previously or, as the group develops, from topics raised by group members. Extensive research on a particular topic is not required.

The actual functioning of a meeting can best be seen by examining its stage. Careful attention to the stages will help to ensure the effectiveness of the meeting as experienced by the group members.

Beginning the Meeting

As do other structured group encounters, the support group begins with a welcome by the facilitator and a brief discussion of the topic, with the assurance that the topic can be changed if group members feel that a different one is more pressing.

To establish group cohesion and to demonstrate the collegiality of the group process, all group members should have the opportunity to talk briefly about themselves and their experiences since the last meeting. This procedure also alerts the facilitator as to what may be affecting particular group members. It is customary for participants to talk about the AIDS-infected child in their care, but they should also be encouraged to recount other aspects of their lives to the other group members.

The affective tone of the meeting is created by this activity; the facilitator can influence this tone through questions directed to the group member who is speaking and by comments to the group. Unless there is a critical and pressing issue affecting one or more of the group members, they will generally take the facilitator's lead and include discussion of the selected topic during this activity.

Working with the Group

The facilitator's objectives during the working stage of the meeting include promoting connections, reducing isolation, and helping members to discover commonalities, through the process of group members sharing with each other; the facilitator's role during this stage is simply that of a guide. The facilitator stays with the issues generated by group members in the course of the discussion; it is the agenda of the members, rather than the agenda of the facilitator, that takes precedence.

Closure

The facilitator should provide sufficient time for group members to clarify any issues or questions that were left unclear in the working stage discussion. It is important for the facilitator to sum up the focus of the support group meeting and to solicit suggestions from members about future topics. Final housekeeping details, such as the date of the next meeting, should precede the social activities that are a part of the end of every meeting.

Summary

Support groups for foster and adoptive parents caring for children with AIDS are one critical feature of a supportive helping network designed for the needs of these unique families, which bring a positive influence to bear on permanency planning for children with AIDS. Although the implementation of these support groups can be complex, the benefits to children with AIDS and to the families who care for them far outweigh the investment they require. Support groups are an invaluable resource for caregivers and help to retain nurturing families for children with AIDS. Development of group supports for biological family caregivers, which are similar to those available for foster and adoptive parents, will further advance the permanence goal for children with AIDS and the continuum of comprehensive care for these children.

18

Informing Agency Decision Makers: AIDS Education for Senior Management and Boards

GARY R. ANDERSON

KATHLEEN McGOWAN[1]

BECOMING INFORMED ABOUT HIV INFECTION AND AIDS AND THE MULTI-faceted effect of this illness on the individual, family, and community is crucial for agency constituencies, such as staff members, caregivers, and clients. Often overlooked or avoided are the senior decision makers of the agency and the agency board of directors—a key audience. In many child-care agencies, the board of directors is the policy-setting group that often initiates as well as oversees the agency's services, and it is important that board members be knowledgeable about AIDS, "to create an environment within the board that is knowledgeable and sensitive to HIV-infection issues so that consideration of agency policy is conducted within an informed context" [Child Welfare League of America 1989]. Although this chapter primarily discusses work with board members, similar issues and actions apply to senior management, who may be

[1]The authors wish to acknowledge the helpful observations of Myrtle Astrachan, Associate Director, Beech Brook, Ohio; William Brown, Executive Director, Sophia Little Home, Rhode Island; Paul Gitelson, Associate Executive Director, Jewish Child Care Association, New York; Donna C. Pressma, Executive Director, Children's Home Society of New Jersey; and Nora Schaff, Director of Foster Care, St. Christopher-Ottilie, New York.

targeted with staff members (see chapter 14), with board members, or as a separate group of agency decision makers who would benefit from discussion of AIDS.

Educational Content

The Child Welfare League of America (CWLA) recommended that members of agency boards be provided with *(1)* basic information related to infectious diseases and specific information about HIV infection; *(2)* prevention education information and its appropriateness to clients served by the agency; *(3)* the psychosocial dynamics that are experienced by infected children, infected family members, other clients and care-givers; and *(4)* legal issues pertinent to HIV infection and the provision of agency services [CWLA 1989].

AIDS education can be presented in five clusters: *(1)* an overview of AIDS, including the incidence of AIDS and demographics; *(2)* psycho-social factors; *(3)* issues of particular relevance to the child welfare system; *(4)* legal issues; and *(5)* the response of a particular agency to the AIDS crisis [McGowan 1987].

AIDS Overview

It is important that accurate, up-to-date facts about AIDS be pre-sented because medical information is essential to understanding those exposed to the virus, those who are infected, those who are ill, and those who will care for them. In the initial segment of board education, medical information should be presented by appropriately experienced medical professionals. It should include an overview of the body's im-mune system, definitions and distinctions between HIV infection and AIDS, diagnostic criteria for HIV infection and AIDS, risk of infection and transmission of HIV, descriptions of HIV testing and its various outcomes, and a review of AIDS prevention measures.

Although this discussion would cover a range of populations, there are some differences in how AIDS affects children and adults. Time should be devoted to pediatric AIDS: a definition of pediatric AIDS, common illnesses of pediatric AIDS, transmission of HIV to children, and risk of infection. The important age group of adolescence should not be overlooked; although many of the experiences of adolescents will be similar to those of adults, the particular vulnerability of teenagers should be highlighted.

Statistics and demographics on the illness are usually limited to information only on cases diagnosed as full-blown AIDS.[2] Because the Centers for Disease Control (CDC) does not receive reports of the incidence of HIV infection and reports only those cases that meet its case definition for AIDS, it is useful to add to AIDS statistics reputable current and future projections of the number of persons with HIV infection in the United States.

Psychosocial Factors

Understanding the psychodynamics of adults and children with AIDS, as well as the community aspects of AIDS, is also important. This discussion should examine the emotional responses of persons with HIV and those close to them; the psychological dynamics, particularly coping strategies and defense mechanisms; the social effect of the illness and the risk of discrimination and ostracism; and the search for understanding, meaning, and spiritual/religious resources.

Board members may be particularly interested in and benefit from a discussion of the dynamic power of drug addiction for the life of an individual and family, because this risk factor is most germane to children and HIV infection. As in staff member education, board members and managers should be asked to explore their own feelings about AIDS; comfort with AIDS information and understanding and empathy for persons with HIV will strongly influence both management and board support for HIV-infected employees and for creating needed services [Kirp 1989].

Child Welfare Issues

The effect of HIV infection on the child welfare system will become evident when discussing medical information. Existing and projected statistics regarding the number of children with AIDS and HIV infection should be presented, highlighting the dramatically increasing number and the spread of incidence beyond major metropolitan cities. The needs of children and their families can be clearly identified: in-home services to support families and prevent placement in foster care or unnecessary hospitalizations; day care and preschool programs for children with

---

[2]Current statistics are reported monthly in the *HIV/AIDS Surveillance* report published by the Division of HIV/AIDS of the CDC. Other resources are noted in Appendix D.

special needs; foster care for children and adolescents whose parents are unable to care for them; residential services for children and youths, particularly those who are dually diagnosed as having emotional and developmental disabilities; adoption for children who are orphaned or freed for adoption by parental consent or inability to provide care; and medical support, hospitalization, and hospice care. This range of services is not only within the expertise of child welfare agencies, but many are the domain of child welfare agencies only. Agencies already offer these services to the general population and will face the challenge of serving HIV-infected children and youths and their families and/or developing those services that are missing from a reasonable continuum of care.

Legal Issues

Issues that have been addressed by local, state, or federal statutes pose a complex variety for board and management consideration. The legal ramifications of serving, or not serving, clients with HIV are central. Other issues include personnel policy formulation, confidentiality, program policies and procedures, training, insurance implications, and liability. Along with senior management personnel, no agency constituent group will have a greater interest than board members in these issues because of the responsibilities and legal obligations inherent in the functions of board members.

Eligibility for and Access to Services

The courts, the U.S. Department of Justice, and the U.S. Department of Health and Human Services have concluded that HIV-infected individuals, even those who are asymptomatic, can be considered handicapped and covered by Section 504 of the Rehabilitation Act. A September 1987 memorandum from the Office of Legal Counsel of the U.S. Department of Justice gave the following opinion:

> Section 504 protects symptomatic and asymptomatic HIV-infected individuals against discrimination in any covered program or activity on the basis of any actual, past or perceived effect of HIV infection that substantially limits any major life activity—so long as the HIV-infected individual is "otherwise qualified to participate in the program or activity" [Horowitz 1989a].

Even though it is beyond dispute that Section 504 and parallel state and local discrimination laws apply to HIV-infected individuals, they apply only if benefit or program participation denials are based solely on the disease. The validity of other exclusions may be defendable [Horowitz 1989a].

Personnel Policy Formulation

Section 504 and state and local legislation and court decisions support nondiscrimination for employees on the basis of HIV infection. The residential group care guidelines drafted by the Child Welfare League of America [1989] recommend:

> A strong, clear, and generic personnel policy conforming to all levels of governmental laws and ordinances regarding handicapping conditions, disabilities, antidiscrimination, and communicable diseases, is required for all child welfare agencies.

Knowledge of the provisions and rationale of these laws and ordinances would prepare board members to review and decide upon agency policies proposed by personnel managers and legal counsel. Management may face a range of personnel decisions including an employee's refusal to serve HIV-infected clients, or clients who are perceived as having HIV; an employee's refusal to work with a colleague perceived as having HIV; and HIV-infected employees experiencing a range of medical conditions while desiring to maintain employment and benefits.

Confidentiality

Board members will need to know confidentiality requirements as addressed by federal, state, and local laws and regulations. At the present time, these laws vary widely, and it is difficult to generalize, which is in part due to the absence of federal government rulings on confidentiality, discrimination, and testing. The implementation of confidentiality—involving record keeping, interagency and intra-agency communications, and case decision making—will be shaped by law and regulation, as well as by professional codes of ethics. As these are clarified and expanded, ongoing interpretation will be necessary.

Program Policy and Procedures

Many agencies offer a range of services and programs for children and families, and the effect of, and provisions for, serving HIV-infected clients may well vary greatly. The formal establishment of an agency's policy with regard to HIV-infection, incorporating the above-mentioned issues, should be reviewed and approved by an AIDS-knowledgeable board of directors.

Training

Training for staff members on AIDS and HIV infection and programs and the necessary interpersonal skills and universal infection-control procedures is advised and is often mandated by regulatory and public health bodies. The board should be aware of the educational needs of the agency staff and strategies for meeting these needs. Board members should also be prepared to deal with staff members' anxiety as to serving children and parents with HIV infection or AIDS—for example, reluctance to make home visits, or pursuing excessive precautions during client interviews. Staff members unfamiliar with, and frightened by, this illness may challenge agency decisions to serve HIV-infected clients. Board members working with the senior agency staff will have to take into account this fear and provide multiple training sessions to allow ventilation of fear and to offer comforting information.

Insurance

Insurance issues include the availability of insurance, the limits of coverage, and the cost of premiums for protecting caregivers who are directly assisting HIV-infected children in foster homes, group homes, and residential settings and shelters and for staff members providing services in their offices or the community. Insurance and legal experts can advise board members, who might also benefit from consultations with agencies and institutions who have already dealt with these issues, particularly those with specialized HIV programs for children and families.

Liability

Whether or not an agency is providing specialized programs for HIV, concern about financial and legal risks is an issue that board members should discuss in the context of knowledge about HIV infection, particularly with regard to transmission and prevention. Strategies for reducing legal risk by instituting educational initiatives, writing and abiding by appropriate policy statements reviewed by legal counsel, and providing a consistent quality of service to clients are important for consideration, implementation, and maintenance [Horowitz 1989b].

Agency Response

Each agency must decide its level of participation in responding to the AIDS crisis, from educating only staff members to the establishment of a variety of specialized services and programs and leadership roles in the community, region, or beyond. Determining a response is a logical outcome of board members' knowledge about HIV/AIDS, statistics concerning incidence and future projections, client needs and service options, and legal matters. Accurate data are continually needed, and a plan should be developed for updating information and discussing changes in medical care, client needs, programs, and laws. An agency that has chosen at one time not to provide a specific service for HIV-infected children may later institute a program as the number of cases in the community increases or needs become more clearly identified.

This process of considering agency action can be initiated by asking the following questions:

> Is the provision of services to children with HIV in accord with the mission of the agency? For example, a board member of an agency that began a specialized program for caregivers of HIV-infected children told the new program director that it was consistent with the agency's history, for the agency had been founded over one hundred years ago to serve children who were dependent because of a cholera epidemic in the city.
> How will potential services support and/or enhance already existing services for children in the community?
> Based on knowledge about HIV infection and the spread of AIDS, how should this particular agency respond?
> Does the agency need to develop an AIDS-specific program or can it build into already existing programs the necessities for serving families affected by AIDS?

In addition to the foregoing components, management and board members should consider the social, political, and economic issues raised by the AIDS crisis. Agency decisions will be made in the context of larger societal attitudes and governmental policies; consideration of specialized programs to serve HIV clients will particularly reflect how decision makers feel the community will perceive the agency. Ability to pay for services for HIV-infected children and families is, of course, among the paramount management and board concerns.

Educational Strategies

The desire for AIDS education may be expressed by individual board members, an agency executive or management group, or inquiries about agency policy from front-line staff members that provide a stimulus for supervisors and managers to respond. Ideally, presenting an agency policy on AIDS or proposing a program to serve HIV-infected children and their families would follow board member and management education. In fact, some board members may be unwilling to consider a policy or program unless educational efforts have reduced their fears and concerns. HIV policy and programs require strong board and management approval and support in the face of probable objections from inside and outside the agency. These decisions are securely made only in light of knowledge about HIV and when the services offered are within agency expertise.

When formal educational sessions have not been feasible, however, a number of alternate, effective means to increase knowledge and facilitate agency action are possible. In fact, the very development of a policy statement can stimulate an informative discussion. Board members can be asked to join senior management and other staff members in drafting a proposed policy, and interim reports on the evolving policy would be made available to all board members. Similarly, a service for HIV-infected clients proposed by an agency executive or board subcommittee could be a vehicle for further board member and senior management education. A continuum of arrangements, at the direction of the agency executive, medical director, board president, or subcommittee, could present HIV content to board members and senior management personnel:

1. Schedule an intensive, half-day or full-day seminar for board members and senior management personnel to discuss their responsibilities and interests. Several agencies could consider a collaborative effort to carry out this educational plan (refer to Figure 1).

2. Use thoroughly competent facilitators to explore board and management attitudes toward the type of clients served and problems addressed by agency services, focusing particularly on drug-addicted clients.

3. Arrange for members to attend national conferences or regional seminars to gain information that they can report back to the board.

4. The board president may designate two or three board members as those who will receive specific training on AIDS and HIV infection and in turn formally and informally bring their colleagues on the board up to date.

5. Invite and encourage board members and senior management staff members to attend HIV/AIDS seminars for agency personnel.

6. Utilize the presentation of agency policy guidelines or

9:30–9:45	Introduction to Topic
	History of Agency Response to AIDS
9:45–10:45	Panel Presentation I
	• Medical Expert
	• Social Service Expert
	• Public Policy Expert
	• Other Experts (e.g., Pastoral Care)
10:45–11:00	Question-and-Answer Period
11:00–11:15	Break
11:15–11:30	Video Segment
11:30–12:15	Panel Presentation II
	• Director of a Children's Agency
	Serving HIV-Infected Children
	• AIDS in the Workplace
12:15–12:30	Question-and-Answer Period
12:30–1:15	Luncheon
1:15 –1:30	Video Segment
1:30 –2:00	Small Groups: Self-Reflection Exercises
	(See Appendix B)
2:00 –2:15	Presentation: Managing Fear
2:15 –3:00	Large-Group Discussion
	• Agency Mission
	• Agency Next Steps

Figure 1. Sample Management/Board Education Day Agenda.
Adapted from Management Meeting, New York Foundling Hospital

educational plans as an opportunity for board and management education.

7. Incorporate AIDS information as a regular agenda item in regularly scheduled board meetings.

8. Report on similar agencies in the region or around the country that have responded to the AIDS crisis.

9. Provide pertinent reading material/news clippings for board members.

As with other agency educational initiatives, board and management education is most effectively presented when speakers have had direct contact with children and families and are able to communicate lively, illustrative case examples. An ideal for training is the use of parents and children directly affected by HIV infection, though videos may be a useful alternative (recruiting parents with AIDS as presenters is often difficult because of the stigma they experience, and revealing themselves is a heroic act). They must be supported and confidentiality maintained so they can continue to live their lives as normally as possible. It may be difficult to assure confidentiality in some settings, a factor that should be considered before inviting a person with HIV to speak out.

Using persons with HIV/AIDS as presenters, therefore, or even persons affected by HIV infection in their families, is risky when board members are in the early stages of achieving some comfort with the topic. Personal experience with AIDS often seems to be the most powerful means of developing compassion toward those afflicted with this disease. As AIDS spreads both geographically and throughout the population, it is likely that board members and management staff members will know some individuals with AIDS. Board members might be encouraged to become involved as volunteers in a variety of HIV-related organizations. This awareness through life experience, educational initiatives, or powerful illustrative stories creates empathy.

Knowledge, interest, and need to know about HIV infection will be uneven among board members. Some will have a strong interest in HIV and will already have thoroughly educated themselves outside the agency arena; others' interests may be limited to financial and liability questions. HIV education should begin with the areas of interest to board and management members, recognizing that certain board committees may have greater interest and need to know about HIV than the group as a whole.

In many agencies, board members and senior management personnel have already played a key role in responding to children and families with HIV infection. Individual board members and administrators have early and quickly educated themselves about HIV and AIDS and have challenged their associates to create new policy and new programs for HIV-infected children. Some board members and administrators have given support and garnered resources for special programs and services within their agencies. This opportunity exists; it need not await staff members' suggestions or anxieties.

Conclusion

For a number of reasons it may be difficult to implement AIDS education for board members and management personnel. Impediments might include insufficient time to include it in agendas, the belief that HIV/AIDS is not applicable to the agency, or hesitancy because serving clients with HIV is a financial and public relations risk. Another impediment may be personal fear and prejudice producing a degree of discomfort that causes avoidance of the whole subject.

Due to limited time and the number of concerns that might demand attention, lengthy, detailed seminars for all senior decision makers may be impractical and poorly attended. As noted earlier, however, HIV issues can be raised in other ways with board and management members. Unfortunately, it may require a small crisis—the first HIV-positive child in care—to assign AIDS education the priority it should have.

Given the widespread concern about AIDS and the already existing number of HIV-infected adults and children, it is difficult to justify avoiding some form of AIDS education on grounds of irrelevance. Even geographic areas with low incidence reports and with no identified HIV-positive children or youths cannot be assured that this condition will continue. In fact, the experience of other agencies in higher-incidence locations presents an opportunity to prepare for HIV issues. Because AIDS is linked with drug use, a growing national problem, and with ensuing parental illness, the involvement of child-care agencies is inevitable. Since AIDS issues may be more strongly related to the focus of some board committees than to that of others, educational efforts may vary from committee to committee. A case can often be made for confronting AIDS issues by means of interviews with local health and social service personnel or clients, surveys, site visits, focus discussion groups, and HIV article and news-clipping examination.

Because risks are involved in serving HIV clients and responding to

HIV-infected employees, pioneering programs for HIV-infected children often experienced an initial fear of being stigmatized as the "AIDS Agency" and encountering an ostracism that would harm their other agency programs. The fear proved unjustified. In fact, agencies have often enhanced their reputations by their compassionate and competent steps to serve those in need [Kirp 1989]. Rather than a financial liability, serving AIDS clients may attract new resources. Agencies serving children are not unfamiliar with serving "risky" clients. Sufficient medical information is available to permit limitation of legal liability for transmission of HIV. The greatest liability risk for an agency may be created by failure to provide education, supervision, and quality services.

Every agency has a mission statement. These statements of high purpose may be ancient altruistic phrases that are little known or adhered to by agency staff members. The AIDS crisis calls upon senior management and board members to bring their mission statements of compassion and service to life.

REFERENCES

Child Welfare League of America. Serving HIV-Infected Children, Youths, and Their Families: A Guide for Residential Group Care Providers. Washington, DC: Child Welfare League of America, 1989.

Horowitz, Robert. "A legal perspective on the provision of services." In Serving HIV-Infected Children, Youths, and Their Families: A Guide for Residential Group Care Providers. Washington, DC: Child Welfare League of America, 1989a.

Horowitz, Robert. Speech. Office of Human Development Services Federal Grantees Conference. Washington, DC, May 1989b.

Kirp, David L. "Uncommon decency: Pacific Bell responds to AIDS." Harvard Business Review 3 (May–June 1989): 140–151.

McGowan, Kathleen. Proposed Child Welfare Agency Educational Plan Regarding Acquired Immunodeficiency Syndrome (AIDS). Unpublished paper, September 1987.

19

Prevention Education For Adolescents

A. DAMIEN MARTIN

THE HETRICK MARTIN INSTITUTE, INC. (HMI), FORMERLY THE INSTITUTE for the Protection of Lesbian and Gay Youth, Inc., is a not-for-profit organization to protect the interests of gay and lesbian youths and their families, to prevent their exploitation, and to promote their physical and mental well-being. Founded in 1979, HMI started an AIDS prevention and education program in 1984. It was one of the first agencies in New York City that tried to develop a systematic program for adolescents and, in this case, specifically for gay and lesbian adolescents. It soon expanded its program to include the training and instruction of other youth-serving agencies and workers in its curricula and strategies.

Since its experience has been primarily with gay and lesbian youths, this paper often uses gay and lesbian youths as examples. HMI has discovered, however, that many of the principles upon which its program is based apply to other groups of adolescents as well and that many of the problems it faced in developing and carrying out its program were also experienced in other agencies. To vary a metaphor from the author's religious training as a child, the substance remained the same although the appearances changed.

HIV infection and AIDS are easily prevented. Simple precautions ranging from avoidance or modification of certain sexual acts to refraining from exchanging needles in drug use can prevent this dread disease. Yet most of those who work with adolescents recognize that, while actual prevention is simple, leading adolescents to practice those preventive techniques is not.

A basic principle underlying HMI'S efforts is that education, and especially education planned for identified groups, is more than a matter of disseminating information. Instead, it is a process in which the characteristics of the target group, the context in which the program will take place, the information to be disseminated, the goals of the program, and the characteristics of those who will do the training must interact [Martin and Hetrick 1987]. Each of these factors must be articulated as part of the development, the presentation, and the evaluation of any HIV educational program for any group.

The following goals for HMI's HIV prevention program are adapted from an earlier work [Martin and Hetrick 1987]. Again, while the needs of gay and lesbian adolescents are highlighted, these are appropriate goals for any AIDS/HIV prevention program.

1. To provide the adolescent, especially the gay or lesbian adolescent, with the opportunity to interact with peers in other than sexual situations.

2. To prevent the development of those sexual and social behaviors that have been identified as predisposing and enabling factors for HIV infection by fostering the acquisition of interactive social behaviors that promote positive relationships rather than just sexual contact.

3. To provide general health information related to sexual activity, but especially health information related to HIV infection.

4. To provide such information within a context that will be appropriate for this population.

Group Characteristics

All educational programs for children and adolescents involve three separate but related concepts: maturation, development, and socialization. Maturation can be viewed as a comparatively automatic and predictable sequence of biological potential. Development can be seen as "a set of sequential changes from simple to more complex structures within the boundaries set by both biological and social structures." Thus, the concept of development stresses an interaction between both social and biological factors. Socialization, however, ". . . refers to the ways in which individuals learn skills, knowledge, values, motives, and roles appropriate to their position in a group or a society" [Bush and Simmons 1981].

An AIDS educational program for any group must, of course, include consideration of all three concepts of maturation, development, and socialization. For example, it may be more effective to teach the use of condoms before puberty rather than waiting for adolescence, when the young person must also be dealing with the emotional, physical, and social changes that are a defining characteristic of adolescence; a program for normal ten-year-olds will be different from a program for developmentally disabled young adults. While acknowledging the importance of all three concepts and their interaction and recognizing the basic simplicity of the information to be presented in HIV prevention programs, this paper concentrates on the socialization aspects of AIDS and HIV prevention programs for adolescents, particularly on those aspects that, while creating problems for the educator, must be addressed [Hetrick and Martin 1988].

When we speak of the characteristics of a particular population, we may mean intrinsic characteristics, characteristics related to the social situation within which the group finds itself, or some combination of both. For example, institutionalized youths may have certain characteristics related to their social situation; institutionalized developmentally disabled youths may have the same characteristics complicated by their condition; the stigmatization of gay and lesbian individuals has specific effects on homosexually oriented adolescents that are of the utmost importance in any AIDS prevention program addressed to these young people [Martin 1982a,1982b; Hetrick and Martin 1984; Martin and Hetrick 1988; Hetrick and Martin 1988].

Articulation of the special characteristics of a group, whether intrinsic or derived through social imposition, and how those characteristics may contribute to high-risk behaviors within the group carries special dangers, however. First, there is always a danger of stereotyping; second, it is easy to confuse culturally induced factors with ideas of intrinsic nature. Therefore, while we can make some general statements about adolescents, they are severely limited by the adolescent's membership in other groups. A black youngster in an economically depressed neighborhood will share certain issues with a white youngster of his or her own age in an affluent neighborhood but will also have other, different issues to deal with. A young gay person, white or black, will also share issues with the other adolescents but will face special differences that must be addressed. Indeed, a major issue in most HIV prevention programs for adolescents is the non-recognition of gay and lesbian youths as part of every adolescent group. The assumption is almost automatic that the young people being addressed in a classroom or educational setting are heterosexual. Such assumptions about any group limit the effectiveness of these programs, as well as doing a disservice to the young people involved.

Similarly, while we can make some general statements about groups, there is variation here as well. Thus, while blacks in general are economically less well off than whites, there are wealthy, middle-class and working-class blacks, and there are very poor whites; while gay youngsters tend to be sexually active sooner and with greater frequency than their heterosexual counterparts, not all gay and lesbian youngsters are sexually active.

Group membership and its characteristics are an extremely important aspect of HIV prevention programming. Again, the basic underlying principle is dealing with those issues that lead to the high-risk behaviors in the first place. For example, a major factor limiting success in our HIV prevention programs lies within the area of self-image as determined by group image [Hetrick and Martin 1984; Sophie 1988; Colgan 1988; Stein 1988; Smith 1988; Martin and Hetrick 1988; Hetrick and Martin 1988]. The internalized self-hatred that comes about because of racism, ethnocentricity, and homophobia are almost insurmountable difficulties in teaching young people how to take care of themselves. HMI serves many young people who, because of their religious training, believe that they are "abominations," condemned to hell for their homosexuality. Their hatred of themselves and their group leads to a "what's the difference, I deserve anything that happens to me" attitude that must be addressed successfully before any amount of instruction in safer sex techniques will help.

This particular difficulty illustrates, however, how issues can be addressed on many levels in an HIV prevention program. All HMI programs, including counseling and socialization programs, deal with self-concept, but it is also incorporated into our HIV curriculum as well. For example, in group discussions following films like "Lady Sings the Blues" and "The Boys in the Band" that focus on racism, homophobia, and self-hatred, we address links between prejudice and self-destructive behavior and, almost incidentally, what the techniques are for protecting oneself, such as not sharing needles and safer sexual behavior.

Such curriculum and program development is not possible, however, unless one has first specified the major and minor characteristics of the group to be addressed and how these characteristics may affect the likelihood of an individual's indulging in high-risk behaviors.

Curriculum is but one aspect of an HIV prevention program that can and will be affected by a specification of the major issues for the group. There are two distinct populations served by HMI: those young gay and lesbian people who are still living at home and going to school or working, but who must deal with their growth within the framework of a stigmatized social identity, and street youths, many of whom are homeless and involved in juvenile prostitution, the majority of whom are gay. For the former group, cognitive, social, and emotional isolation are the major factors leading to high-risk behaviors; for the latter group, survival is the major factor in their sexual and drug behaviors. While commonalities exist in these two populations, the emphases in HMI's educational and service programs are far different. For those who are not on the streets, socialization and counseling programs are the foundation of our preventive work; for street youths, basic services ranging from food and clothing to shelter referral are the core of our program. For example, a basic service provided to street youths is the opportunity to take a shower and get some clean underwear and clothing. We have found that these young people are much more amenable to discussions of the use of condoms, possible alternatives to their lives, safer sex practices, and so forth after they have showered and changed clothes. Again, the major issue here is not so much the provision of condoms or information to either population, but the specification of the related needs of the client and the discovery of a group-appropriate context for the delivery of that information.

Program Context

A basic concept in systems theory is that any system, defined here as a process in operation, is a subsystem of another system and also serves as the context for still another system. Thus, a school system exists within the system of the dominant culture but serves as the context for the individual classroom. This idea of hierarchically integrated systems is important to an understanding of the kinds of difficulties facing those who wish to develop HIV prevention programs. For example, HMI, as a gay- and lesbian-identified private agency, has more freedom to use sexually explicit materials in its curriculum than an agency operating under a religious umbrella group may have. The religious agency may conform more to the prescriptive norms of sexual socialization, however, thus receiving more general support in the media, government agencies, and other powerful representatives of the larger culture. Space limits the degree to which the complexities of the effects of these systemic relationships on HIV education can be discussed. The following discussion highlights some examples within the area of program content, but it must be recognized that the issues are far more complex than the discussion here.

Content

Sex is a difficult topic for discussion in our culture unless it is placed in the context of drama or comedy. Off-color jokes and sexual representations on television and the movie screen are common, but rational discussion, especially in an educational environment, is difficult if not often impossible. This situation is doubly true when the discussion should include such issues as homosexuality, condoms, premarital sex, and other cultural "hot potatoes." Since AIDS and AIDS prevention programs must address sexual issues, one is immediately faced with difficulties in content.

Discussion of sex is further limited by the ideological and political restraints imposed by various levels of our society. For example, the Helms' amendment limited by law the subject matter of federally funded AIDS education programs to content that conformed to certain religious concepts of sexual morality. A combination of political and religious forces has tried to limit sexual instruction to "Just say no" or "Chastity is the only truly safe behavior." Youth workers recognize that this position is inadequate for many reasons. First and foremost, almost all of the research in the field indicates that adolescents are sexually active, even adolescents operating within religiously oriented environments. Second, the information is not true. Certain sexual practices, such as mutual masturbation, are as safe as chastity within the framework of AIDS transmission.

The conflict lies in a difference in goals. In the one case, the religious goal may be to socialize the young person against any sexual activity except that in heterosexual marriage and to use fear of AIDS as a tool in achieving that goal. For another educator, the goal may be to give young persons sufficient accurate information to handle their sexual behavior in a safer manner. Both are based on value systems; both aim to influence sexual behavior. (The conflict between the two would be a suitable subject for another paper.) The main point here is that health education must be primarily dependent on our level of knowledge. The issue is similar to that posed by the creationism versus evolution controversy. Since our western traditions of religion depend primarily upon revelation, I believe that they should not have veto power over health policy or health education. This belief does not mean that such considerations cannot be presented, or that individuals may not make decisions based only on religious belief—nor does it mean a value-free system of education. It means a complete presentation of issues, information, and educational strategies. It means that religious groups should not have the power to limit in any way the presentation of the best and most recent health information, especially in publicly funded health education programs. The alteration and modification of sexual behavior through the expansion of individual perceptions of sex as more than just intercourse is a primary tool of HIV prevention in those programs that have been demonstrated to work within the gay and lesbian community. Yet such discussion is extremely difficult within the context of classrooms or other settings for adolescents.

This circumstance becomes a major problem for the AIDS educator. How does one give accurate information within a context that limits information for ideological reasons? There is no simple answer to this, of course, but one possibility lies in the greater use of community-based organizations rather than the present reliance on school systems. Community-based organizations, while not completely independent, are usually not under the control of bureaucracies such as boards of education. In addition to possessing greater knowledge of the needs of the particular populations they are serving, they have more freedom in decision making for their own programs. For example, as a community-based organization, HMI is able to develop materials, hold discussions, and present information that can be sexually explicit as well as supportive of our young people. It has developed comic books, posters, and curricula, all of which would have been banned by the Helms' amendment.[1] Other organizations, not directly involved in service delivery to

[1] The Hetrick Martin Institute, Inc., will be pleased to share its materials with other agencies or groups. Please write to Andrew Humm, Director of Education, The Hetrick Martin Institute, Inc., 401 West Street, New York, NY 10014; (212) 633-8920.

gay and lesbian youths, have been able to use these materials for their own educational purposes.

Greater use of community-based organizations is but one possibility, and one that avoids the more basic issue. Young people have the right to obtain accurate information, especially information that may determine whether they live or die. It is the professional and ethical obligation of all youth-serving professionals to advocate for young people in all settings and all situations. All HIV education programs must have an advocacy component. A program that teaches, incorrectly, that the only safety against AIDS lies in heterosexual monogamous marriage is unethical, dangerous, and cruel to all young people but especially to gay and lesbian youngsters. Again, ours is a culture that avoids certain conflicts. We will use religious belief as a shield against discussion of the effects of certain educational programs and strategies, placing them above defense or attack; the result is an abdication of our responsibility to the youths we are serving. This factor has been recognized in some circles and, at the time of writing this paper, there is a lawsuit by several agencies against federal restrictions on content in federally funded AIDS education programs.

Advocacy must go beyond the young people, however. The teacher or AIDS educator in certain settings runs risks if he or she addresses certain issues. We must develop support systems for those educators and youth-serving professionals who are placed in the position of confronting suprasystems such as the administration of the agency or school, hostile community groups, or even political forces within the government. For example, a colleague of mine, experienced both in working with street youths and in HIV education, was recently ordered by the agency for which she works to teach that chastity was the only sure protection against AIDS. To refuse meant she risked her job; to acquiesce meant she had to teach something she felt to be professionally and ethically incorrect. She had very little support within the agency or outside because this order was felt to be solely an intra-agency problem. To her credit she refused to follow orders. While she has not yet been fired, she is suffering severe stress on the job.

Advocacy, of course, need not only be confrontational. Education, especially professional education, is an avenue for advocacy. Community-based groups, universities, or national organizations such as the Child Welfare League of America can play a major role in affecting school and community boards, large service organizations, school systems, and other youth-serving systems.

Educational Strategies

The following are just a few suggestions derived from HMI's experience.

The preceding discussion has highlighted problems and issues in the delivery of an HIV/AIDS education program. The core of any program, of course, is the faculty or staff members who interact with the young people. There must be ongoing teacher- and youth-serving professional training, which must focus not only on keeping up to date on AIDS, but on all the issues discussed above. The training cannot and should not be solely didactic. Support groups, bereavement, and burnout counseling, as well as the above-mentioned administrative and professional support are essential, especially for those who work with special populations like homeless street youths. It is difficult to deal with the illness and death of a young person with whom you have worked intensively; it becomes even more difficult to continue working.

With the focus on AIDS and HIV infection, we sometimes forget other health issues, especially those related to sex. Syphilis, gonorrhea, hepatitis B, yeast infections, and all the other maladies are still with us. HIV prevention should always be carried out within the framework of a larger, more comprehensive health education system and should include ongoing screening for sexually transmitted diseases both as a preventive measure and as a means of identifying youngsters at special risk. If a young person, whether homosexually or heterosexually oriented, has syphilis, we can be pretty sure that young person is not practicing safer sex techniques. Similarly, the young woman who becomes pregnant is not practicing safer sex techniques.

All information should be incorporated into activities and materials that are meaningful for the adolescent group with which one is working. The comic books described above address issues that are extremely important to our clients: isolation, family difficulties, violence. These themes serve as the context for the inclusion of more directly related HIV and AIDS materials. The more that health information can be incorporated into socialization activities, the better. If an organization offers other services, such as individual counseling, its personnel should be trained to integrate HIV prevention information with all their activities, including intake, and such integration of health information, including HIV-related information, should occur on levels of agency or organization functioning.

Commercial films can be extremely useful even though they may not deal directly with HIV/AIDS. Very often, as described above with "Lady Sings the Blues" or "The Boys in the Band," commercial films can serve as springboards to discussion of issues related to the likelihood of high-risk behavior. For example, at HMI, in a recent discussion of a film on a woman's discovery of her lesbianism, the young people discussed such issues as coming out, parental responsibility, and the ethical issues involved in lying about one's sexuality. This discussion then led into specific discussions of HIV/AIDS issues but, again, always within a context meaningful to the young people. Discussions of "Boys in the Band" often end by examining the health implications of promiscuity both for the promiscuous male and for his monogamous male partner, possible ways to protect oneself and the relative safety of the precautions, and so forth. These discussions can take place while examining related issues, such as alcoholism and depression [Kus 1988].

Conclusion

This discussion has attempted, in a limited fashion, to examine some of the issues in developing an HIV/AIDS education program for adolescents. While many of the examples are drawn from our experience with gay and lesbian youths, the underlying principles apply to all youth programs.

Since neither a cure nor a vaccine seems feasible in the near future, prevention is the primary strategy at present. Prevention will not come about solely by throwing condoms at the issue, by giving classes on safer sex, or by talking about responsibility. It will occur when we help our young people to deal with what leads them to high-risk behaviors.

REFERENCES

Bush, D. M., and Simmons, R. G. "Socialization processes over the life course." In Rosenberg, M., and Turner, R. H., Social Psychology: Sociological Perspectives. New York: Basic Books, 1987: 133–164.

Colgan, P. "Treatment of identity and intimacy issues in gay males." In Coleman, E. (editor), Psychotherapy with Homosexual Men and Women: Integrated Identity Approaches for Clinical Practice. New York: Haworth Press, 1988: 101–124.

Hetrick, E. S., and Martin, A. D. "Ego-dystonic homosexuality: A developmental view." In Hetrick, E. S., and Stein, T. S. (editors), Innovations in Psychotherapy with Homosexuals. Washington, DC: American Psychiatric Press, 1984: 2–21.

Hetrick, E. S., and Martin, A. D. "Developmental issues and their resolution for gay and lesbian adolescents." In Coleman, E. (editor), Psychotherapy with Homosexual Men and Women: Integrated Identity Approaches for Clinical Practice. New York: Haworth Press, 1988: 25–44.

Kus, R. J. "Alcoholism and non-acceptance of gay self." In Ross, M. (editor), Psychopathology and Psychotherapy in Homosexuality. New York: Haworth Press, 1988: 25–42.

Martin, A. D. "Learning to hide: The socialization of the gay adolescent." In Feinstein, S. C., Looney, J. G., Schwartzberg, A., and Soroskey, J., (editors), Adolescent Psychiatry: Developmental and Clinical Studies, Volume X. Chicago: University of Chicago, 1982a: 52–65.

Martin, A. D. "The minority question." etcetera 39 (1982b): 22–42.

Martin, A. D., and Hetrick, E. S. "Designing an AIDS risk reduction program for gay teenagers: Problems and proposed solutions." In Ostrow, D. (editor), Bio-behavioral Control of AIDS. New York: Irvington Publishers, 1987: 137–152.

Martin, A. D., and Hetrick, E. S. "The stigmatization of the gay and lesbian adolescent." In Ross, M. (editor), Psychopathology and Psychotherapy in Homosexuality. New York: Haworth Press, 1988: 163–184.

Smith, J. "Psychopathology, homosexuality, and homophobia." In Ross, M. (editor), Psychopathology and Psychotherapy in Homosexuality. New York: Haworth Press, 1988: 59–74.

Sophie, J. "Internalized homophobia and lesbian identity." In Coleman, E. (editor), Psychotherapy with Homosexual Men and Women: Integrated Identity Approaches for Clinical Practice. New York: Haworth Press, 1988: 53–66.

Stein, T. "Theoretical considerations in psychotherapy with gay men and lesbians." In Ross, M. (editor), Psychopathology and Psychotherapy in Homosexuality. New York. Haworth Press, 1988: 75–96.

20

HIV Testing and Counseling: Crisis and Coping for Adolescents and Adults

ROBIN JAMES

HIV TESTING POSES A HOST OF ETHICAL AND CLINICAL DILEMMAS WITH regard to policy and practice. Deciding between individual privacy and autonomy and societal need to know and duty to warn, together with determining harm and best interests for all parties, have led to a number of policy viewpoints and suggestions ranging from mandatory testing and disclosure of test results to total anonymity and individual freedom to share or retain HIV status information. This chapter describes HIV testing for adolescents and adults and the associated clinical issues and reflects and responds to many of the thorny questions surrounding HIV testing at the present time.[1]

This procedure is known by a number of names: the HIV test, the AIDS antibody test, or, simply, the AIDS test. The most accurate designation is the HIV test, because the test identifies the presence of the human immunodeficiency virus in the blood sample, which does not indicate whether the person has the disease AIDS. There is no test for AIDS, which is also called HIV disease.

The term "HIV disease" indicates that the disease is present in a

[1] For additional information, see the HIV Testing and Counseling section of the Bibliography in Appendix D.

continuum: exposure, infection, and progression to the possibility of developing symptoms. It is a chronic illness; if diagnosed early, however, medical and therapeutic interventions can alleviate some symptoms and delay others. The most recent data indicates that it may take as long as ten years from exposure to the onset of symptoms. During this time, however, individuals are able to pass the infection on to others through the transmission of infected blood products or some body fluids, such as semen and vaginal fluid.

HIV testing is encouraged or requested in order to learn one's health status for peace of mind, for decision making with regard to pregnancy planning, and for early diagnosis and medical intervention. Ideally, persons learning that they are infected will use this information to reinforce the need for protection against transmission to others and for self-protection against additional exposure to the virus.

> John, a 17-year-old intravenous drug user who has abstained from drugs for one year, decides to be tested because he is in a steady relationship, and he and his girlfriend are considering having a child. He feels healthier than ever, which he attributes to being drug-free, in love, and back in school. Though he has been feeling good, he has been using condoms since he got clean. He clearly recognizes that his past drug use and sexual activity may have placed him at risk. He has met other people in his recovery program with whom he identified, and they are HIV-positive. He tests HIV-positive. Because of his good health, he has tremendous difficulty in believing that he is positive. He still felt that he was so young, used drugs for only three years, and that the disease would not get him.

HIV Testing

The location and services provided by an HIV test site are discovered through several means. In New York City, information is provided by the City Health Department's AIDS hot line, by a range of social service agencies that display posters, or by individual professionals who possess information regarding the test site and services. Ads are also placed in community newspapers and on subways and buses. Persons who come to the site are either self-identified as at risk for HIV infection or are influenced by a professional or family member who believes the person to be at risk.

Linda, a 16-year-old, comes into an anonymous counseling and testing site with her maternal grandmother. Linda's mother has recently died from AIDS-related complications. Linda had just visited the sexually transmitted disease (STD) clinic, where she is being treated for syphilis. In the initial counseling session, it is learned that Linda has been sexually abused by her stepfather, who, the grandmother says, is a drug user and is "not looking well."

Although HIV testing is a voluntary procedure, some people do come for testing under pressure. Sometimes coercion comes from a misinformed therapist who thinks that the client is at risk when in fact there is no risk. Some programs, particularly drug programs, insist that a person be tested to be eligible or to continue to receive services. Some circumstances may lead a child welfare agency to push for testing. For example, if the biological mother has died of AIDS, there is pressure to have all of her children in foster care tested in the belief that they are at high risk.

Whether voluntarily or in response to external encouragement, persons requesting testing should seek testing sites and agencies that have a commitment to respect confidentiality, and that provide intensive, thorough counseling services associated with the testing.

Confidentiality

The New York City Department of Health anonymous testing sites assign a three-digit number to persons who request an appointment for testing. First and last names are not recorded or used. When persons come for their first interview, the receptionist refers to them by number only. They often tell the counselor their names (both first and last). The counselor may use the first name in the interview, but the counselor explains why numbers are substituted for names and educates the individual about confidentiality. They are warned that HIV status is special information and cautioned concerning the possibility of discrimination: "You need to know that it is important to protect this information and think about whom you want to talk to about HIV." Although concern for confidentiality encourages individuals to be tested, persons who come to the test site still need to be cautioned about sharing this information.

If, after counseling, persons are going to be tested, the three-digit number is replaced by a six-digit number, which goes on the case record, the appointment card, and the blood sample. In addition, zip code, gender, race, and age are recorded as a cross-reference for proper identification without disclosing identity.

This care about identification and cautions concerning sharing information do not mean that persons have to endure this process alone; many come to test sites accompanied by friends and family members. This practice is encouraged, especially for clients at high risk. Clients are asked if they want the other person to join them for either pre-test counseling or discussion of the test results. Counselors recommend that adolescents come to receive their test results together with a supportive person. For example, a child-care worker could accompany a teen. The worker would be excluded from part of the interview, but to bring a friend or a support person along is highly recommended at the time of the test results. Clients are generally counseled individually, and most of the session is spent with the individual alone; counselors leave some time for the other person to be brought in and to do whatever is necessary—usually education of the other person.

One of the more difficult challenges to confidentiality occurs when clients test positive for HIV. The counselor will discuss how to tell one's sexual partners or others who have been placed at risk or potentially will be at risk. Clients are informed of the health department's Contact Notification Assistance Program (CNAP)—in which a counselor will anonymously contact partners whom clients feel they cannot contact: "If Joe finds out I'm positive he is going to kill me." The counselor will tell these persons that they have been placed at risk. The client's identity is never revealed, even to the point of disguising it with misinformation.

Clients who test positive and indicate to the counselor that they intend to continue high-risk behaviors and not to disclose their status to sexual partners are confronted by the counselor. Although the clients' identity will remain confidential, the counselor will tell them the consequences of continuing high-risk behaviors, sometimes asking in frank language why the clients want to harm someone else.

Pre-Test Counseling

Counseling is a required part of the testing process. In addition to required pre-test counseling and an in-person interview when receiving the test results, clients are also encouraged to talk to the site counselor or to call the Health Department's AIDS hot line between the time of the test and receiving the result. Support groups are available for clients after they receive test results. Many clients are also encouraged to have a counselor independent of the test site counselor.

Test site counseling includes education about the meaning of the test, the nature of HIV illness, future risk reduction, and treatment options. At the first (pre-test) appointment, clients are given a booklet that describes the HIV test and what a negative, positive, or inconclusive result would mean and also discusses discrimination issues (for example, who should or should not be told about the test results). The booklet has seven pages, in Spanish- and English-language editions. There is also an audiotape in Creole; the receptionist will set up the tape recorder in a listening room for clients.

After reading the booklet in the reception room, clients are invited by a counselor to a private office for a pre-test interview that generally begins with an introduction by the counselor:

> Hello, my name is Linda Smith. We will be going through a counseling session in which we will talk about risk assessment, risk reduction, what the test means, answering questions that you might have. Then, if you feel that you would like to take the test—I am not the person who will draw the blood—I will take you to another room.

If clients are anxious, however, the counselor may engage them immediately in an interactive process and leave introductory comments and gathering required information for later in the interview or for a second interview.

In the first pre-test interview, the counselor will often ask the clients what has brought them to the test site. Clients usually want to know if this is a test for AIDS: "Does this mean that I have AIDS?" It is important, therefore, that they learn the meaning of the test and that it will not tell them whether or not they have AIDS.

The assessment of risk of infection is also crucial. The counselor will ask, "What have you done that might have put you at risk? Have you ever used intravenous drugs? Have you ever had sex with someone who is using intravenous drugs? Are you sharing needles?" Clients are asked about their sexual behaviors. The questions are guided by an intake form. The counselor may say, "We know this may be embarrassing, but you aren't going to tell me anything that I haven't heard before and I assure you that everything you say is confidential." Clients have as a rule felt free to discuss behaviors in this confidential setting.

If clients' descriptions indicate the absence of high-risk behaviors, testing will be subtly discouraged: "Now that I have told you about behaviors that put a person at risk of acquiring HIV, and you have described and we have discussed your behaviors, do you really feel that you want to be tested today?" If the client asks for the counselor's opinion, a general response might be, "From what you have told me, you have not been exposed to the virus. You have come here, which is great, but it is not a waste of our time if you choose not to test. There is no pressure to be tested—education is the most important part of our work." Preventive education about HIV risk reduction is an important topic in these interviews.

> A maternal grandmother, her two granddaughters (aged 14 and 16), and the grandmother's daughter (the girls' aunt) reported to the test site counselor that the granddaughters' mother had recently died of AIDS. Their family physician sent them all in to be tested. The adolescents were seen individually, alone, to assess potential risk and how they were handling the loss of their mother. Neither girl was engaged in risk behaviors, and both were already involved in individual counseling. The site counselor discussed condom use if the girls became sexually active and gave them her number in case they had any questions. The counselor met with the whole family to discuss modes of HIV transmission, to evaluate household exposure, and to reassure them that testing was not necessary. A letter to this effect was given to the grandmother to show to the family physician.

AIDS prevention and risk reduction education focuses on sexual practices and drug use. If clients are sexually active and are not using condoms, they are asked if they know that condom use reduces the risk of HIV infection, and the counselor explains why condoms are effective and demonstrates how to use them. The use of condoms to prevent unwanted pregnancies and increasingly prevalent sexually transmitted diseases is also noted. Clients are encouraged to avoid intravenous drugs and, if involved with drugs, to use clean needles. Assistance in accessing drug treatment programs is offered.

After initial assessments of risk and prevention education, the features of the test are discussed.

> When you come back here in two weeks, I will say one of three things to you. Either the test results were negative, the test results

were positive, or the test results were inconclusive. If you were negative that means that, at the time you were tested, there was no trace of the antibodies for the HIV virus in your blood, but if there was a risk exposure within the past six months then perhaps you will need to be retested. The test is only definitive if there were absolutely no risk behaviors within the past six months. If your test was positive, that means that antibodies were present in your blood, and I would recommend that you be retested, because there is the chance of an error, although this has never happened in our experience. If the results were inconclusive, a retest is needed. We don't really understand why some tests are inconclusive, but a certain percentage of people do test inconclusive.

If clients are at high risk, based on the assessment of risk behaviors, the counselor will talk at great length with the clients about what they will do if they test positive. This discussion includes asking clients to anticipate how they will feel if informed that they are positive. Role-plays will be used to increase their understanding of possible responses to a positive test result. It is the counselor's aim to prevent someone from learning the test outcome while totally unprepared for a positive result. Counselors take as much time as is necessary to help clients arrive at some stage of preparation for this possibility.

Most clients who have experienced high-risk behaviors have thought about the possibility of a positive test outcome for some time before the test. This self-preparation differs from characteristic magical thinking—that they will be the ones who will be negative. It is still important and sometimes difficult to get clients to talk about this possibility, but the counselor insists on their talking about their reaction and explains that the insistence is due to the potential trauma of learning of one's positive status.

During the pre-test interview, the counselor begins to plan with the clients what they will do if they test positive. This front-loaded discussion of test outcomes is important because at the time they are told of a positive test they may not hear anything else that is then discussed. Counselors have seen the trauma and anguish of individuals who received no pre-test counseling, were tested by insurance companies or private physicians, and were informed of the positive results over the telephone. A number of persons who have had this experience have contacted the test site for counseling.

The pre-test interview usually lasts for 60 to 90 minutes. For adolescents, this interview may be longer, or several pre-test interviews may be scheduled. The counselor may delay the testing and offer additional sessions by asking, "Do you still want to be tested today or do you want some time to think about this information?"—thus affording an opportunity to talk with them after they have had a chance to assimilate the information and to think about what they want to do and whether they can deal emotionally with the information.

As the pre-test interview concludes, the counselor must make a judgment about the clients' ability to take and effectively respond to the HIV test. If the counselor does not feel comfortable about the individual's receiving the test, a recommendation can be made not to test. The counselor will ask the client to return for another interview at a later date and will explain why this delay is desirable.

> From what you have told me today, it is my feeling that today is not the right day to be tested. I think you need to think about this more, talk to a friend about it, bring a friend with you. Perhaps you should get engaged in regular counseling before you get tested because there are a lot of issues here.

Circumstances that lead to a decision to delay testing include a history of suicidal attempts or ideation, affect that appears to be disconnected and not related to the seriousness of the issues being raised, or a high-risk client who has no support group. The judgment that the clients will hurt themselves or others is the most serious objection to having a test.

If the counselor believes that clients can handle the test, they walk together to a nearby office and the clients are introduced to the phlebotomist, the lab technician who draws the blood. The phlebotomist is handed a laboratory slip that contains the client's birth date, zip code, case number/six-digit number, gender, race, and a rating of risk based on the interview. Before testing, clients sign an informed consent form with their identification number.

The worker will not stay during the blood drawing, unless requested. The procedure requires less than five minutes; blood is drawn from the arm (intravenous), not from a finger prick, in a standard small blood drawing similar to other blood test procedures that clients may have experienced. Clients are then given a card with an appointment time assigned by the worker at the end of the interview and are reminded that no test results will be given over the telephone.

The pretest counseling must raise a number of issues: (1) the meaning of the test and its possible outcomes, (2) the importance of confidentiality, (3) risk assessment based on a discussion of client behaviors,

(4) risk reduction and prevention education, and (5) the exploration of possible responses to the outcome of the test. A variety of psychosocial issues are also addressed, based on individual circumstances.

A middle-aged woman and her second husband come in for the HIV test. Her first husband was an intravenous drug user. With her second husband she has had two sons, the first, ten years old, is in perfect health. The second son, less than two years old, had been hospitalized for pneumonia three times in the past 18 months and showed other signs of immunosuppression. He is now hospitalized and diagnosed as having PCP, a pneumonia related to HIV infection. At no time in the past have the physicians talked with the parents regarding the possibility of the mother having HIV. In view of their son's diagnosis, they are now requesting testing. Interviewed individually and together, they expressed their overwhelming sense of guilt and their sadness. They reported feeling helpless and betrayed by a past that they thought they were through with. The mother has been tested and is HIV-infected, and in counseling they are beginning to consider the implications for her and the family; however, they continue to focus primarily on their hospitalized son. The father will soon be tested.

Louis, a 15-year-old foster child, comes in for the "AIDS test." His agency counselor had insisted that he be tested because he has had unprotected sex with a man. Louis considers himself to be heterosexual. In the pre-test interview he was highly agitated and said that he felt all alone. He resented his agency counselor's insistence that he be tested. The HIV counselor talked with Louis about risk reduction and proper condom use. With Louis present, the HIV counselor arranged an appointment for Louis at an adolescent health program and tried to reach his agency counselor to coordinate services. Louis became distracted as the interview progressed and, saying he had to go to court with a friend, he walked out of the interview. He did not return or follow through on referrals.

Post-Test Counseling

The laboratory test used to identify the presence of HIV antibodies is called the ELISA test. If the first test of the blood sample results in a positive or inconclusive finding, the sample is retested with the ELISA test. If the results are again positive or inconclusive, the Western blot test is used. If the results are still inconclusive after the Western blot, the immunofluorescent assay (IFA) test is used. The IFA clarifies the Western blot test, but this assay is still considered experimental and does not always render a clear result.

After the drawing of blood there is approximately a two-week wait before the client returns to receive the results. It is often an anxious two weeks. Clients are encouraged to call their counselor or the AIDS hot line if they have any questions or concerns they would like to discuss. A number of clients have maintained contact with staff members during this interim period.

Ninety-five percent of the clients who have been tested return to receive the results. After presenting their six-digit number to the receptionist, clients are normally reunited with their pre-test counselor, who takes them to the same room.

Positive Test

The session begins with a request for the client's birth date and zip code to confirm that this individual is the right person—an important verification, when identifications are made through numbers. Once the person has been identified, the counselor immediately tells the client the result: "Your test result was positive."

To learn that one's test was positive provokes much anxiety. Clients are shown the laboratory paper with the results, eliminating any mystical fantasy that there is a secret code. Clients are not given this paper.

Typical responses have included crying hysterically, going blank and numb, ranting and shouting—"I'm going to die now!"—and questioning—"Did the test tell you how long I have?" Some clients try to bolt out of the office. Counselors have been known to throw themselves in front of the office door to stop them; it is undesirable to have a client leave with that degree of panic.

Some clients report that they were prepared for this and have a plan of action/treatment. Most clients, however, are "freaked out." This reaction has been particularly true for pregnant women or for those who have recently given birth. Counselors will talk with a client as long as necessary until he or she can begin to address the next steps in his or her life. The counselor has to feel that, when this client leaves the office, the pain and stress will be accompanied by a plan of action. A doctor's appointment may be made while the client is still in the office, as would appointments for counseling. Other first steps would include discussing nutrition and lifestyle changes (cautioning against drinking alcohol and smoking, and encouraging safer sex practices). The clients are given a packet of resource information to take with them.

> We know you are probably in shock and cannot hear everything that we say. That is why I am giving you all of this information to take home with you and read. Reading this may help you when you have calmed down and are ready to take further action.

Clients are informed that there are open-ended, drop-in, confidential support groups for persons who are HIV-positive. These groups are held at the test site and at other community agencies and may range in size from eight to 40 people. There is also a group for the seronegative sexual partners of HIV-positive persons.

As noted earlier, if someone accompanies the client, the client first has a private interview. If the client wants the other person to come into the room later, the counselor tells the client that the counselor cannot tell the other person the test results; if the client wants the other person to know, the client must tell him or her. A number of clients who test positive will return to the test site with their partners after sharing the information with them. There may be three or four post-test counseling sessions. Requesting retesting often assures the counselor of seeing the client again.

Negative Test

"Your test result was negative." When the result is negative, the clients are generally greatly relieved. Some clients want proof that it is really their test result; they are shown the results. The counselor reinforces the point that there is a six-month period during which HIV infection would not necessarily appear on the test. The counselor also has to impart some unfortunately confusing information about negative seroconverting to positive. If high-risk behavior has occurred in the last six months, the clients should be retested accordingly.

Post-test counseling includes prevention education: "You are negative now but it is your responsibility to stay negative." Potential obstacles to using safer sex and talk about drug treatment, if appropriate, are also discussed. Clients are given condoms and a fact sheet that explains the test results.

The counselor may be confrontational with clients who test negative but continue high risk-behaviors: "We don't want to see you again and tell you that you are positive." Psychosocial impediments to risk reduction are identified and discussed. Counselors have observed that a small number of clients seem to be trying to become positive. In one case, a 19-year-old woman had unprotected sex with her boyfriend while he was in the hospital for an AIDS-related illness; when she was tested a second time, she had converted from a negative to a positive test result. Counselors want to make sure that if a person becomes infected, the change is not due to ignorance. Ongoing counseling is encouraged for clients who seem unwilling to change their risky behaviors.

Special Issues in Testing

Testing raises a number of cultural issues when personal behaviors, risk-reduction practices, and relationship elements are addressed in counseling. Persons coming to be tested are from a range of cultures, ethnic groups, and races, posing a challenge to provide counseling and informational materials in the language that is most comfortable for the client. Sensitivity is particularly required when discussing safer sex with women who express a fear of being rejected or physically abused by boyfriends or husbands if safer sex, such as condom use, is requested. Some men are extremely reluctant to admit or discuss their bisexuality because of family and community condemnation of homosexuality. The sensitivity of the topics and the diversity of cultures require that counselors must be prepared to recognize and respect clients' values and to understand the necessity of developing a sense of trust.

Counselors also need preparation for working with adolescent clients.[2] Although there are many similarities between an adult's and an adolescent's experience and their reaction to testing, teenagers have a harder time taking in the information and truly believing that HIV could happen to them. Adolescents feel less vulnerable than adults. Consequently, the shock, denial, and disbelief are greater. When adolescents test negative, they tend to believe that they can continue high-risk behaviors and fantasize that they will remain immune. Knowledge of

[2]HIV testing of younger children should be done in a medical facility as part of a complete medical workup. Pre-test and post-test counseling with caregivers is essential, because the ramifications of having a child test positive are far-reaching; for example, this information may be the first indication to the biological mother that she has HIV.

adolescent development is an important part of test site counselor training.

Initial preparation of test site counselors requires a five-day training course. After this orientation, they go to their assigned test site and join experienced counselors, observing sessions. This apprenticeship will continue for as long as necessary for the new counselor to be comfortable and knowledgeable in conducting interviews. There is no pressure for the counselor in training to acquire this level of comfort quickly. Each counselor is supervised by an experienced senior counselor/supervisor. The educational backgrounds of counselors vary; they often have backgrounds that are similar to the clientele who live near and use the testing site.

Conclusion

The decision to receive testing for the HIV virus confronts individuals with issues of physical and mental health, mortality, discrimination, and possible ostracism from family, friends, and society. The sophistication required for coping with this information is complicated and difficult for adults, even with careful counseling. The challenge for adolescents and children is even more intense, requiring additional supports. HIV testing should take place only after careful pre-test counseling, informed consent, and post-test counseling, regardless of test results. These crucial services should be provided by a well-trained and supervised counseling staff sensitive to client concerns and with high respect for client confidentiality.

21

Grief Education: Educating about Death for Life

KENNETH J. DOKA

To speak of grief education seems almost ludicrous. One might as well speak of education for breathing, for at first glance, both seem so natural that the very concept that one need "educate" persons about them seems pedantic. Why do we need to educate people on what to feel? Why not simply recognize that they will feel grief?

Yet, in many ways, that assumption frames the problem. First, emotion has both an internal and a social component. Our feelings and reactions have to be interpreted. As Hochschild [1979] states, even emotions are governed by social norms or "feelings rules" that tell how one is "expected" to feel. Hence, according to Hochschild, we spend much time on emotion work, trying to evoke the emotions we perceive as socially desirable and suppress those that we believe are negatively sanctioned. Thus, even grief is governed by social norms that define who, how, and when one should grieve.

This attitude then becomes the core of the problem. The social perception of appropriate grief is often at variance with the personal experience of the bereaved. Both public and professional perceptions underestimate both the duration and symptomatology of grief [Doka and Jendreski 1985]. Thus, grief is frequently complicated by the fact that the bereaved often experience reactions, typical of grief, that they perceive as troubling and inappropriate, spending their energy trying to suppress such reactions rather than exploring and resolving them.

This response is often exacerbated in AIDS deaths, particularly deaths of children experienced by surviving foster parents and social work staff members. AIDS is, by the fear and panic it generates, a disenfranchising death, which often isolates survivors. Survivors of AIDS losses frequently and prudently fear sharing that loss with others, and grieve alone. This inability to seek or find support complicates grief. And the problem may be especially severe for social workers and foster parents, who are often dually disenfranchised, suffering both the isolation of AIDS and the ambiguous status of their "role right" to grieve [Anderson et al. 1989].

Information, then, about grief can play a significant role in grief resolution, with two basic functions. First, information about symptomatology and the nature of grief can be validating, can reassure survivors that their experiences and reactions are both normal and natural, setting a context for eventual resolution. Once, a graduate student, widowed a year earlier, questioned me about my lecture statement that it takes years to resolve grief. He later told me that he took a photocopy of my sources and showed it to friends who were pressuring him into involvements and commitments he was not yet ready to make. Education about grief let him understand that his reactions were not unusual or abnormal.

Second, grief education can have interventive value as well, clarifying strategies and resources as individuals seek, in their unique ways, to cope with a loss.

This chapter offers a basic understanding of the nature of grief education: its contents, target audience, appropriate times for grief education, and models and resources for grief education—not as a panacea, but as part of an agency's services and support to its clients and staff.

The Content of Grief Education[1]

One problem in grief resolution is that our image of grief shows it as a minor difficulty, quickly resolved. Even our media images of grief either ignore it or identify intense reactions with weaker characters and point to rapid resolution [Wass 1985]. It is little wonder that even profes-

[1]Sections on the symptoms and process of grief have been adapted from the author's entry on grief in the *Encyclopedia of Death* (Oxford University Press, in press).

sional groups such as the clergy often underestimate the effects of grief [Doka and Jendreski 1985]. Hence simply informing bereaved persons about the multiplicity of patterns and symptoms that accompany loss can often have great therapeutic value, reassuring them that their responses and experiences are not a cause for alarm.

The bereaved may need to learn that the symptoms individuals experience in grief are intensive and can vary from person to person. Physical symptoms can include headaches, exhaustion, dizziness, muscular aches, menstrual irregularities, sexual impotence, loss of appetite, insomnia, breathlessness, tremors and shakes, and pains. While physical symptoms are typical and may not be a cause for concern, it is important to encourage bereaved persons to report them to a physician who is aware both of the loss and the nature of grief.

Bereaved persons may also experience affective symptoms: guilt, anger, anxiety, hopelessness, sadness, shock, yearning, numbness, blame—even relief and emancipation. As in many situations of emotional crisis, these feelings, even seemingly inconsistent ones (such as relief and sadness) can be experienced simultaneously.

Grief can be manifested cognitively as well. There can be a sense of depersonalization, inability to concentrate, a sense of disbelief and confusion, and idealization of the deceased. These cognitive symptoms can impair performance in work or school. A number of studies have also shown that many bereaved persons experience a vague sense of the deceased's continued presence, or even have fleeting auditory, visual, olfactory, or tactile hallucinatory experiences [Hoyt 1980; Lindstrom 1982]. Though some bereaved persons may find this experience strange, most interpret it positively as a sign of reassurance that the person will be near them, or is happy, and/or as a sign to continue life. In some cases, however, these experiences can be perceived negatively and can inhibit grief resolution. An example of this was a six-year-old boy ridden with guilt who saw, on occasion, images of his father beckoning him to dangerous places.

Behavioral symptoms of grief can include loss or changes of patterns of conduct, changes in interaction patterns and responses to others, crying, withdrawal, avoiding reminders of the deceased, seeking or carrying reminders of the deceased, and overactivity.

Grief education programs can also remind people that, despite current images, grief may persist for a considerable period of time. It may take as long as three to five years to resolve a significant loss, and some recent research indicates that a continued sense of loss, an "empty space," can last indefinitely [McClowry et al. 1987]. Many bereaved persons experience grief as a roller coaster, a series of highs and lows that tend to be intense at first and diminish over time. Many bereaved persons more typically experience a wide range of intense symptoms in the first six to 13 months, symptoms that gradually diminish. It is not uncommon for them periodically to experience painful episodes at other times, particularly at holidays, significant dates in the relationship, or at the anniversary of the death.

Grief education programs can reaffirm that each individual experiences grief uniquely, varying in symptoms, intensity, pattern, time, and resolution. A number of factors influence the nature of a grief reaction: the bereaved's unique relationship to the deceased; the strength of the attachment; the degree of ambivalence and unfinished business in the relationship; the circumstances of the death, including the length and nature of the illness, the preventability of the death, and the conditions of the death (e.g., what happened at the time of death, where was the bereaved, and so on); reactions to previous loss; the personality of the bereaved, including coping behaviors, ability to express emotions and to seek and receive help, and social variables such as the strength and nature of the family system; the presence and nature of informal or formal support systems, cultural and religious beliefs and practices, and beliefs about appropriate gender-related behaviors; and general health and lifestyle practices.

Education programs may also reinforce the understanding that the ways in which bereaved persons resolve grief are also highly individual. The bereavement process was once seen as a series of general stages, beginning, for example, with shock and ending with recovery and resolution. More recent work has emphasized that the bereaved must complete certain tasks, such as accepting the reality of the loss; experiencing and resolving the emotions associated with the grief; readjusting to life without the deceased; withdrawing emotional energy from the deceased and reinvesting it in other ways and/or finding creative ways to retain the memory of the deceased (e.g., dedicating oneself to fulfilling the deceased's ideals); and perhaps reassessing and rebuilding faith or philosophical systems challenged by the loss [Rando 1984; Worden 1982; Doka in press].

Discussion of grief resolution should also include strategies and resources for resolving grief. Individuals often need just supportive environments in which they can verbalize feelings, consider coping strategies, and assess ways in which they are resolving their grief. When these networks are not normally available, or individuals feel a need for more intensive work, counselors and self-help groups may be indicated. Since both the dread of AIDS and the unique role of foster parent (and caseworker) may cause reluctance to join established groups, agencies may wish to develop their own groups. Books on grief are an important resource too, reassuring the bereaved that their reactions are normal, offering insights, and encouraging hope of eventual resolution. Grief education programs can suggest resources, and agency libraries can provide them.

In summary, then, grief education programs should include basic information about the symptoms of grief, the process of grieving, factors that affect grief reactions, and strategies for grief resolution. Such programs should emphasize that each individual's reaction is unique, that there is no single right way to feel or to resolve grief.

Models of Grief Education[2]

Toward whom then should grief education be directed? A general answer is a society in which death and grief are denied. Agencies involved in the AIDS crisis have neither the time, resources, or mission for such educational endeavors; however, they should offer education to staff members, foster family members, and, when possible, biological parents.

Staff education is essential in any agency grief education program, for three reasons. First, and most obviously, staff members will be providing care for bereaved foster parents and biological parents. They have to understand how grief may affect these bereaved persons, perhaps even influencing their interaction with each other and the agency. For example, a parent's or foster parent's natural anger at loss may be displaced on the agency, often on one worker. A splitting of anger in which one worker is blamed while others are exempted can be destructive to staff relationships. Second, the staff will need education to provide support, empathy, and counsel for the bereaved. Finally, education

[2]Two book services specialize in books on loss, grief, and death: Center for Thanatology Research and Education, 391 Atlantic Avenue, Brooklyn, New York 11217-1701 (718-858-3026); and The Compassion Book Service, 216 Via Monte, Walnut Creek, California 94598 (415-933-0830). Media are regularly reviewed by the journal, *Death Studies*.

may help staff members to understand their own grief over present or previous loss. These grief reactions may be multifaceted. In crisis situations where strong emotion peaks, bonding can be intense and rapid [Fulton 1986]. Hence, staff members may be highly vulnerable to grief over the loss of a child, and perhaps even the loss of contact with foster or biological families. Failure to resolve this grief can lead to burnout and can complicate interaction, perhaps raising countertransference issues with their clients. One young man, for example, away at a school of social work when his mother died, was highly sensitive to any perceptions of a child "abandoning" the mother, and frequently projected his complex of feelings on clients, insisting on contact with biological parents even in situations where it was inappropriate. Only when he came to terms with his own loss was he able to avoid the countertransference.

In-service educational programs should not be limited to the professional staff. All staff members, including clerical and secretarial, can benefit both personally and professionally. All staff members who have contact with families may have a supportive role; participation in the education can build morale and a team sense. In agencies regularly involved in AIDS work, grief education should be offered periodically to the staff. These programs might emphasize personal grief awareness, as well as provide workers with the basic skills they need as they interact with clients.

For three reasons, grief education should also be offered at regular intervals to foster parents of children with AIDS/HIV infection, as part of regular foster parent training and in advance of loss. First, it may help foster parents to come to terms with their present feelings as well as unresolved feelings from previous losses. Failure to resolve previous losses can complicate subsequent grief. Second, foster parents may be experiencing anticipatory grief. Anticipatory grief is a grief reaction to a loss that has not yet been experienced, but is expected [Fulton and Fulton 1971; Rando 1986]. Since a diagnosis of AIDS is often perceived as terminal, it is highly likely that foster parents may be experiencing anticipatory reactions even as they bond with and care for their foster children. Grief education then can assist them in identifying, understanding, and coping with these reactions. Finally, there is much that can be done in the period before and at the time of death, such as participating in care, saying goodbyes, finishing unresolved interpersonal and financial business, enhancing interaction, and making therapeutic decisions about care, treatment, and rituals that can facilitate subsequent bereavement [Rando 1984]. Grief education can help with suggestions and choices.

Agency programs should also be offered to foster parents after the death, a time which can be very isolating. A child in their care has died, and they may experience a deep sense of loss, perhaps complicated by the reality that these foster parents are experiencing a diminution of ties, either gradually or abruptly, with their social worker and other agency staff members who may have been a significant part of their social support network—a network that may have already been diminished by their decision to accept a child with AIDS. Post-death programs then can offer not only education and support but also a vital continued connection to the agency.

While agency programs may naturally focus on these two groups, they should not ignore the needs of others. Biological parents may also need education and support. Special programs and groups can be periodically offered to biological and foster siblings. Furthermore, in any of these offerings, persons can be encouraged to bring friends and other family members who may have been touched by the life and death of the AIDS-affected child, and who may also need assistance in learning both how to cope with their own loss and how to support the foster or biological parents.

In fact, all foster and biological parents, not only those with HIV-infected children, can benefit from grief education. Grief is ubiquitous to foster care. Foster families, biological families, and foster children will all experience grief as they deal with cycles of separation from each other. Grief, after all, is a reaction to loss, and not all losses occur through death.

Not only the audience, but also the model of grief education can vary. Some programs may be primarily informational. In a seminar-like approach, a group leader discusses the nature of grief, inviting responses, questions, and participation from the audience. This non-threatening approach can convey essential information to a fair-sized group, albeit with certain supports. Opportunities such as coffee breaks should be built into the program for informal interaction and for individuals to approach the group leader privately. There should also be opportunity for follow-up. The group leader may refer members of the audience to a therapist when their needs are too intense and immediate to be met by this approach.

Grief education can also be offered naturally in the context of a grief support group. At regular intervals, a leader may present particularized discussions on topics such as getting through the holidays. This approach has the advantage of allowing intensive interaction and providing ongoing support.

Education can also be provided through print and other media. Each agency should give thought to maintaining a small library of professional resources for the staff, as well as self-help books for clients. Budget permitting, agencies may consider a series of videos, too. Varied video programs may be suitable for the aforementioned individuals and even for children. Excellent videos are available both on grief and on the particular problems of AIDS. This approach should be used within a context that allows support; for example, social workers should provide opportunities for clients to discuss any books they have read or videos they have viewed.

Grief education in whatever format, then, can be a vital part of agencies' efforts as they respond to the AIDS crisis, but they have also to recognize the limits of educational programs. First, there must be an understanding that the line between education and counseling can be thin. Agencies cannot offer one without at least providing access to the other, for educational offerings may identify and uncover needs that indicate more intense work. Finally, grief education programs will not end the pain of loss. At best, they may help people to understand their pain and perhaps, we hope, give them the means to begin to heal the hurt.

REFERENCES

Anderson, G. R., Gurdin, P., and Thomas, A. "Dual disenfranchisement." In Doka, K. (editor), Disenfranchised Grief. Lexington, MA: Lexington Press, 1989.

Doka, K. "Grief." In The Encyclopedia of Death. New York: Oxford University Press, in press.

Doka, K., and Jendreski, M. "Clergy understanding of grief, bereavement, and mourning." Research Record 2 (1985): 105–114.

Fulton, R. "Unanticipated grief." In Corr, C., and Pacholski, R. (editors), Death: Completion and Discovery. Lakewood, OH: Association for Death Education and Counseling, 1986.

Fulton, R., and Fulton, J. "A psychosocial aspect of terminal care: Anticipatory grief." Omega 2 (1971): 91–99.

Hochschild, A. R. "Emotion work, feeling rules, and social support." American Journal of Sociology 85 (1979): 551–575.

Hoyt, M. "Clinical notes regarding the experience of 'presences' in mourning." Omega 11 (1980): 105–111.

Lindstrom, B. "Exploring paranormal experiences of the bereaved." Paper presented at the Fifth Annual Conference of the Association of Death Education and Counseling, 1982.

McClowry, S. E., Davies, B. B., May, K. A., Kulenkamp, E. J., and Martinson, I. M. "The empty space phenomenon: The process of grief in a bereaved family." Death Studies 11 (1987): 361–374.

Rando, T. Grief, Dying and Death: Clinical Interventions for Caregivers. Champaign, IL: Research Press, 1984.

Rando, T. Loss and Anticipatory Grief. Lexington, MA: Lexington Press, 1986.

Wass, H. "Depiction of death, grief, and funerals on national television." Research Record 2 (1985): 81–92.

Worden, W. Grief Counseling and Grief Therapy. New York: Springer, 1982.

22

Advocating for AIDS Children: A Call to Action

ELISABETH KUBLER-ROSS[1]

FAMILIES WHO ARE CARING FOR CHILDREN WITH HIV/AIDS NEED MUTUAL support, feedback, nurturing, and the exchange of ideas. In talking together about the turmoil, the problems, and the blessings, a number of common issues are often raised. Because of these important concerns, we are starting a task force, a forum, for national advocacy for children with AIDS; they need advocates to take them out of institutions and hospitals, and to prevent experimentation and the creation of a new American business out of children with AIDS. It is not early any more; it is high time to do something nationally. The people who can most effectively speak for these children are the biological parents, guardians, and foster and adoptive parents who know the needs of the children because they live with them.

The Need for Permanence

The first, and most urgent, problem is to get children out of the hospital. Keeping children with HIV/AIDS in hospitals when this is not

[1] The author wishes to acknowledge the invaluable assistance provided by a number of committed and loving foster parents, adoptive parents, and guardians of children with HIV infection or AIDS, particularly Peggy Marengo, Alison Smith, Brother Toby, Sister Marti, and Jim and Joy Jenkins. Their stories and counsel, shared here to help and encourage others, are further evidence of their devotion to these special children.

medically necessary is a national problem and tragedy, particularly when there are hundreds of families across the country ready to adopt a baby.

Several years ago, I met a child with AIDS who had been in a hospital for two years, in a pediatric unit but isolated from the other children. There was no bonding, no one permanent love object; nursing shifts changed and hospital personnel peeked in, said "Hello," and left. This child didn't walk or talk or socialize, had never been outdoors in her life, and had never seen grass or a butterfly. She was exposed to various infections and germs in the hospital. The hospital had received hundreds of thousands of dollars for the child, over $1,000 a day, and didn't want to lose such a fantastic income. Hospital personnel also wanted to perform all kinds of experiments with the child, including repeated bone marrow tests; there was no patient advocate to say enough is enough. How can this child not be chronically traumatized? I told the hospital administration that I was going to tell her story to all the newspapers, naming the hospital. It took another four months before this baby was finally able to go to a foster family. Their loving care and dedication would be tested by this child, who was then showing signs of brain damage. Three months later, when I next saw the child, she was a healthy, normal child—not medically healthy but developmentally catching up at unbelievable speed.

If children are not moved into foster homes as soon as possible, by the time they do get there they may be emotionally and socially traumatized, even brain-damaged, and it will be extremely difficult to teach them basic developmental skills, such as standing up and walking. When they linger in institutions and are then transferred to group homes, where there isn't one permanent love object, children do not develop to their potential, and they are cheated out of their short, beautiful lives. The two-year-old child just described now has a real life. If she dies in six months, she will have had a real family and touched many lives, rather than vegetating in a hospital.

Overhospitalization, even in a good hospital, complicates the medical and developmental conditions of children. One child had many medical difficulties, including diabetes, epilepsy, and a heart condition, none of which required the 20 months she spent there. Her adoptive parent, Sister Marti Aggeler of the Starcross Community in Sonoma County, California, also thought that she had orthopedic problems, but there was in fact nothing wrong with her except that she had spent most of her life in bed. The hospital was trying to provide quality care, but a hospital cannot be a home, and this child had never been outside. Now she does not like to go inside. Brother Tolbert "Toby" McCarroll, of the Starcross Community, observed: "She swings, she likes to play with butterflies, look at kites, all the kinds of things that should be a child's legacy."

There are several obstacles to rapid provision of a permanent, loving home for a child. One is the child welfare goal of family reunification. One foster parent who adopted her foster son said:

> The priority of reunification, in our experience, means that not only children who can be reunified are being worked on but children for whom there is no hope of reunification are being left in limbo for 12 to 18 months, while they wait out this period during which reunification is to be taking place. Everybody is in limbo. This is a serious difficulty for children. Children with serious health problems should have a different agenda. They don't have 18 years of life to work things out. They need a home, and they need it quickly. If there isn't hope, a permanent home in which the baby can bond should be found, not a temporary shuffling around, because the children do not have time to wait.

Brother Toby, an adoptive parent, said:

> Every AIDS baby is unique—the system needs to customize to these babies. There has to be a humane approach to get children freed for permanency—so children can grow up in a permanent, stable home where bonding can take place, where the child owns one of us— so when the time comes for dying they do not reach out to a strange hand. I guess that is the ultimate right of any child—not to die among strangers.

It is my experience that hundreds of families are willing to care for children with AIDS; they may not be in the places where professionals typically search, but they are out there. The stumbling blocks to placement must be found and eliminated. The first priority is service to the biological family, but if that doesn't work, the obstacles should be cut through to reach a permanent placement.

Permanency is so important because insecurity and stressful separations are harmful to children. One foster parent told of a time a year before, when she had to go away from her foster daughter, who has AIDS, for three days. In that three-day period, the little girl had high temperatures, several episodes of hyperventilation, and almost had to be hospitalized. The foster mother concluded that this reaction showed what stress can do to anybody with AIDS, and she expressed her sorrow for adults with AIDS who experience rejection by their families.

Permanency creates a consistent, loving relationship that grows and facilitates the careful medical and nutritional supervision that may save a child's life. Better nutrition boosts the immune system and improves the ability to fight illness. One foster mother said she gives her HIV-positive foster children only distilled water, with vitamins and minerals, and maintains high fluid input to counter recurrent bouts of diarrhea. She feeds the children a high-protein formula, because of thrush, a common ailment, and avoids sugar or whole milk because these foods seem to stimulate thrush. Her four-year-old with AIDS was accidentally given a glass of whole milk by a babysitter; by morning thrush had spread outside the foster child's mouth, and it took two weeks to get the outbreak under control. The same child was exposed to chickenpox for five minutes in a child-care setting. A year and a half later, new eruptions still break out into large lesions. Her teeth had no enamel and disintegrated easily; abscesses formed, and her condition worsened because a dentist refused to treat her. Eventually all of her teeth were extracted, and it has not been possible to fit her with dentures. This attentiveness to nutrition, diet modifications, and long-term physical problems, as well as sensitivity to body temperature changes indicating the onset of potentially deadly infections, require a consistent, permanent caregiver.

Another obstacle to permanence is the lack of communication between professionals responsible for the care of children with AIDS. Sister Marti described the following situation:

> We were negotiating with an agency—a terribly overburdened agency that was having trouble coping anyway and then AIDS came along—for six months about taking a particular baby who was in the hospital. The social worker finally discovered that the baby had actually died five months before. The system was so clogged that the social worker had not been advised. This can't be allowed to happen—we have to cut through whatever allows this situation.

Lack of AIDS education poses an additional obstacle to permanent care for children with AIDS. Many social workers have very little information about AIDS. One foster mother reported that her worker refused to make home visits for fear of AIDS. Many foster parents, finding themselves in the position of having to educate themselves, often have to educate their workers. Biological and foster parents can be an extremely valuable resource to social service and medical personnel by providing day-to-day information about children's needs and behaviors. Educated social workers become more astute and better able to work in behalf of children and parents, but there is no guarantee that every AIDS child will get an educated worker. It should be an agency's responsibility to educate both its staff and its foster parents.

In addition to the previously cited obstacles, sometimes it seems that professionals move more slowly when planning for children with AIDS. Unfortunately, sometimes it looks as though this slowness is due to an attitude that says the child is going to die soon anyhow, so why go to the trouble of working in the child's behalf.

Stigma and Discrimination

Not all the infants who test positive for HIV antibodies will develop AIDS. Some will become seronegative—losing their mother's antibodies and not developing their own HIV infection. Even when they become negative, however, they will experience ostracism like children with AIDS. Neighborhood children will be prevented from playing with them. They will not be encouraged to attend schools and play with peers. Many children will test negative and remain well, but they will bear the stamp and label of AIDS children. How will their families cope with their heartbreak when they see other children playing on the playground and know their child is not welcome to join them?

Stigma and fear of rejection may include one's own family members, in addition to the community's reaction. One mother, who adopted a boy who tested positive for HIV, told the following story:

> My parents told me a long time ago they had unconditional love for me. My husband and I called my parents and told them we were going to become foster parents and adopt a baby, and they were pretty excited. I told them that our child was biracial—had a white mother and a black father—but I didn't tell them about the AIDS. My parents are from a small community and don't have the same opportunity for education as in a lot of the big urban areas. So we sent pictures back. In the first pictures there was one of the baby with a pacifier in his mouth; my father is not one to believe in pacifiers or thumb-sucking, so he wrote back saying get rid of that pacifier! We didn't have to worry

about that because the baby threw it out of the crib two weeks after he
was home.

In October the baby and I went to see my parents, so I could
introduce them to the baby. My parents live on a farm about 22 miles
from the nearest airport. They had had company the first night for
dinner, so after the company left and my mother was clearing away the
dishes and my father was playing with the baby and holding and
cuddling him and making goo-goo noises to him and was going on
and on about what a beautiful baby he was, I decided to drop the big
bombshell. I said, "Before we go any further into this visit, there are
some things I have to tell you about the baby. You know that he was a
drug-addicted baby, and you can see he was a mixed baby." My father
said "That's OK, so what?" He continued to hold and pat and carry on
with the baby. "I didn't tell you that his mother has AIDS and he
carries the AIDS antibodies and we don't know how long we will have
him but you know he is our son." My father held him out at arms
length and said, "Jesus Christ!" I was very worried. I have got to get 22
miles to the airport and it was cold outside, and I didn't have anyone
to pick me up and take me to the airport, and here's my father holding
the baby at arm's length, and I'm thinking "Oh no, he is going to drop
him!" My father's eyes started to go up and I looked at my father and
looked again and there was a tear in the corner of his eye. Now this is a
man who never shows any kind of emotion, and he says, "Oh, my
God!" and he held onto the baby and hugged him as close as he could
and said, "You poor, poor thing, if I had known that you had had such
a hard start in life I would have never made them take away the only
thing that meant anything to you—that pacifier—how could I do that
to you!" My parents came and spent two weeks with us in February,
and we never had to worry about the baby—my parents got up with
him, took him for rides in the carriage—it is just wonderful the way
they reacted [Jenkins 1988].

Overcoming Fear

My dream of taking care of AIDS babies in my home went down the
drain because of the objections of the community [Kubler-Ross 1987].
These objections were based on fear and ignorance, not knowing that if
you adopt or get near a baby you can't get AIDS. You can conduct
educational AIDS programs in a community—you can tell people that
they cannot get AIDS by hugging and kissing babies or by sharing the
same room or meals—but fear closes their ears. The issue is fear. They

still say that if you need an ambulance, we will not respond because we do not want to contaminate our ambulance; if you bring your child to the school, the doors will be locked because we do not take AIDS children. This situation is still true in my community and in communities all across the United States.

Fear can change to caring when one meets children in need. Many people who are now willing to care for children with HIV/AIDS may have been afraid a short time ago—it may take a long time for information to sink in and change attitudes. Brother Toby tells the following story:

> We had a local government official who, when he heard we were going to be taking babies with AIDS, called them rattlesnakes, and said that a little rattlesnake can kill you just as well as a big rattlesnake. After we had a baby with AIDS, he came knocking at the door and I was afraid of what he would do, because he wanted to see the foster baby. He went up, looked in her crib, and started to cry—and this man has now become one of our supporters. When they see the babies, they change their attitudes, and that is why we cannot hide these babies any more.

An adoptive mother said:

> The babies are not freaks. A lady we have heard on the television and radio several times called the babies freaks—said they have huge foreheads, their noses and their upper lips are separated by a great distance, and their eyes are misplaced. They are not freaks. You cannot call any human a freak—they are beautiful people. Everyone is different. They don't have an arm growing out of the middle of their forehead.

Even if children did have arms growing out of their foreheads, we would still love them. We are all brothers and sisters and can take care of each other lovingly. Some babies may live long and others may have only a few months, but if people are willing to love unconditionally and love these babies they will be blessed beyond any description. I cannot tell you what joy and happiness they can bring into a family. As an adoptive father said, "People tell us the baby is lucky to have a loving family. We tell them we are the lucky ones."

Not only is there the fear of AIDS, there is also the fear of death.

Children in families with an AIDS baby who is dying can see that death does not have to be a nightmare. It can be a lovely shared experience. They can hold and love and hug a baby who can literally fall asleep in the arms of a parent or brother or sister. A child can die within the family; we grown-ups make a nightmare out of it, but not the children—they are our teachers.

It has been one of my dreams to take mothers with AIDS together with their babies into my home, so that when these mothers are very ill, I could care for them and their children. Although the mother may not be able to stand up, or cook, or care for her needs, she would still be able to rock the baby. The mother could be cared for until she died, and she could die in peace because she would know that her baby is in a loving environment, where the baby is hugged and touched and some bonding has already taken place before the mother dies.

Conclusion

My dream to use my home has been changed to national advocacy. Starting small with family after family will have a ripple effect. If enough people care for AIDS babies, showing that it can be done and can be a positive experience, many others will be willing to care for an AIDS baby, and, when there is an avalanche of HIV-infected babies, hundreds of families will be ready.

The biological, foster, and adoptive families already caring for children are the best recruits and advocates for children. This network of families, in cooperation with the human resource and child welfare systems, can together learn about this disease, exchange information on helping children, and create a range of home environments for children. Children with AIDS are everyone's problem. Brother Toby, an adoptive parent of children with HIV/AIDS, mentioned earlier, noted that he receives calls from a variety of locations: "The calls we get now are not from the big cities; they are from towns in Iowa and Idaho and places like that; the mothers who are intravenous drug users often go home, and home is all across this nation."

Working for permanence and fighting discrimination will require new partnerships and national action. Caring for all children requires unconditional love; AIDS education for adults will eliminate fear and encourage families all across the country to open their hearts and homes to children with AIDS.

REFERENCES

Jenkins, Joy, and Jenkins, Jim. Personal conversation, 1988. (They are co-founders, together with all those who contributed to this chapter, of The Children with AIDS Project of America, 4020 N. 20th Street, Suite 101, Phoenix, Arizona 85016; telephone 602-843-8654.)

Kubler-Ross, Elisabeth. AIDS: The Ultimate Challenge. New York: Macmillan Publishing Company, 1987.

The references to and quotes from Brother Tolbert McCarroll and Sister Marti Aggeler in this chapter reflect experiences and commentary also reported in *Morning Glory Babies: Children with AIDS and the Celebration of Life* (New York: St. Martin's Press, 1988).

23

Present and Future Challenges in Caring for Children with HIV and Their Families

GARY R. ANDERSON

JEAN EMERY

IN 1980, AIDS AND HIV WERE UNKNOWN. IN 1982, THE FIRST CASE OF AIDS in children was described. By 1985, there were no specialized child welfare programs for HIV-infected children. Coordinated pediatric health care, social service, and child welfare service programs barely existed. Educational initiatives for children and their families were few in number and untested. Misinformation was too often the order of the day. Now, at the beginning of the 1990s, AIDS more often confronts Americans through media reports and—particularly in higher-incidence geographic areas—firsthand or secondhand contact with a person with HIV or AIDS.[1]

In part, awareness has grown because of the increasing number of persons with HIV infection—5,000,000 people worldwide, including 1,500,000 in the United States. Projections have forecast high future expenditures and demand for a range of services as the cumulative total of Americans with AIDS reaches 450,000 by 1993, and 1,000,000 by 1998

[1] In 1985, the International Conference on AIDS had two papers on pediatric HIV infection; the 1988 conference had 213 papers, most still addressing medical issues rather than a comprehensive approach to the crisis.

[Altman 1989]. This chapter explores the implications of this continuing epidemic for services to children and their families and identifies issues that will have a prominent place in a child welfare agenda.

Practice Issues

As individuals and agencies have responded to the needs of children with HIV infection, a number of future issues affecting frontline service delivery have been identified: education and prevention, recruitment and respite care, permanency planning and adoption, and professional survival.

Education and Prevention

Because there has been incremental positive movement in placing a true and responsible picture of this complex disease before the public, future planners may not face the same degree of ignorance and fear as has been evidenced in the past. Nonetheless, the need for professional and community education will remain a high priority, necessitated in part by evolving information and the need for repetition to create a level of acceptance of the difficult issues involved with AIDS—sexual activity, drugs, and death. As people encounter colleagues, neighbors, friends, family, and clients with HIV, their need and desire to acquire information will increase dramatically.

Educational initiatives require attention to questions of effectiveness: .

> How can attitudes and behaviors be changed, particularly with regard to people involved in high-risk behaviors, such as sexually active adolescents, and the intravenous drug-using (IVDU) population, particularly if either are women of childbearing age?
>
> How can people be encouraged to be properly cautious but not irrationally fearful, when working with or caring directly for persons with HIV infection?
>
> How can giving information be structured to reinforce HIV knowledge and assure its retention?

The urgency of HIV/AIDS education and prevention, particularly for adolescents, is increasingly being noted:

By 1990, every junior and senior high school student in the U.S. should receive accurate, timely education about sexually transmitted diseases. Congress should assume a greater leadership role in addressing AIDS by setting up a National AIDS Committee; supporting a massive media campaign which includes the promotion of condoms among sexually active youth; assisting in the development of curricula and school programs especially in high HIV prevalence areas; and recognizing that subpopulations of adolescents, including minority youth and youth in detention, may be particularly high risk and should be targeted for immediate and intensive intervention [Shafer 1989].

Another significant population of adolescents are homosexual teenagers who share the same sense of immortality, invulnerability, and impulsiveness as their heterosexual counterparts but experience particularly dangerous sexual encounters [Gross 1987].

Equipping child welfare agencies to provide HIV prevention and sex education is a priority in work with high-risk children and youth and biological families. Education is the primary means of prevention; creativity is required, and model programs should be identified and tried in new settings (for example, using teenagers as educators, as in the TEENS Teaching AIDS Prevention [TAP] Project in St. Louis, Missouri, or the PEER program of Terrific, Inc. in Washington, DC). Prevention education strategies may be complicated by conflicting societal values, for example, with regard to condom use, or whether to instruct on how to clean needles or the provision of clean needles [Verhovek 1989].

Recruitment and Respite

Service providers have faced the challenge of recruiting caregivers to help children and their families. Empowering extended family members and recruiting day care providers, foster parents, and a variety of health and social service professionals to provide assistance to children living with their families will continue and intensify as the need for services increases, fueled by rising numbers of children with HIV and their increased longevity. Recruitment efforts will require considerable energy and creativity and an honest discussion of the satisfactions and difficulties of caring for children and family members with HIV/AIDS (see, for example, the video "With Loving Arms"). Retention of qualified caregivers must receive close attention and must be part of the recruitment plan.

Respite care is important for biological families (including the extended family) caring for HIV-infected children as well as for foster parents and other caregivers. Many biological and foster parents also care for noninfected children and other family members and are faced with community and, sometimes, employment obligations that combine to tax their physical, psychological, and financial resources severely. Respite care reduces the number and intensity of stressors associated with caring for children with special needs so that quality care can be consistently given, decreasing the possibility of multiple placements of children and helping to avoid possible child abuse or neglect.

Respite care can be provided in a variety of ways: (1) by formalizing and funding informal babysitting arrangements for foster parents [Gurdin 1989]; (2) by using professional community organizations such as homemaker, visiting nurse, and home health care services; (3) by using beds in transitional care residences (for example, St. Clare's, Newark, New Jersey; Incarnation House, New York; Herbert G. Birch Residential Children's Center, Brooklyn, New York); and (4) by recruiting volunteers for families or by establishing a foster parent network.

In 1989, two demonstration programs were funded by the federal government:

1. Project HARP (HIV/AIDS Respite Program) provides respite care for 20 foster families from child welfare agencies in Brooklyn, New York. Respite care providers (RCP)—trained volunteers recruited from the community—will (1) assist the foster parent in hospital and clinic waiting rooms; (2) provide relief to the foster parent when the child is hospitalized; (3) facilitate play groups/structured recreation; or (4) if a licensed foster parent, take children to their homes for part of a day or an overnight stay. The respite service prevents a crisis in caregiving by providing support before the foster parent is overwhelmed. The program will also include the biological children and non-HIV-infected foster children of foster parents, freeing the foster parents to care for the HIV-infected child without feeling that their biological child is being neglected. Foster parents and RCPs, it is hoped, will get to know each other, increasing the parent's comfort when the child is supervised by the RCP and encouraging continuity of relationships by using the same volunteer with the same family to the extent possible [Shapiro 1989].

2. The Central AIDS Board of the Massachusetts Department of Social Services (DSS), responsible for departmental policy and place-

ment, testing, and clinical trial decision making, noted the need for respite care. With federal assistance, a Child Care AIDS Network (CCAN) will formalize an informal foster care network to provide reimbursed respite care. First, foster families with HIV-infected or high-risk children, who are licensed for more than one child, have been identified and invited to join the network. The network proposes a "respite exchange" in which a foster family is provided up to ten days of respite care a year per family in exchange for providing ten days of respite care for other foster families. After network invitations are mailed, a pre-respite survey, completed by the participating foster family to give a family profile, is used to match a family requesting respite with a family offering to take in another foster parent's foster child(ren) for a brief stay. Foster parents who, for example, are going on a trip for three days will call the network, tell the coordinator how many foster children need respite placement, for how long, the children's special needs, and if they have a particular network family with whom they would like to exchange. The coordinator will match a foster parent with another network foster parent; these two foster parents will communicate regarding the children's needs; the placement will be reviewed by a departmental nurse, and homefinders and social workers will be notified. After care is provided, a bill will be submitted to the network office, the respite foster parent will receive payment equal to the child's daily and supplemental board rate, and the relieved foster parents will not experience a reduction in their usual monthly board payment. The Foster Parent Association is planning a similar exchange for children who are not at high risk or HIV-infected. There are further plans to extend respite programs to biological parents. Also projected will be a CCAN column in a DSS newsletter for DSS staff members and network families; support groups combining recreation and training; and increased recruitment efforts focusing on religious, school, and health communities in Boston [Stoleroff 1989].

Respite programs for children with HIV are relatively new and untested. In addition, varying existing program structures, geographic and demographic compositions, and incidence rates of HIV will shape and require creative responses to the need to sustain caregivers. Respite efforts will have to be extended to biological families caring for children with HIV and to those guardians and caregivers who are not affiliated with child welfare agencies. Guidance may come from existing respite care programs serving special populations, such as developmentally disabled children and adults.

Permanency Planning and Adoption

Children with HIV pose a special challenge for permanency planning, calling first for increased efforts to offer services to biological families in order to keep families intact or in kinship homes. When it is necessary to place a child in foster care, biological parents may have difficulty maintaining contact with their children. This problem is particularly possible when the parents are sick, often due to their own HIV infection. Efforts to reach out to families must be initiated and, in some cases, an open, involved relationship between foster parents and biological parents may be encouraged.

Foster care programs report that HIV-infected children are frequently not returning home after foster care placements, often due to parental incapacity because of HIV illness; the tenets of permanency planning, based on the best interests of the child, would dictate that a permanent home for the child should be achieved. Usually this goal would involve asking the foster parents to consider adopting the child in their care, since their home is often the only one the child has ever known. There was a time when this response was not believed to be a very common course of action with HIV-infected children, since it was thought that most children would die quickly and few foster parents, or others, would be willing to adopt them. Both of these beliefs are proving unfounded. It seems that medical interventions and loving environments providing consistent physical, nutritional, and emotional care often lead to children living longer than expected when first diagnosed in the hospital. If the experience with children proves to be similar to that of adults with HIV infection, the potential for longer life spans seems even more probable with increased availability and use of azidothymidine (AZT), which until the autumn of 1989 was experimental and its use with children limited [Lambert 1989b]. Also, a number of foster parents and families from communities across the United States have expressed a desire to adopt HIV-infected children.

There are several obstacles to adoption. One obstacle is that foster parents who adopt HIV-infected children may lose the network of services provided when they were members of a child welfare system, even though they receive an adoption subsidy that reduces the financial disadvantage of adoption. If adoption is going to be encouraged as one way of achieving permanence for HIV-infected children, the provision of long-term post-adoption services, in addition to subsidies and medical insurance, must be considered. In fact, comprehensive services for all families—foster, adoptive, and biological—caring for HIV-infected children are needed.

The time-consuming process of adoption is another obstacle. Sometimes a dying biological parent will plan ahead for the adoption of her or his child. More likely, the adoption process involves an extended period of time in which a biological parent's voluntary surrender of parental rights or a court case leading to a court-ordered termination of parental rights is sought. For children who may have a limited life span, this time of legal limbo and the energy required to secure the adoption may be discouraging to prospective adoptive parents.

Some foster parents do not want to adopt their foster child but are reluctant to have the child leave them. This reaction is not a new phenomenon in family foster care. They are attached to the child and recognize that the child considers their home as his or her only home. It is a difficult decision to move any child, let alone an HIV-infected child, from a long-term, stable foster home to a preadoptive home that may or may not be successful. Such movement must be carefully considered case by case, with the recognition that there may be a place for long-term foster care for HIV-positive children.

Living, Dying, and Burning Out

HIV-infected children are living longer than originally expected, presenting the challenge of helping children and their caregivers to live with HIV rather than to cope for a few months before the child dies. As younger children grow older, caregivers are faced with increased involvement in the larger social world of the preschool and school-age child. The child welfare system and the educational system will increasingly intersect as HIV-infected children attend day care or reach school age and enroll in and attend local schools. Biological, foster, and adoptive parents will need special support from school officials, child welfare workers, and community families to minimize discrimination and to help HIV-positive children make these transitions. The goal is to provide an environment in which children can have the normal experiences they need as they grow up and learn. Advocacy with schools in children's behalf and involvement in the AIDS education initiatives of primary schools will become essential tasks. With youths, sensitive assistance will be needed as adolescents face decisions about their future relationships and work in light of their HIV infection.

While it is acknowledged that some children are living longer than expected, children and their biological parents *are* dying. Ethically and clinically complex decisions will be confronted more and more frequently, such as whether or not to use extraordinary life support measures, or whether to hospitalize the terminally ill child or maintain the child in the home.

> Tommy, aged 11 and diagnosed with AIDS, had been placed in foster care at age eight after his mother, an intravenous drug user, had died of AIDS. During his placement he had a variety of physical ailments and his medical condition slowly deteriorated. He experienced several hospitalizations. Social workers and a pastoral worker visited frequently and established a close relationship with Tommy and his foster mother. When his condition worsened and became life-threatening, a hospital bed was brought to the foster home and Tommy was maintained at home, with the approval of his doctor. The pastoral worker visited more frequently and spent considerable time sitting with Tommy and watching videos with him. Tommy knew he was terminally ill and the worker talked with him about what he wanted them to do for him before and after his death. With his foster family by his side, one night he died, several hours after the pastoral worker had been with him. The director of the foster care program called all of the foster families in the HIV-positive foster parent support group and told them about the death. The agency helped plan the funeral and Tommy was buried in one of several cemetary plots that had been purchased by the agency to prevent a pauper's burial in the city's potter's field [Bear 1989].

AIDS is also causing the deaths of parents, brothers, sisters, and extended family members of children who may not have AIDS. Caregivers and child-care workers will confront AIDS-related grief as a number of children and youths currently in foster homes, group homes, or residences may not be HIV-infected but will be losing loved ones to the disease. The death of parents with AIDS will also create an increasing number of orphaned children, many of whom will not be infected with the virus, who will need a home [Lambert 1989a].

The need to sustain staff members and caregivers after they have been recruited has already been noted in relation to respite care. In addition to agency and institutional leaders identifying and preparing new caregivers—a "second generation" of leaders and service providers to begin, shape, and maintain efforts to help HIV-infected children and their families—current caregivers need continued help and relief. At this writing, the authors have not heard of an HIV-infected child in foster or residential care being abused or neglected; however, hospital experience with boarder babies and foster care experience with neonatally crack-addicted infants can serve as a warning. Medical personnel and care-givers have noted that many crack-addicted babies have troubling behavioral traits, including difficulty in accepting comfort, hugging, and closeness. They appear to smile less, demand more, and are irritable [Blakeslee 1989]. In addition, many children who have experienced early separations, neglect, or institutionalizations may be distrustful of adults and display angry, rejecting postures. With caregiver sleeplessness due to dealing with persistent illness, the stress of caring for a child with severe and chronic diarrhea, and possible weakening of social supports due to fear of discrimination, the need for consistent and readily available agency supports is self-evident.

Programmatic Actions

A range of creative programs that can intervene at various stages in the life of a child is needed. Unprecedented cooperation between child welfare providers and other systems that serve children and families is also required.

Continuum of Care

A comprehensive continuum of care for HIV-infected children and families is both in their best interests and cost-effective. The continuum should include services to prevent the breakup of the biological home by offering these families and extended family caregivers services similar to those available to foster families: meeting concrete needs, education about HIV infection in children, training in child care, support, respite, financial assistance, coordinated health care services, and social work/nurse/health educator/pastoral care worker visits. Families need qualified case managers to coordinate, monitor, and evaluate the delivery of services and advocate for needed services that should be accessible so that multiple visits at widely separated sites are not imposed upon already stressed families. If children cannot remain with their parents, efforts must be made to locate appropriate relatives for kinship care. Placements within or near the parents' communities would facilitate visits and continuing contacts. In addition to foster care placements, other settings may have a limited but important role for some HIV-infected children, such as transitional residences that provide temporary group home care while a foster home is being located, and hospices. Many services, such as hospice care and care for more medically needy children who at present are hospitalized for long periods of time, can be accomplished in specially equipped and trained foster homes. The continuum of care should strive for a range of services and settings to afford children "the least restrictive, most nurturing and family-like environment available, preferably in proximity to the parent's home and consistent with the best interests and special needs of the child" [Novello 1988].

Creative Care

Assisting children and their families will require creative responses and program modifications, such as placing HIV-infected mothers and children together in the same foster home; placing siblings in separate foster homes in the same apartment building; including biological parents and foster parents together in support groups; using camp (e.g., Camp Sunburst in California) and retreat experiences for families and children; planning with critically or terminally ill parents for the foster care, guardianship, or adoption of their children, if and when necessary; and open adoptions and open foster care placements. The creativity of the child welfare system and others will also be challenged by the need to find homes for uninfected siblings of infected children, whose parents have died of AIDS [Norwood 1988]. The New York City Health Department estimates that 20,000 "AIDS orphans" will need foster care or adoption in New York by 1995 [Lambert 1989a].

Cooperation and Collaboration

One of the greatest opportunities and challenges in serving HIV-infected children and their families is the coordinated involvement of multiple major service delivery systems, as, for example, child welfare agencies; drug treatment agencies; educational institutions; hospitals and medical personnel; public health agencies; black and Hispanic community organizations; homosexual organizations; "AIDS agencies"; national organizations such as the Red Cross, National Urban League, and the National Hemophilia Association; agencies and networks that serve women; and religious institutions and agencies. Collaboration within large social service and medical organizations, such as the Massachusetts Department of Social Services Board, mentioned earlier, to facilitate policy implementation and decision making is also required [Herskowitz and Pontes 1989].

The Child Welfare League of America has called for an office for HIV-infected women, children, and their families, funded by Congress, to coordinate education/prevention, services, and research [CWLA 1989a]. The Pediatrics AIDS Coalition, comprising 20 national organizations committed to sound federal legislation that addresses the needs of children and their families affected by HIV, and co-founded by the Child Welfare League of America with the American Academy of Pediatrics, is advocating the establishment of pediatric AIDS Resource Centers [Pediatric AIDS Coalition 1989]. Included in these requests is the desire for annual reports to Congress by the Secretary of the Department of Health and Human Services on federal efforts to combat pediatric AIDS.

HIV infection requires coordinated services across human service systems and professional boundaries in order to muster the financial and other resources and services for assisting HIV-infected children and families and to work together to prevent the spread of HIV infection and to discover a cure. Few programs for children have been launched without the combined financial support of governmental, private foundation, and individual financial support. This patchwork of financial resources should be expanded, enriched, and coordinated not only to fund programs but also to make medications, medical treatment, and home care affordable and available, regardless of the stage of the infection [Boland 1989].

Advocacy Agenda

A comprehensive continuum of services, creatively designed and delivered, will be the result of individual, organizational, and community advocacy. Public policy issues identified by the Department of Health and Human Services (DHHS) Secretary's Work Group on Pediatric Infection Report [Novello 1988] included recommendations for immediate action to address the pediatric HIV crisis:

1. Encouraging DHHS agencies to work collaboratively with state and community agencies to support the development of family-centered, community-based, coordinated systems of care for children with HIV infection

2. Distributing up-to-date information on HIV-related counseling and other essential HIV-related services to all organizations and individuals in contact with youths at risk

3. Encouraging states and localities to explore every possible option and strategy for recruiting foster parents for HIV-infected children

4. Developing special education and prevention programs in settings other than schools for hard-to-reach adolescents, including minorities, drug abusers, runaways, street youths, and homeless teenagers

5. Requiring all federally funded clinics for sexually transmitted disease, family planning (Title X), or other medical clinics to offer HIV counseling and testing to all women, with special outreach efforts to women of child-bearing age who are at risk for HIV infection

Medical treatment and research were discussed in the report:

> Despite the challenges, research has progressed to the point that clinicians can now offer a variety of therapies to children with HIV infection. These include treatment with azidothymidine (AZT); intravenous gamma globulin; antimicrobial therapy for various opportunistic infections; adjunctive therapies, including nutritional support; and therapies aimed at the various consequences of the disease, for example, interventions for children with developmental delay, and respiratory therapy for children experiencing the consequences of the various lung diseases associated with pediatric HIV disease.

The report also noted, however: "To date, few of these therapies have been rigorously evaluated for efficacy in children; other than microbial therapy for documented infection, the precise therapies that should be applied to HIV-infected, symptomatic children remain matters for further studies."[2] These studies are under way, with interim reports given at the Surgeon General's Conference in Los Angeles in September 1989, for publication in 1990.

[2] In October 1989, the widespread use of AZT—in a reformulated berry-flavored liquid—with children was approved by the federal government. This approval, based on AZT's success in slowing the progression of AIDS in adult patients and in samples of children involved in medical center studies, will increase its availability and use for children, together with continuing attempts to minimize side effects and enhance treatment value [Pizzo et al. 1988; Lambert 1989b].

A number of perennial but crucial public policy issues should be addressed. Some are detailed in the Child Welfare League of America's *Residential Group Care Guidelines* [1989b]:

Prevention and education initiatives to assure full, age-appropriate sex and HIV education content

Early, voluntary, confidential HIV testing with professional and culturally sensitive counseling of high-risk women and children

Antidiscrimination regulations and laws to make it illegal to refuse service delivery based on HIV infection

Expanding the funding base and establishing prevention as well as service delivery as priorities

Pressing questions—Who will provide health care, counseling, and testing services for the rising number of AIDS patients? Who will educate millions of adolescents? Who will care for battle-weary caregivers? Who will be the new recruits to join the small group currently caring for AIDS patients?—require immediate attention and future preparation [Altman 1989]. As the disease gains momentum, and as awareness has grown, some people may tire of hearing about AIDS; complacency, indifference, or denial are threats to a necessary commitment to prevent HIV infection, find a cure, and assist HIV-infected children and families [New York Times 1989].

Conclusion

Notable efforts have been made to respond to the needs of HIV-infected children and their families, a number of which are described in this volume. These programs and services offered by competent and dedicated people are consistent with the mission and historic actions of people who care about the welfare of children. This terrible illness has caused tremendous suffering for many people; the challenge to caregivers, however, has just begun. The need to maintain, expand, and replicate quality efforts is great. There is room for many more creative ideas and actions. To accomplish goals for children, vocal public concern and increased funding from a variety of sources are necessary. Continuing compassion and commitment on the part of individual private citizens and professionals is called for. Hope for a better life for persons with HIV infection and for a cure for AIDS must be translated into a response to human pain and action in behalf of children and families.

REFERENCES

Altman, Lawrence. "Some optimism amid grim predictions as 87-nation AIDS meeting opens." New York Times (June 5, 1989).

Bear, Susan. Personal interview. New York Foundling Hospital, July 1989.

Blakeslee, Sandra. "Crack's toll among babies: A joyless view, even of toys." New York Times (September 17, 1989).

Boland, Mary. Draft. Report to Members of the Finance Work Group. Surgeon General's Conference, September 1989.

Child Welfare League of America. Testimony Before the Subcommittee on Human Resources and Intergovernmental Relations—Hearing on Pediatric AIDS. February 1989a.

Child Welfare League of America. Residential Group Care Guidelines. Washington, DC: Child Welfare League of America, 1989b.

Gross, Jane. "AIDS threat brings new turmoil for gay teenagers." New York Times (October 21, 1987).

Gurdin, Phyllis, Leake and Watts Children's Home. Respite Care Guidelines for HIV Seropositive Children. Draft, June 1989.

Herskowitz, Julia, and Pontes, Kenneth. "Pediatric AIDS: A child welfare response." Massachusetts Department of Social Services Report, May 30, 1989.

Lambert, Bruce. "AIDS legacy: A growing generation of orphans." New York Times (July 17, 1989a).

Lambert, Bruce. "AIDS and children: Longer, but troubled, life." New York Times (November 7, 1989b).

New York Times. "Complacency seen in battle on AIDS." (November 3, 1989).

Norwood, Chris (co-chair, National Women's Health Network). AIDS Orphans in New York City: Projected Numbers and Policy Demands. Unpublished report, September 1988.

Novello, Antonia, Chair. Secretary's Work Group on Pediatric HIV Infection and Disease. Final Report. Department of Health and Human Services, November 18, 1988.

Pediatric AIDS Coalition. "Agenda for the 101 Congress." Newsletter. Pediatric AIDS Coalition, 1331 Pennsylvania Avenue, N.W., Washington, DC 20004. January 23, 1989.

Pizzo, Philip A., Eddy, Janie, Falloon, Judy, et al. "Effect of continuous intravenous infusion of zidovudine (AZT) in children with symptomatic HIV infection." New England Journal of Medicine 319 (14) (October 6, 1988).

Shafer, Mary-Ann. University of California at San Francisco, Workbook for the Fifth National Pediatric AIDS Conference and the Follow-up to the 1987 Surgeon General's Workshop on Children with HIV Infection and Their Families, September 1989.

Shapiro, Janet. Project Coordinator, Project H.A.R.P. (HIV/AIDS Respite Program). Brookwood Child Care, Brooklyn, New York. Interview, July 1989.

Stoleroff, Jane. Program Coordinator, Child Care AIDS Network (CCAN), Office of Special Projects, Massachusetts Department of Social Services. Interview, August 1989. Also involved with these initiatives are Pamela Whitney, Program Administrator for CCAN; Sara Sneed, Resource Coordinator; Ken Pontes, Chair of Central AIDS Board, Director of Family Life Center, Office of Special Projects, Central Office, DSS; Linda Spears, Director of Special Projects, DSS; and Marie A. Matava, Commissioner of the Department of Social Services, State of Massachusetts.

Verhovek, Sam H. "Religious sect fights L. I. school district over class on AIDS." New York Times (November 12, 1989): A40.

APPENDICES

APPENDIX A

Glossary

GLOSSARY REFERENCES WERE DRAWN FROM *Dorland's Illustrated Medical Dictionary,* 27th Edition, Philadelphia, PA: W. B. Saunders, 1988; *Medical Answers About AIDS,* by Lawrence Mass, New York: Gay Men's Health Crisis, 1988; *Questions and Answers on AIDS,* by Lyn Frumkin and John Leonard, Oradell, NJ: Medical Economics Books, 1987; *The Truth About AIDS,* by Ann Fettner and William Check, New York: Holt, Rinehart, and Winston, 1984.

A special note of appreciation is offered to Dr. Virginia Anderson, New York City Health Department, who reviewed this glossary and adapted it to the purposes of this volume.

Acute: Illness exhibiting a rapid onset and a short course with pronounced symptoms.

AIDS (Acquired Immune Deficiency Syndrome): A severe infection of the immune system caused by human immunodeficiency virus (HIV), which results in an acquired defect in immune function that reduces the infected person's resistance to opportunistic infections and cancer.

AIDS Arteriopathy: Destruction of the walls of blood vessels that carry oxygen-rich blood away from the heart, a condition caused by HIV.

Alveolar Septa: Dividing walls (septa) which bound a small saclike dilatation in the lungs (alveolus); oxygen from the lungs enters the blood stream via the alveolar septa, and carbon dioxide is diffused from the

323

blood. In AIDS, the alveoli become thick and infected, resulting in pneumonia or respiratory failure.

Anemia: A condition caused by reduction in the size and number of red blood cells as a result of blood loss, of impaired production of or destruction of red cells.

Antibiotic: A soluble substance, derived from a mold or a bacterium, that inhibits the growth of other organisms and is used to combat disease or infection.

Antibody: A protein in the blood produced in response to exposure to specific foreign molecules; antibodies neutralize toxins and interact with other components of the immune system to eliminate infectious microorganisms from the body.

Antigen: A foreign or altered protein that stimulates antibody production.

Antiviral: A subtance that attacks a virus and stops or suppresses viral activity.

ARC (AIDS-Related Complex): A variety of chronic symptoms and physical findings that occur in some persons who are infected with HIV but do not meet the Centers for Disease Control's definition of AIDS; symptoms may include chronic swollen glands, recurrent fevers, unintentional weight loss, chronic diarrhea, lethargy, minor alterations of the immune system/T-cell abnormalities (less severe than those that occur in AIDS), and oral thrush. ARC is an irreversible condition which eventually progresses to full-blown AIDS.

Assay: A laboratory test designed to determine the amount of a chemical, biological, or pharmacological substance present in the specimen.

Asymptomatic: Term describing an infection, or phase of infection, without obvious signs or symptoms of disease.

AZT (Azidothymidine): A synthetic thymidine/deoxythymidine analogue that inhibits HIV; this antiviral medication blocks viral production and slows the clinical course of HIV infection; it may have serious, toxic side effects and lose efficacy over time.

Bacteria: Microorganisms composed of single cells that are capable of independent reproduction; some bacteria cause disease in human beings (*see also* Virus).

B Cells: White blood cells, called lymphocytes, derived from bone marrow; immune cells which circulate in the blood and produce antibodies to detect foreign material; B-cell clones produce specific antibodies to a wide range of infectious agents. When the immune system is disturbed, B cells produce antibodies against the self, as in autoimmune disease.

Biopsy: The removal and microscopic examination of tissue from the living body, performed to establish a precise diagnosis.

Broviac Catheter: A flexible tube inserted into blood vessels for infusing fluids or drawing blood.

Candidiasis/Candida: A yeast-like infection caused by *Candida albicans*, which affects mucus membranes, the skin, and internal organs, and has become a common problem for immune-depressed people. Such oral infections are called thrush and exhibit creamy white patches of exudate on inflamed and painful mucosa. Common sites are the mouth, the esophagus, nailbeds, axilla, umbilicus, and around the anus. Rarely, the infection may occur systemically and affect the heart and the lining of the brain and spinal cord.

Cardiomyopathy: A general diagnostic term that describes decreased contractibility of the heart muscle; the etiology may be obscure.

Casual Contact: Refers to day-to-day interactions between HIV-infected individuals and others in the home, school, or workplace; it does not include intimate contact, such as sexual or drug-use interaction, and it implies closer contact than chance passing on a street or sharing a subway car.

Cellular Immune Deficiency: Reduction in the number or ability of T cells in the body's immune system to respond to infectious agents.

Centers for Disease Control (CDC): A federal health agency, a branch of the Department of Health and Human Services, that provides national health and safety guidelines and statistical data on AIDS and other diseases.

Central Nervous System (CNS): That body system consisting of the brain and spinal cord.

Cofactor: A factor, other than the basic causative agent of a disease, that increases the likelihood of developing that disease; cofactors may include the presence of other microorganisms or of psychosocial elements, such as stress.

Contagious: Term describing disease that can be transmitted by an infectious agent from one person to another. HIV is not contagious during the activities of daily living, but it is contagious during sexual intercourse and intravenous drug use. Using the word "contagious" to describe HIV may be misleading because the word is often used to imply disease transmission from casual or household contact.

Cortical Atrophy: Wasting away of the outer layer of an organ or body structure (as distinguished from the internal substance).

Cryptococcosis: A disseminated opportunistic fungal infection affecting the respiratory tract, seen in AIDS patients. The fungus *Cryptococcus neoformans* enters the lungs and spreads to the lining of the brain (meninges); the resulting meningitis with headache, blurred vision, confusion, depression, agitation, or inappropriate speech is the most common clinical presentation and is frequently fatal.

Cryptosporidium: A parasitic protozoan found in the intestinal tract of reptiles, birds, and mammals; it can cause an infection called cryptosporidiosis in immunocompromised patients. Prolonged, debilitating diarrhea, weight loss, fever, and abdominal pain may occur; spread of the infection to the trachea and bronchial tree is rare.

Cytomegalovirus (CMV): This virus is a member of the herpes family; CMV infections may occur without any symptoms in more than half of the population. Infection may also result in mild flu-like symptoms of aching, fever, mild sore throat, weakness, diarrhea, and enlarged lymph nodes. Severe CMV infections can result in hepatitis, mononucleosis, or pneumonia, especially in immune suppressed people. CMV is shed in body fluids such as urine, semen, saliva, feces, and sweat. CMV retinitis, an infection of the retina, causes severe visual impairment and blindness. Infection of the brain may cause dementia, and infection of peripheral nerve roots may result in intractable pain.

Dysplasia: The disorganized growth of cells during exfoliation or repair of tissue with loss of cellular maturation.

ELISA: An acronym for "enzyme-linked immunosorbent assay," a test used to detect antibodies against HIV in blood samples.

Encephalopathy: Also called AIDS dementia (AD), AIDS-dementia syndrome (ADS), and AIDS-dementia complex (ADC); although there may be other causes such as herpes simplex, cytomegalovirus, or toxoplasmosis, the most common cause is believed to be direct involvement of the brain by HIV, resulting in sensory disturbance, personality changes, memory and judgment impairment, and/or loss of intellectual, social, or occupational abilities.

Enterocolitis: Inflammation of the small intestine and colon, which may be caused by the protozoa cryptosporidium, CMV, or other infectious agents, resulting in diarrhea.

Epidemiology: Study of the frequency and distribution of specific diseases.

Epstein-Barr Virus (EBV): A herpes virus that causes one of the two kinds of mononucleosis; the other is caused by CMV. The virus lodges in the nose and throat and is transmitted by kissing. EBV lies dormant in the lymph glands and has been associated with Burkitt's lymphoma, a cancer of the lymph glands—the clearest link to date between viruses and cancer.

Esophagitis: An inflammation of the esophagus.

Focal Glomerulitis: An inflammation of the blood vessels of the kidney (renal glomeruli); the adjective focal means that some glomeruli are affected while others are spared.

Frank AIDS (Full-Blown AIDS): Those cases of infection with HIV which meet the Centers for Disease Control's definition of AIDS; that is, opportunistic infection, AIDS-related cancer, wasting, or encephalopathy is present.

Glomerulosclerosis: Destruction of renal glomeruli and their replacement by scar tissue.

Hemophilia: A rare hereditary bleeding disorder leading to spontaneous or traumatic hemorrhage; inherited by males through the maternal X chromosone, resulting in a deficiency in the ability to make one or more blood-clotting proteins (Factor VIII deficiency).

Hemophilus influenzae: A bacterium that produces a serious form of meningitis, pneumonia, or ear infections, especially in infants and young children.

Hepatosplenomegaly: Enlargement of the liver and spleen.

Herpes Simplex Virus (HSV I): The virus that causes cold sores or fever blisters on the mouth or around the eyes. Like all herpes viruses, the virus may lie dormant for months or years in nerve or lymph tissue and flare up again under stress, trauma, infection, or immunosuppression; there is no cure.

Herpes Simplex II (HSV II): The virus that causes painful sores on the anus or genitals, but can be transmitted to the face or mouth.

Herpes Zoster Virus: This virus causes the painful infection shingles— small, blister-like clusters surrounded by reddened, swollen, and itchy skin, usually found along a nerve root.

HIV (Human Immunodeficiency Virus): The name proposed for the causative agent of AIDS by a subcommittee of the International Committee on the Taxonomy of Viruses; sometimes called ARV (AIDS-related virus), HTLV-III (human T-cell lymphotropic virus Type III), or LAV (lymphadenopathy-associated virus), it has a selective affinity for helper T cells. HIV-1 is the first AIDS-related retrovirus identified as the AIDS agent in the United States; a variant, HIV-2 retrovirus, has been identified in Africa.

HIV Wasting Syndrome: A syndrome of profound, involuntary weight loss that appears to be associated with HIV infection.

Humoral Immune Deficiency: Reduced resistance to disease associated with deficiency of B-lymphocyte antibodies.

Hypergammaglobulinemia: An excess of antibodies called gamma globulins, or immunoglobulins, in the blood; it is observed frequently in chronic infectious diseases.

Hypoxia: A reduction of the oxygen supply to tissue below physiological levels despite adequate perfusion of the tissue by blood. Anemic hypoxia refers to the reduction of blood's oxygen-carrying capacity due to a deficiency of red blood cells.

Immune System: White blood cells that recognize foreign agents or substances, neutralize them, and recall the experience later when confronted with the same challenge.

Immunoglobulin: A protein with antibody activity that, when given to a person who has been exposed to a transmissible agent, may be capable of minimizing the risk of acquiring the disease produced by the agent.

Immunosuppression: The decreased ability to fight infectious diseases because of a deficient immune system.

Incubation Period: The time interval between initial exposure to a virus or pathogen and the appearance of the first symptom or sign of infection.

Infection: The state or condition in which the body (or part of it) is invaded by an agent (microorganism or virus) that multiplies and produces an injurious effect (active infection).

Inflammation: A localized, protective response elicited by destruction of tissue, which serves to destroy, dilute, or wall off both the injurious agent and the injured tissue; in acute form, this response results in pain, heat, redness, swelling, and loss of function.

In Situ Hybridization: An assay method that uses complementary protein with an indicator to amplify or make visible a protein of interest; the label is identified in the cell, hence the term "in situ."

Interferon: A naturally existing antiviral substance secreted by an infected human cell to strengthen the defense of uninfected neighboring cells.

Intravenous: Into a vein.

IVGG: Intravenous gamma globulin.

Kaposi's Sarcoma (KS): An atypical form of cancer—a proliferation of blood and lymphatic vessel wall tissues forming tumors in various organs; these tumors are typically present with hard, non-painful, purplish plaques on the skin or mucous membranes; KS is rare in children.

Lactate Dehydrogenase: An enzyme that occurs in the cytoplasm of nearly all cells, is involved in reactions, such as glycolysis—the conversion of glucose; widespread in tissues, particularly kidney, skeletal muscle, liver, and myocardium (the middle and thickest layer of the heart wall composed of cardiac muscle), and elevated when tissue is injured; identification of its various types is used for clinical diagnosis.

Latency: The period of time between contracting a disease and showing the first symptoms. Viruses that are not replicating or producing infectious particles are dormant or latent; immunodeficiency may activate latent viruses.

Lymphadenopathy: Enlarged and/or enlarging, hardening, painful, or otherwise prominent lymph nodes/glands in the neck, armpit, or groin. If continuing for more than three months and in different locations, it is diagnosed as persistent generalized lymphadenopathy (PGL).

Lymphocytes: White blood cells found in lymphoid tissue and blood; originating in bone marrow, they are involved in the immune activity of the body as either T or B lymphocytes.

Lymphocytic Pneumonia: A chronic form of pneumonia associated with an increase of the interstitial tissue of the alveolar septa and impairment of oxygenation of red blood cells; also called lymphoid interstitial pneumonia.

Macrophages: Cells that are able to ingest and destroy microorganisms.

Malnutrition Cachexia: A profound and marked state of general ill health evidenced by weakness or emaciation, attributed to unbalanced, insufficient, or defective assimilation of food, or to soluble substances produced by macrophages that destroy cells.

Microcephaly: A small head, usually associated with mental retardation.

Microencephaly: A small brain.

Microglial Nodules: Collections of microglia; which, as interstitial cells in the central nervous system, behave as brain macrophages.

Mitogen Stimulation: A process utilizing a substance that induces cell proliferation in response to antigen stimulation, leading to lymphocyte transformation, which is decreased in immunodeficient patients.

Mucous Membrane: A moist layer of tissue that lines body cavities having an opening to the external world; for example, the lining of the mouth, nostrils, vagina, anus, or rectum.

Mycobacterium Avium Intercellulare: Microorganisms situated between the cells of any structure; its HIV clinical manifestations may include systemic infection and may cause persistent diarrhea.

Neonatal: Concerning the first 28 days of life after birth.

Nephrotic Syndrome: Loss of protein in urine as a result of kidney disease; in HIV infection, focal glomerulosclerosis can occur.

Neuronal Loss: Death of neurons—the information-processing cells of the nervous system, which can never be replaced; in the brain, this condition leads to dementia.

Opportunistic Diseases or Infections: Diseases caused by ubiquitous agents that may be frequently present in our bodies or environment but cause disease only when the immune system becomes depressed; healthy persons with normal immune functions do not get opportunistic infections.

Pandemic: Pertaining to or affecting all the people; widely epidemic.

Parenteral Alimentation: The injection of nutriments through subcutaneous, intramuscular, or intravenous routes rather than through the alimentary canal.

Pathogen: Any disease-producing microorganism; *pathogenic* means that a disease produces symptoms attributable to a causative agent.

Pentamidine: An antimicrobial used in the treatment of PCP.

Peribronchiolar Areas: Lung tissue situated around the small subdivisions of the bronchial tree (air passages).

Persistent Generalized Lymphadenopathy (PGL): Chronic, diffuse, non-cancerous lymph node enlargement that has been typically found in those with immune system dysregulation; frequent and persistent bacterial, viral, and fungai infections indicate that full-blown AIDS has occurred.

Pneumocystic Carinii Pneumonia (PCP): A parasitic infection of the lungs caused by airborne protozoa, present almost everywhere, that are normally destroyed by healthy immune systems; the most common opportunistic infection in AIDS patients; once it has developed, the person is susceptible to recurrences, and the outcome is often fatal. Frequently treated with trimethoprimsulfamethaxazole (Bactrim) or pentamidine isethionate (in an aerosolized form); these medications may be prescribed prophylactically with possible side effects.

Prophylaxis: Any substance or steps taken to prevent something from happening (for example, vitamins, condoms, vaccines); pentamidine or

AZT may be given to asymptomatic patients, for example, to prevent or slow the development of full-blown AIDS.

Pyogenic Bacteria: Bacteria that produce pus, which is a liquid inflammation polymorphonuclear product made up of white blood cells and a thin proteinaceous fluid.

Retrovirus: A type of virus common in mice but until recently unknown in humans; refers to a large group of RNA viruses that carry reverse transcriptase; the AIDS virus is a retrovirus.

Rhonchi: A sonorous sound, produced in the lower airways, as an abnormal respiratory sound indicating disease in the bronchial tubes.

Rosette Technique: An assay for human lymphocytes (*E rosetta* refer to T cells surrounded by a ring of red blood cells; or *EAC rosettes* refer to red cells and antibodies that designate B cells).

Salmonella Enteritis: An inflammation of the intestine, chiefly the small intestine, due to salmonella microorganisms; may result in pain, nausea, vomiting, or diarrhea.

Salmonella Sepsis: The presence in the blood or other tissues of this pathogenic bacterial microorganism or its toxins/poisons.

Seroconversion: The initial development of antibodies specific to a particular antigen.

Seropositive: In the context of HIV, the condition in which antibodies to the virus are found in the blood.

Staphylococcosis Aureus: A species of staphylococci (bacteria), which causes serious suppurative (pus-producing) infections and systemic disease; the organism produces toxins that cause food poisoning.

Streptococcus Pneumoniae: Bacterium that cause serious pyogenic disorders, such as meningitis (inflammation of the membranes of the brain and spinal cord), septicemia (blood poisoning), empyema (accumulation of pus in a body cavity), peritonitis (inflammation of the membrane lining of the abdominopelvic walls), pneumonia (most common), and ear infections in children; a vaccine is available for some strains.

Syndrome: A group of symptoms and signs that, when considered as a whole, constitute an illness.

Tachypnea: Rapid respiration with quick, shallow breathing.

T Cells: White blood cells formed in the thymus and part of the immune system; the normal ratio of helper T cells to suppressor T cells is about 2:1; this ratio becomes inverted in AIDS patients because the number of helper cells is dramatically decreased; also called T lymphocytes.

Thrombocytopenia: A decrease in the number of blood platelets, which have a role in blood coagulation.

Thrush: A common fungus—*Candida albicans*—leads to candidiasis of the mucous membranes of the mouth, characterized by the formation of whitish spots there; often accompanied by fever and gastrointestinal irritation, it may spread to the groin, buttocks, and other parts of the body.

Toxoplasmosis: A disease due to infection with the protozoa *Toxoplasma gondii*, which frequently causes inflammation of the brain (encephalitis) or the heart (myocarditis).

Vaccine: Material composed of an agent or agents that stimulate immunity, thus protecting the body against future infection with that agent.

Villus Atrophy: Flattening of the mucosal lining of the intestines.

Virus: An acellular protein, much smaller than a bacterium, that can reproduce only inside a host cell; some viruses cause disease in human beings.

Western Blot Technique: A test that involves the identification of antibodies against specific protein molecules; it is believed to be more specific than the ELISA test in detecting antibodies to HIV in blood samples; it is also more difficult to perform and considerably more expensive. Before an individual is diagnosed as HIV-infected, Western blot analysis is required as a confirmatory test on samples found to be repeatedly reactive on ELISA tests.

Window Phase: The length of time needed for the body to develop antibodies after exposure to an infectious agent such as HIV; this interval is different from an incubation period and generally occurs one to six months after contact.

APPENDIX B

Resources for HIV/AIDS Education: Cases

PATRICIA BECKLER

THE FOLLOWING CASE DESCRIPTION HAS BEEN USED IN AIDS TRAINING programs for social workers, foster parents, adoptive parents, and respite caregivers from child welfare agencies in New Mexico. It is a compilation of numerous cases and realistically reflects some of the many issues families face in their environment.

An eco-map is presented [Figure 1] that provides a visualization of the relationships between the case family and larger societal systems [Hartman 1978]. Each circle represents a resource connected to the child and family. An unbroken line between the family and a resource indicates a supportive connection. A dotted line means that the connection is tenuous and stressful. The case discusses the family's relationship with each resource.

This is the story of Anna B. and her family. Anna is a two-and-a-half-year-old Hispanic child who has HIV. She is currently in a foster home with parents who are in the process of adopting her. Her mother, Mrs. B., used the child welfare system to make a permanent plan for Anna, to be carried out upon her mother's death.

Mrs. B was three months pregnant when she found out that her husband, R., had AIDS. They had been separated for several months when he and his doctor informed her that she was a possible carrier of the virus. They were also concerned about the child that she was carrying and the possibility that the virus could be transmitted to the baby.

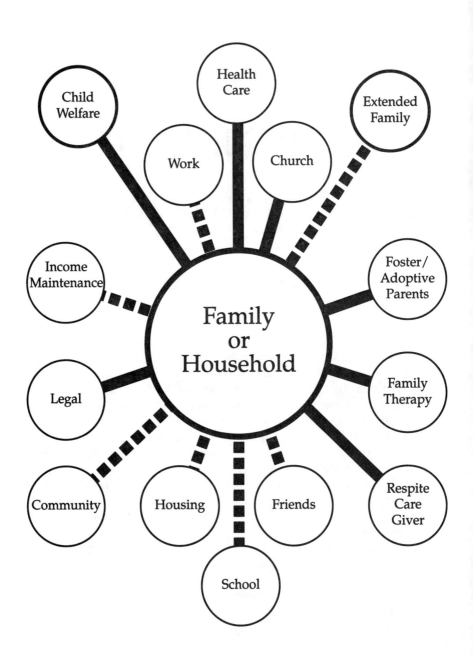

Figure 1. Eco-Map

When Mrs. B. heard this, she panicked and disappeared for two weeks. She left her son from a previous relationship, Jose, age five, with her parents, saying that she would return in a day or two to pick him up. Mrs. B. was prone to drinking binges and had left for periods of time in the past, but her parents reported she had never before disappeared for so long.

When Mrs. B. returned, she contacted the local AIDS testing center. She knew that she had to take the HIV test, but she was not ready to handle the results. She had a very supportive counselor at the testing center; she was told that she would experience a grieving process if she tested positive, and they discussed her ability to build a resource network. When they jointly agreed that she was able to handle the test results—a process that included a screening for assessment of her risk for suicide—the results were given to her. The test was positive, and she knew that in the coming months she would have to make many decisions. With the counselor's support, she made plans to get help in making and carrying out those decisions.

One of the first decisions Mrs. B. faced was the question of continuing the pregnancy; she knew the risk of infecting yet another human being. Like most who face this decision, she had to examine her personal values and her cultural and religious beliefs. Her Hispanic Catholic background led her to seek advice from the Catholic priest in her parish; she saw him three times before making the decision to continue the pregnancy. They discussed the shame and guilt that she felt about the possibility of infecting the child. She questioned what would happen if she died first. She also had heard from a friend that children born of a parent who has HIV do not always get the virus. This information rekindled her hope that the baby she was carrying would not become infected with the virus, and she learned that the risk of transmission ranged from 30 to 50 percent.

Mrs. B.'s family were greatly upset by her behavior. When she had returned, she had told them her diagnosis; she was ashamed and worried about their reaction, fearing they would reject and abandon her. They wept and expressed disbelief, and then became angry and demanded to know how she had gotten the HIV infection. She told them about R.'s diagnosis and said that she believed it was most likely due to his intravenous drug use. The parents blamed R. and were much affected in another way by the news: their daughter was the only one of their children on whom they depended for their own care. They were both elderly, and, because of their medical conditions, Mrs. B. had already been helping them. They were both worried about what would happen to them; the possibility of having their child die first was doubly painful.

The family was in crisis. Mrs. B.'s two brothers, who were both alcoholics and unmarried, offered no support. The parents were unsure about seeking support from their extended family; they too feared rejection. Mrs. B.'s mother decided to tell her own sisters and brothers, who did become very sympathetic. She said many times that she wished this were happening to her instead of to her daughter. Both parents supported her decision to continue the pregnancy but were uncertain about their role in helping her negotiate care for herself and the baby; they worried about who would take care of the parents (themselves), as well as of her and the baby, as the disease progressed. They often felt helpless.

At the time of Anna's birth, Mrs. B. could not afford medical care but had been followed up by the public health department. She checked into a hospital emergency room for delivery. She told the doctor of her medical condition. The doctor and the staff members were most supportive. They had bilingual personnel, including a medical social worker who helped break through the language barrier; they were sensitive to the risks associated with infected blood and took precautions in their own behalf. They made plans to help Mrs. B. with the issues that she would face in testing the baby for HIV, and they did everything they could to help her with the bonding process, because they knew that her diagnosis and the resulting physical and emotional issues could negatively affect the bonding process.

Baby Anna, like many other children born of HIV-positive parents, tested positive at birth. Because of the mother's antibodies, however, she would have to be tested at six-month intervals to determine whether she did indeed have HIV. This uncertainty was difficult for Mrs. B., for her parents, and for the extended family. Mrs. B. was ready for discharge from the hospital within three days of the delivery; the baby was not ready and needed more extensive observation. Mrs. B. had difficulty returning to see Anna during the first few days and, in anger and frustration, again fled, leaving Anna in the hospital. The grandparents feared that Mrs. B.'s shame might put her at risk for suicide.

Her disappearance precipitated a referral to the Human Services Child Protection Unit. When she returned, in two weeks, she was told by the hospital social worker to meet with a Ms. Martinis. She stormed out of the hospital, feeling very angry, and went to the human services agency. Ms. Martinis was able to meet with her and discussed the agency's concern for Anna, for herself, for her son Jose, and for the extended family. The worker told her that she would be a case manager for her in receiving and linking her to services that she would need in the coming months as her disease progressed. They discussed the need for a permanent plan for both children in case of her death. She agreed to services for herself and her family, but she felt that her family would be more reluctant than she was to accept the services. The worker and she discussed the traditional cultural differences for her family of origin; her parents believed that help should come not from an agency but from family resources.

She had had a job as a part-time waitress before her diagnosis. She returned and informed her employers, who were at first supportive, placing her in another position as a hostess. Afraid of losing business, however, they laid her off. She lost both a source of income and important relationships with her co-workers.

She was forced to apply for government assistance to help with her medical expenses and the support of her two children. She had two different experiences with this system. Her first income maintenance worker was well educated about HIV and helpful, understood the cognitive, physical, and psychological stresses accompanying AIDS, and, when Mrs. B. was too exhausted or too ill to make an office appointment, the worker would make a home visit. This worker was transferred. The second worker became angry at her lack of follow-through on getting verifying documents to the worker; assistance was cut off for one month.

Her medical condition began to deteriorate. She was referred to an in-home, family-based team at another agency, where a social worker discussed her fear of what would happen to both her parents and her children, and the effect of the losses of body functioning and control over her life that she was beginning to experience. They discussed her fear of loneliness and how she was to handle the intensity and variability of her feelings. They talked about her ability to live with as much dignity as possible and about her making decisions as long as she could. The old family issues about alcohol also needed discussion with her family; her parents agreed to join her with the family-based social worker for this discussion. This social worker helped her to talk about the sad ending of her life, including how to discuss her death with her parents and children.

As Mrs. B.'s disease progressed, she needed respite care when she was sick and medical follow-up for both herself and the baby. The family-based team provided her with a respite caregiver who came into her home and helped with the daily work that she was no longer able to complete. The respite caregiver and the family-based social worker supported Jose, who often seemed to be overlooked as he faced the impending death of his mother and sister. This attention helped him to deal with some of his fears about himself, AIDS, and the future.

Through discussion with her case manager and family-based social worker, Mrs. B. decided to place Anna with foster parents who might eventually adopt the child. She feared that, as her disease progressed, she would have memory losses and that she would not be able to care for her children. Jose's father could care for him during these times and at the time of her death, but there were no resources within either her's or her husband's family. Although her parents and extended family were unhappy about this decision, feeling that something should be done within the family, they acknowledged they were unable to take care of Anna. The foster parents made the commitment to take the baby for short-term care when Mrs. B.'s medical needs were overwhelming. If Anna outlived her mother, the foster family was willing to adopt her.

The foster parents, the Garcias, discussed the baby's needs with Mrs. B. and the obstacles to bonding. When the baby received medical treatment and had to be hospitalized, they told her how afraid they felt. They saw the baby regress after she was hospitalized, unable to sit up and walk. They also told her of the frustrations of community reactions and their extended family criticism for taking a child that might have AIDS. Mrs. B. saw that the foster parents felt as she did as they too lived with the uncertainty of this disease.

During Mrs. B.'s illness, her friends kept in contact with her. Calling frequently, they asked if they could do anything to help her. But a number of friends were reluctant to allow their children to play with Jose or Anna, which was disturbing to Mrs. B., who was surprised to note who stood by her and who gradually faded away.

Jose's school became a source of contention for his mother. Wanting to protect him from discrimination, she asked him to tell no one about her illness, which was a difficult burden for him. He felt lonely and began to have difficulty concentrating in class. Referred to the principal, Jose was disciplined by isolating him from others, which made his mother more unhappy about increasing Jose's loneliness. The foster parents contacted the school system to enroll Anna in an infant stimulation program, but the school refused. As a family advocate, the case manager helped the foster parents and Mrs. B. to appeal the school's decision successfully.

Mrs. B. developed a positive relationship with the local legal aid lawyer and child welfare judge and sought their help with a permanent plan for the children. They devised a will that allowed for Anna's adoption after her mother's death. They also helped her to spell out a plan for her family to visit Anna in the adoptive home. She felt a great deal of support from them, including their advocacy in the family's behalf with the school system.

Mrs. B. lived in a federal housing project. Her neighbors seemed supportive, but the project director was nervous about her presence. Until the time when she could no longer live by herself with in-home support, the director frequently commented on the effect of the disease on the others in the project. She felt that the message was "We can't force you to leave but it would be best if you choose to leave." One month she lacked enough money to cover the rent and was harassed for making a late payment.

She was unable to keep her diagnosis a secret, and her community responded in a variety of ways. Some people tried to raise some money to help her with medical bills; others shunned her and her family. Some referred to her house as the "house of AIDS." Some parents wanted to keep Jose out of school and Anna out of her early childhood program.

Mrs. B. died a short two years after her diagnosis. Jose went to live with his father, and Anna's foster parents began adoption proceedings. Anna's grandparents and extended family maintained regular contact with her through the cooperation of the foster/adoptive family.

REFERENCE

Hartman, Ann. "Diagrammatic assessment of family relationships." Social Casework 59 (8) (1978): 465–476.

Case Vignettes[1]

1. You are the coordinator of the agency's day treatment program for mentally retarded adults and have been concerned about the un-

[1] Created by Terry McKeon, Senior Director of Programs, and Gary Anderson, Child Welfare Consultant, for an AIDS Policy Training Day for supervisors, managers, and senior staff members, Catholic Guardian Society of Brooklyn and Queens, New York

usually high rate of sick time being used by one of your instructors, John L., during the last several weeks. Another reason for your concern is the persistent rumor among the staff for the last two months that John has AIDS. Already one of his assistant instructors has requested a transfer to another classroom because of "personality differences." You decide to have a conference with John to discuss his absenteeism. He tells you during the conference that his doctor has been treating him for chronic fatigue and a skin rash that are all related to his recent diagnosis of AIDS-related complex. He adds that his health has improved over the last week, and his doctor feels that he is able to work a full schedule.

Would you discuss the following issues with John and, if so, what would you say?

> Job security
> Confidentiality
> The persistence of the rumor
> Treatment options
> Infection control

2. The mother told the social worker that her young son had first tested positive for HIV infection. She finally worked up the courage to have herself tested, and now she knows that she has the virus, too. She hasn't seen her boyfriend for several months. She wants to tell her parents because she really needs their help; she needs a lot of help with her son, and she is worried about her future. What should the social worker do to help?

3. You are a social worker at the agency's preschool for developmentally disabled children, from birth through five years of age. You have reviewed referral materials on a three-and-a-half-year-old youngster, Derek L., whose speech is impaired, and note that the medical report shows he is positive for the AIDS virus. When he came into the school for a screening, his mother reported that he has a chronic yeast infection in his mouth. Would you recommend Derek for acceptance into the program? Who would have to be informed of his illness? As a member of the treatment team, what would be your recommendations in regard to infection control and confidentiality?

4. Mrs. Jones, a newly licensed foster mother, knew that her foster child was born to a drug-addicted mother, but she hadn't counted on the little girl getting sick so frequently in her first year of life. In addition to stubborn colds, there had been several long episodes of diarrhea. Now,

Mrs. Jones is worried that the girl may have AIDS, and she wants to have her tested immediately. She wants a long conference with her worker to discuss these concerns and the child's future. What issues can the worker expect, and how will the worker respond to Mrs. Jones' questions?

5. Shirley M. is a resident in one of the agency's supportive apartments for adults who are minimally retarded. She is employed and enjoys an active social life. You are the coordinator of the apartments, and Shirley comes into your office very upset. Apparently, a friend of hers just told Shirley that one of Shirley's former boyfriends died of AIDS. Shirley explains why she is so upset: "I'm afraid and I want to take the test right away so I know that I don't have AIDS." What information would you offer Shirley?

6. Near tears, the teenager has told you that she has just received doubly bad news: she has HIV and she is pregnant. She doesn't want you to tell anyone, and she doesn't know what to do. What should you do in this case?

7. You are the manager of a group home for young adults who are mentally retarded and you are becoming increasingly concerned that they do not have enough information about AIDS. What are the most important facts that you want them to know?

8. You have just learned that one of the children enrolled in the family day care program is HIV-positive. There are several other children in the provider's home. What should you do with this information and the child?

Rank Order Exercise for AIDS Training[2]

As the director and manager of a foster care department, you have only one vacancy. You have to choose among the following cases. You can choose only one child to be placed; be prepared to discuss the reason(s) for your selection.

1. An eight-year-old Latino girl contracted HIV after being sexually abused by her stepfather, who is an intravenous drug user. After a report was made to central registry, the mother reluctantly signed place-

[2] Adapted from a management training program for New York Foundling Hospital, courtesy of Susan Bear, Director of Foster Care

ment papers. The mother continues to live with her husband—the girl's stepfather—and one other child.

2. A 14-year-old white girl runaway from Indiana has been homeless in New York for two years. She contracted HIV either through needle sharing or sexual activity. She has been using drugs for three years. Thus far, her parents have not been located.

3. A one-month-old interracial boy was born with HIV, as well as addicted to crack. His father, who is now deceased as a result of AIDS, was white and bisexual. His mother, who is black, began using crack after learning her partner was dying from AIDS. She was six months pregnant at the time. She is now hospitalized with the disease. The paternal grandparents are interested in caring for the child. They are 65 and 62. The grandfather is retired, and the grandmother works part-time.

4. A 17-year-old Latino boy contracted HIV through a blood transfusion after being injured in a car accident. His parents died in the same accident. There are no other known living relatives. He is a senior in high school and recently received a scholarship to attend college.

5. A two-and-a-half-year-old black girl was born with HIV as an indirect result of her father's hemophilia. Her mother has symptoms, but not full-blown AIDS. Due to financial hardships as a result of enormous medical expenses, the family has decided that the daughter would best be served through placement. Two older siblings, who are healthy, are temporarily staying with the maternal grandparents.

APPENDIX C

Directory and Resources[1]

Contents

I. Agencies

WHEN SEARCHING FOR COMMUNITY AGENCIES SERVING CHILDREN WITH HIV infection and their families, *public child welfare agencies* or *social service departments* are often a resource. For example, in Maryland, information and assistance can be obtained from a central office:

Social Service Administration
Attn: Gerri Robinson
311 West Saratoga
Room 551
Baltimore, Maryland 20201

---

[1] This directory/resource list is not exhaustive, nor is it intended to be an endorsement by the author or the Child Welfare League of America of all programs or videos noted herein.

or from county offices, for example, in Baltimore County (301-361-3000) or Prince Georges County (301-341-6720). Or from private agencies under contract with the public social service department to serve a specialized population:

>Kennedy Institute
>Specialized Foster Care
>Attn: Judy Levy
>707 N. Broadway
>Baltimore, Maryland 21205-1890
>301-550-9411

>Family and Children's Services of Central Maryland
>Attn: Betty Cavanaugh
>204 West Lanvale Street
>Baltimore, Maryland 21217
>301-669-9000

>Villa Maria
>Specialized Foster Care
>2300 Dulaney Valley Road
>Timonium, Maryland 21093
>301-252-4700

Some state public child welfare agencies have established special units, often strategically located to serve children and families. For example, in Michigan:

>Medically Fragile Unit
>Wayne County Children and Youth Services
>(Michigan Department of Social Services)
>Attn: Jerome Sprung
>801 West Baltimore
>Detroit, Michigan 48214
>313-876-6052

City and *state public health departments* are also often a source of information and assistance. For example:

>The AIDS Institute, New York State Health Department
>Empire State Plaza

Corning Tower—Room 717
Albany, New York 12237
518-473-1996
212-268-4510 (New York City)
212-430-3333 (Children and Youth AIDS Hot Line)

Puerto Rico Department of Health
Box 70184
San Juan, Puerto Rico 00936
809-766-1616

Michigan Department of Public Health
Special Office on AIDS Prevention (SOAP)
3423 N. Logan Street
Lansing, Michigan 48909
517-335-8468

The Public Health Foundation of Los Angeles County
13200 Crossroads Parkway North, No. 135
City of Industry, California 91746
213-226-2406

Seattle-King County Department of Public Health
110 Prefontaine Place South, Suite 500
Seattle, Washington 98104
206-587-2797

Children's hospitals and *pediatric departments* of major hospitals and medical centers are also a resource for family members and professionals caring for HIV-infected children. For example:

University of Miami
Department of Pediatrics
1600 N.W. 12th Avenue
Miami, Florida 33125
305-547-6535

Integrated Health Project
Women and Children with AIDS Project
Cook County Hospital
1835 West Harrison Street

CCSN Room 912
Chicago, Illinois 60612
312-633-5080

Maternal Infant Center for HIV
Children's Hospital
3901 Beaubien Blvd.
Detroit, Michigan 48201
313-745-5565

Children's Hospital AIDS Program (CHAP)
Children's Hospital of New Jersey
15 S. Ninth Street
Newark, New Jersey 07107
201-268-8273
201-268-8251 (Caroline Burr, National Resource Center for HIV
        Infection)

This interdisciplinary, case management program is being replicated at Jersey City Medical Center (Jersey City), St. Joseph's Hospital (Patterson), Robert Wood Johnson Medical Center (New Brunswick), and Cooper Medical Center (Camden).

Children's Hospital National Medical Center
Attn: Robert Parrott
111 Michigan Ave., NW
Washington, DC 20010
202-745-4004

A variety of federal offices provide information and support for pediatric AIDS initiatives (for example, Head Start; the Administration for Children, Youth and Families; Administration on Developmental Disabilities; Administration on Native Americans). A number of foundations have demonstrated active interest in services for children and families (for example, Robert Wood Johnson Foundation, College Road, P.O. Box 2316, Princeton, New Jersey 08543-2316; 609-452-8701).

Specialized Agencies/Resources

Ackerman Institute for Family Therapy
AIDS and Families Project

Attn: John Patten and Gillian Walker, co-directors
149 East 78th Street
New York, New York 10021
212-879-4900
[counseling]

AIDS Center of Queens County
97-45 Queens Blvd.
Suite 1220
Rego Park, New York 11374
[counseling and information]

AIDS Interfaith Residential Services
600 West North Avenue
Baltimore, Maryland 21217
301-383-2133
[residential]

AIDS Resource Foundation for Children
182 Roseville Avenue
Newark, New Jersey 07107
201-483-4250
[residential; multiple services; also in Jersey City and Monmouth County]

Aliveness Project
730 East 38th Street
Minneapolis, Minnesota 55406
612-822-7946
[counseling and information]

Baby Moms
Fragile Infant Special Care Program
Department of Social Services
Attn: Marian Collins
P.O. Box 7988
San Francisco, California 94120
415-557-5157
[case management]

Best Nest
1846 Acorn Lane
Abington, Pennsylvania 19001
215-546-8060
    [foster care]

Bethana
Attn: Fred Weaver, Executive Director
1030 Second Street Pike
Southampton, Pennsylvania 18966
215-355-6500
    [information and referral]

BIABH Study Center
Attn: Robert J. Jones
204 Avery Avenue
Morgantown, North Carolina 28655
    [counseling and foster care]

The Herbert G. Birch Community Service, Inc.
Residential Children's Center
145-02 Farmers Blvd.
Springfield Gardens, New York 11434
718-763-3198
    [residential]

Building Transitional and Support Services for Children with
    HIV Project
Attn: Glenanne Farrington or Linda Coon
Illinois Department of Children and Family Services
Springfield, Illinois
217-785-2459; or 312-917-4152
    [Supported by the Administration for Children, Youth and
    Families, DHHS]

Camp Sunburst
148 Wilson Hill Road
Petaluma, California 94952
707-763-4782
    [camping]

The Center
3421 Martin Luther King Jr. Way
Oakland, California 94609
415-655-3435
[counseling, support groups, concrete services, volunteers]

The Center for Attitudinal Healing
Attn: Cheryl Daniels-Shohan, Coordinator/AIDS Project
19 Main Street
Tiburon, California 94920
415-435-5022
[support groups]

Child Care AIDS Network (CCAN)
Attn: Pamela Whitney or Jane Stoleroff
Massachusetts Department of Social Services
Office of Special Projects
150 Causeway Street
Boston, Massachusetts 02114
617-727-0900
[respite and support]

Child Welfare and AIDS Project
Attn: Richard Barth, University of California—Berkeley
Family Welfare Research Group
School of Social Welfare
Berkeley, California 94720
415-643-7020
[Supported by the Administration for Children, Youth and Families, DHHS; training, policy, and information]

Childkind
Attn: Barbara Chamness
4036 Wetherburn Way
Norcross, Georgia 30092
404-246-0819
[foster care; residential]

The Children with AIDS Project of America
Attn: Jim and Joy Jenkins
4020 N. 20th Street

Suite 101
Phoenix, Arizona 85016
602-843-8654
    [advocacy and adoption]

Children's AIDS Program (CAP)
Boston City Hospital
Dowling 5 South
818 Harrison Avenue
Boston, Massachusetts 02118
617-424-5903
    [residential and day care]

The Children's Home
Attn: Sister Mary Patricia Hennessey
P.O. Box 600732
Houston, Texas 77260
    [residential]

Children's Home Society
SMILE
Attn: Sema Coppersmith
800 N.W. 15th Street
Miami, Florida 33136
305-324-1262
    [foster care]

The Children's Place
Attn: Rosemary Crowley
1525 E. 53rd Street, Suite 418
Chicago, Illinois 60615
312-324-2668
    [residential; open August 1990]

Chrysalis
Center for Women
2104 Stevens Ave.
Minneapolis, Minnesota 55404
612-871-0118
    [counseling and support]

Covenant House
460 West 41 Street
New York, New York 10036
212-613-0300
[residential, adolescent services]

Elisabeth Kubler-Ross Center
South Route 616
Head Waters, Virginia 24442
703-396-3441
[information and advocacy]

Families' and Childrens' AIDS Network (FCAN)
Catholic Charities
Attn: Becky Patterson
721 N. LaSalle Street
Chicago, Illinois 60610
312-266-6100
[information and education]

Family Support Service
Yale Child Study Center
Attn: Steven Nagler
132 Davenport
New Haven, Connecticut 06511
203-785-2513
[in-home family-based services]

Farano Center
Community Maternity Services
Attn: Sue Van Alstine, Program Director
25 N. Main Avenue
Albany, New York 12203
518-482-8836
[residential]

Gay and Lesbian Adolescent Social Services, Inc. (GLASS)
Attn: Teresa DeCrescenzo
8235 Santa Monica Blvd.
Suite 214

West Hollywood, California 90046
213-656-5005
    [residential, adolescent services]

Grandma's House
Joan McCarley, Program Administrator
1222 T Street NW
Washington, DC 20009
202-462-8526
    [residential]

Hale House
Mainliner Newsletter
68 Newcombe Avenue
New York, New York 10030
    [Although Hale House works primarily with infants with
    drug problems; its newsletter may be of interest to persons
    concerned about pediatric AIDS, although this is not its
    main focus.]

Hemophilia Council of California
2206 K Street
Sacramento, California 95814
916-448-7444

Hetrick Martin Institute
Attn: Joyce Hunter
110 East 23rd Street
New York, New York
212-473-1113
    [adolescent services]

H.O.P.E. in Kansas
Foster Homes for Children with AIDS
The Salvation Army
Booth Family Service Center
Box 2037
2050 W. Eleventh Street
Wichita, Kansas 67204-2037
316-263-6174
    [foster care]

Incarnation Children's Center
142 Audubon Avenue
New York, New York 10032
212-928-2590
[residential]

Kaleidoscope—Chicago
1279 North Milwaukee, Suite 250
Chicago, Illinois 60622
312-278-7200
[foster care]

Leake and Watts Children's Home
Pediatric AIDS Foster Care (Phyllis Gurdin)
Training and Technical Assistance Project (Diane Berg)
463 Hawthorne Avenue
Yonkers, New York 10705
914-376-0106
[The project provides a newsletter—*Pediatric AIDS Foster Care Network Bulletin*, support groups, and an AIDS Foster Care Hot Line: 914-423-5273.]

Long Island Association for AIDS Care, Inc.
P.O. Box 2859
Huntington Station, New York 11746
516-385-AIDS (2437)
[case management, advocacy]

Minnesota AIDS Project
2025 Nicholet Avenue South
Suite 200
Minneapolis, Minnesota 55404
612-870-7773
[information]

New York Foundling Hospital
18 West 18 Street
New York, New York 10010
212-633-9300
[foster care]

Northern Lights Alternatives/Children's Care Program
150 West 26th Street, Suite 503
New York, New York 10001
212-255-8879
[With educated volunteers, this program seeks to assist children with AIDS and their caregivers through love, care, and community experiences, and to educate the public about the needs of children with AIDS.]

Open Arms, Inc.
Bryan's House
Attn: Stephanie Held, Executive Director
P.O. Box 191402
Dallas, Texas 75219
214-559-3946
[residential]

Pediatric AIDS Program
Attn: Beth Scalco
c/o Children's Hospital
200 Henry Clay Avenue
New Orleans, Louisiana 70118
504-899-9511 (Hospital)
504-866-2994 (Program)
[case management, volunteers]

Pediatric HIV Family Resource Center
Attn: Ertha Drayton or Constance Ryan
New Jersey Department of Human Services
Division of Youth and Family Services
1 South Montgomery
CN717
Trenton, New Jersey 08625
609-292-8510; 609-984-4219
[Supported by the Administration for Children, Youth and Families, DHHS]

Project H.A.R.P. (HIV/AIDS Respite Program)
Brookwood Child Care

363 Adelphi Street
Brooklyn, New York 11238
    [respite]

Project WIN
Project STAR
Attn: Geneva Woodruff
77B Warren Street
Brighton, Massachusetts 02135
617-783-7300
    [case management, counseling]

Rainbow House
Attn: Mary Inzana
2205 Pennington Road
Trenton, New Jersey 08638
609-771-1600
    [residence for adolescents]

St. Vincent's Children's Services
Attn: Sister Elizabeth Mullane
66 Boerum Place
Brooklyn, New York 11201
    [foster care]

South Florida AIDS Network
East Wing, 3rd Floor
1611 N.W. 12th Avenue
Miami, Florida 33136
305-549-7744
    [information and referral]

Starcross Community
Attn: Sister Marti
P.O. Box 14279
Santa Rosa, California 95402
707-526-0108
    [adoption, national network, family services]

Terrific, Inc.
Attn: Debbie Tate, President
1222 T Street, NW
Washington, DC 20009
202-234-4128
   [adolescent education]

TEENS TAP/TEENS Teachings AIDS Prevention
Good Samaritan Project
3940 Walnut
Kansas City, Missouri 64111
816/561-8784
   [establishes local chapters; a pamphlet: *Warning This Brochure May Save Your Life*]

Urban League of Essex Co., New Jersey
Attn: Melvin Brice
3 Williams Street
Suite 300
Newark, New Jersey 07102
201-624-6660
   [foster parent recruitment]

Women and AIDS Resource Network
Attn: Marie St. Cyr
P.O. Box 020525
Brooklyn, New York 11202
718-596-6007
   [information, counseling]

II. National Organizations

AIDS Action Council
729 Eighth Street, SE
Suite 200
Washington, DC 20003
202-547-3101

AIDS Information Sourcebook
Oryx Press
2214 North Central at Encanto

Phoenix, Arizona 85004-1483
[directory of organizations, bibliography]

American Foundation for AIDS Research
1515 Broadway
New York, New York
212-719-0033

American Social Health Association
P.O. Box 13827
Research Triangle Park, North Carolina 27709
919-361-5736
[National AIDS Hot Line: 1-800-342-AIDS
Spanish Access Number: 1-800-344-SIDA
Deaf Access Number (TTY/TDD only): 1-800-AIDS-TTY]

American Red Cross
AIDS Education Office
1730 D Street, NW
Washington, DC 20006
202-737-8300
[pamphlets: *Teenagers and AIDS; Women, Sex, and AIDS; School Systems and AIDS; Children, Parents and AIDS;* publication: *AIDS Prevention Program for Youth—Information for Teachers/Leaders,* 1987 (No. 329516); resource list included]

Association for the Care of Children's Health (ACCH)
3615 Wisconsin Avenue, NW
Washington, DC 20016
202-244-1801
[educational material, video]

The Center for Population Options
1012 14th Street, NW
Suite 1200
Washington, DC 20005
202-347-5700
[adolescence information]

Child Welfare League of America
440 First Street, NW, Suite 310

Washington, DC 20001-2085
202-638-2952
[information and video]

Gay Men's Health Crisis
129 West 20th Street
New York, New York 10011
212-337-3616
[information]

Hyacinth Foundation
National AIDS Hot Line 800-433-0254
[pamphlets/buddy system]

Minority Task Force on AIDS
c/o New York City Council of Churches
475 Riverside Drive
Room 456
New York, New York 10115
212-749-1214
[information]

National AIDS Information Clearinghouse
P.O. Box 6003
Rockville, Maryland 20850
1-800-458-5231
[information]

National AIDS Network
2033 M Street
Washington, DC 20036
202-293-2437
[information]

National Association of Children's Hospitals and Related
    Institutions
401 Wythe Street
Alexandria, Virginia 22314
703-684-1355
[information]

National Association of People with AIDS
P.O. Box 65472
Washington, DC 20335
202-483-7979
[information]

National Association of Social Workers
Publications, P.O. Box 92180
Washington, DC 20090-2180
1-800-752-3590
[annotated bibliography: *AIDS and Ethics*]

The National Coalition of Hispanic Health and Human
Services Organizations (COSSMHO)
1030 15th Street, NW
Suite 1053
Washington, DC 20005
[hot line for Hispanic Leadership 1-800-AIDS-123]

National Education Association
1201 16th Street, NW
Washington, DC 20036
[leaflets: *Learning About AIDS*
Guidelines for Dealing with AIDS in the Schools]

National Hemophilia Foundation
110 Greene Street
Room 406
New York, New York 10012
212-219-8180
[information]

National Institute of Allergy and Infectious Diseases
AIDS Clinical Trials Information Service
P.O. Box 6421
Rockville, Maryland 20850
301-251-5750
[hot Line: 1-800-TRIALS-A (874-2572)]

National Minority AIDS Council (NMAC)
714 G Street, SE
Washington, DC 20003
202-544-1076
1-800-669-5052
　　[technical assistance materials]

San Francisco AIDS Foundation
333 Valencia Street
P.O. Box 6182
San Francisco, California 94101-6182
415-861-3397
　　[AIDS Educator Catalog]

Pediatric AIDS Coalition
1331 Pennsylvania Avenue, NW
Suite 721 North
Washington, DC 20004-1703
202-662-7460
800-336-5475
　　[information]

Sex Information and Education Council of the U.S.
New York University
32 Washington Place
New York, New York 10003
212-673-3850
　　[catalogue of publications, including a consumer bibliogra-
　　phy, and *How to Talk to Your Children About AIDS*]

United States Conference of Mayors
1620 Eye Street, NW
Washington, DC 20006
202-293-7330
[list of School AIDS Education Resources]

U.S. Public Health Service
Public Affairs Office
Hubert H. Humphrey Building
Room 725-H
200 Independence Avenue, SW

Washington, DC 20201
202-245-6867
[*America Responds to AIDS* series of pamphlets]

From a Special Issue of Health/PAC Bulletin (Spring 1988); Minority Organizations Fighting AIDS:

BEBASHI
1319 Locust Street
Philadelphia, Pennsylvania 19107

HERO
101 W. Read Street, Suite 812
Baltimore, Maryland 21201

Hispanic AIDS Forum
140 W. 22 Street, Suite 301
New York, New York 10011

The Kupona Network
4611 S. Ellis
Chicago, Illinois 60653

Minority AIDS Project
5882 W. Pico Blvd., Suite 210
Los Angeles, California 90019

Minority Task Force on AIDS
92 St. Nicholas Ave., Suite 1B
New York, New York 10026

National Native American Prevention Center on AIDS
5266 Boyd Avenue
Oakland, California 94618

People of Color United Against AIDS
2813 SE Colt Drive, No. 432
Portland, Oregon 97202

San Francisco Black Coalition on AIDS
URSA Institute
185 Berry Street, No. 6600
San Francisco, California 94107

III. Videos (please preview before presenting)

1. "With Loving Arms"
   Child Welfare League of America
   1989/Stock No. 3925/$34.95
   c/o CSSC
   P.O. Box 7816
   300 Raritan Center Parkway
   Edison, New Jersey 08818-7816

2. "Pediatric AIDS: A Time of Crisis"
   Available from the Association for the Care of Children's Health
   3615 Wisconsin Avenue, NW
   Washington, DC 20016
   202-244-1801

3. "AIDS: Helping Families Cope"
   National Association of Social Workers

4. American Red Cross
   "Beyond Fear" (English and Spanish language)
   "A Letter from Brian"
   "Answers About AIDS," with discussion guides
   "Don't Forget Sherrie," with discussion guide
   Contact your local Red Cross Office to order or purchase these
      videos.

5. "The Medical Aspects of HIV Disease"
   "The Psychosocial Aspects of HIV Disease"

These two one-hour tapes with study guides are designed for social workers, foster parents, adoptive parents, and respite caregivers. They are interactive guides to the latest medical and psychosocial information on HIV disease. The first covers transmission of the disease and risk prevention for families providing substitute care. The author of this tape is Dr. James Waltner, New Mexico Human Services Department, Coordinated In-Home Care Unit, Santa Fe, New Mexico. The second tape covers psychological stressors including fears, behavior patterns, and issues experienced by children, teens, or adults who have HIV; child welfare responses are identified. The author is Patricia Beckler, ACSW, Assistant Professor, Department of Social Work, New Mexico State University. For information on both tapes, contact Patricia Beckler, Box 30001, Department of Social Work, New Mexico State University, Las Cruces, New Mexico 88003; 505-646-2143.

6. "Talking with Teens"
   San Francisco AIDS Foundation
   P.O. Box 6182
   San Francisco, California 94101
   415-861-3397

7. "Sex, Drugs and AIDS"
   An 18-minute video and film for adolescents narrated by Rae Dawn Chong.
   "The Subject Is AIDS (The message is abstinence)"; revised version of "Sex, Drugs and AIDS" for younger audiences.
   "The ABC's of AIDS"; AIDS prevention film for elementary school-age students.
   "Face to Face with AIDS (Reaching Latino Youth)."
   Select Media, Inc.
   Educational Film and Video
   74 Varick Street, No. 305
   New York, New York 10013-1909
   212-431-8923

8. "Black People Get AIDS Too" (video or film)
   Adult and general audience versions, including high school; also:
   "AIDS—What Everyone Needs to Know"
   Churchill Films
   662 N. Robertson Blvd.
   Los Angeles, California 90069
   800-334-7830

9. "HIV Test Counseling: Avoiding the Pitfalls"
   Network Publications
   ETR Associates
   P.O. Box 1830
   Santa Cruz, California 95061-1830
   1-800-321-4407

10. "The Burks Have AIDS"
    Phoenix/BFA Films and Video
    468 Park Avenue South
    New York, New York 10016

11. "Condoms: A Responsible Option" (video or film)
    Landmark Films
    3450 Slade Run Drive
    Falls Church, Virginia 22042

12. "Choices"
    (AIDS prevention video for young people)
    "The Best Defense."
    (AIDS prevention)
    "Condom-eze" A User's Guide
    Intermedia
    1600 Dexter N.
    Seattle, Washington 98109
    1-800-553-8336

13. "AIDS Alert" (cartoon format)
    United Learning
    6633 W. Howard Street
    Niles, Illinois 60648

14. "AIDS: Everything You Should Know"
    Hosted and narrated by Whoopi Goldberg—for teenagers
    AIMS Media
    6901 Woodley Avenue
    Van Nuys, California 91406-4878
    1-800-367-2467
    In California: 818-785-4111

15. "AIDS in Your School," for teenagers
Peregrine Productions
330 Santa Rita Avenue
Palo Alto, California 94301

16. "The AIDS Movie," for general audiences and teenagers
New Day Films
22 Riverview Drive
Wayne, Indiana 07470

17. "Too Little, Too Late," grief issues
Fanlight Products
47 Halifax St.
Boston, Massachusetts 02150
617-524-0980

18. "One of Our Own"
Carle Medical Communications
Urbana, Illinois

"Superb video dramatizing how corporate executives can responsibly address their fears and concerns when it is revealed that a valued workers has AIDS. The depiction includes early involvement of and support by top management, adherence to legal protections of confidentiality and nondiscrimination in employment, and the creation of humane relationships with an employee with AIDS. Fears of transmission and prejudice are openly faced . . ."
—George Getzel
Media Review in *AIDS Education and Prevention* 1 (2) (Summer 1989)

19. Prevention films and behavior skills training films
AIDSFILMS
50 West 34th Street
Suite 6B6
New York, New York 10001
212-629-6288

APPENDIX D

Bibliography

Contents

I. Children and Youth

A. General Articles, Monographs, and Books

American Psychological Association. Task Force on Pediatric AIDS. "Pediatric AIDS and human immunodeficiency virus infection: Psychological issues." *American Psychologist* 44 (2) (February 1989): 258–264.

Anderson, Gary R. "Children and AIDS: Implications for child welfare." *Child Welfare* 63 (1) (January–February 1984): 62–73.

Anderson, Gary R. *Children and AIDS: The Challenge for Child Welfare.* Washington, DC: Child Welfare League of America, 1986.

Anderson, Gary R., Gurdin, Phyllis, and Thomas, Ann. "Dual Disenfranchisement." In Doka, Ken (editor), *Disenfranchised Grief.* Lexington, MA: Lexington Books, 1989.

Belfer, Myron, Krener, Penelope, and Miller, Frank B. "AIDS in children and adolescents." *Journal of the American Academy of Child and Adolescent Psychiatry* 27 (2) (March 1988).

Blanche, Stephane, et al. "A prospective study of infants born to women seropositive for human immunodeficiency virus type 1." *New England Journal of Medicine* 320 (25) (June 22, 1989): 1643–1648.

Bloom, Al. "Acquired immune deficiency syndrome in childhood." *Public Health* 102 (2) (March 1988): 97–106.

Boland, Mary G. *The Child with HIV Infection: A Guide for Parents.* Newark, NJ: Children's Hospital of New Jersey, 1986.

Boland, Mary G. *Diet Guidelines for the Child with AIDS.* Newark, NJ: Children's Hospital of New Jersey, 1986.

Boland, Mary G., Allen, Theodore J., Long, Gwendolyn I., and Tasker, Mary. "Children with HIV infection: Collaborative responsibilities of the child welfare and medical communities." *Social Work* 33 (6): (November–December 1988): 504–509.

Boland, Mary G., Tasker, Mary, Evans, Patricia M., and Keresztes, Judith S. "Helping children with AIDS: The role of the child welfare worker." *Public Welfare* 45(1) (Winter 1987): 23–29.

Boland, Mary G., and Klug, Ruth Maring. "AIDS: The implications for home care." *American Journal of Maternal Child Nursing* 11(6) (November–December 1986): 404–411.

Boland, Mary, and Rizzi, Deborah. *The Child with AIDS (Human Immunodeficiency Virus): A Guide for Families.* Newark, NJ: Children's Hospital of New Jersey, 1986.

Brown, Lawrence, Mitchell, Janet, DeVore, Sherri, and Primm, Beny. "Female intravenous drug users and perinatal HIV transmission." *New England Journal of Medicine* 320 (22) (June 1, 1989): 1493, 1494.

Chachkes, Esther. "Women and children with AIDS." In Leukefeld, Carl G., and Fibres, Manuel (editors), *Responding to AIDS: Psychosocial Initiatives.* Silver Spring, MD: National Association of Social Workers, 1987.

Children's Defense Fund (CDF). *Teens and AIDS: Opportunities for Prevention*. Washington, DC: CDF, 1988.

Child Welfare League of America (CWLA). *A Guide for Residential Group Care Providers: Serving HIV-Infected Children, Youths and Their Families*. Washington, DC: CWLA, 1989.

Child Welfare League of America. *Attention to AIDS. Proceedings of a Seminar Responding to the Growing Number of Children and Youth with AIDS*. Washington, DC: CWLA, 1987.

Child Welfare League of America. *Report of the CWLA Task Force on Children and HIV Infection. Initial Guidelines*. Washington, DC: CWLA, 1988.

Citizens Committee for Children of New York, Inc. *The Invisible Emergency: Children and AIDS in New York*. New York: Citizen's Committee for Children of New York, Inc., April 1987.

Cooper, Ellen R. "AIDS in children: An overview of the medical, epidemiological, and public health problems." *New England Journal of Public Policy* 4 (1) (Winter-Spring 1988): 121–134.

Council of Family and Child Caring Agencies (COFCCA). *Caring for Children and Families with AIDS: Suggested Guidelines for Voluntary, Not-for-Profit Agencies*. Published by COFCCA, 220 E. 23rd Street, Suite 905, New York, NY 10010. March 1989.

Dokecki, Paul R., Baumeister, Alfred A., and Kupstas, Franklyn D. "Biomedical and social aspects of pediatric AIDS." *Journal of Early Intervention* 13 (2) (1989): 99–113.

Falloon, Judith, Eddy, Janie, Wiener, Lori, and Pizzo, Philip. "Human immunodeficiency virus infection in children." *The Journal of Pediatrics* 114 (1) (January 1989): 1–30.

Garfinkel, F., and Goldsmith, L. "Child welfare agencies. Possible bases of liability for placement of children with AIDS in adoptive or foster homes." *Journal of Legal Medicine* 10 (1) (March 1989): 143–154.

Gelber, Seymour. "Developing an AIDS program in a juvenile detention center." *Children Today* 17 (1) (January-February 1988): 6–9.

Grossman, M. "Children with AIDS." *Journal of Infectious Disease Clinics of North America* 2 (2) (June 1988): 533–541.

Gurdin, Phyllis, and Anderson, Gary R. "Quality care for ill children: AIDS-specialized foster family homes." *Child Welfare* 66 (4) (July-August 1987): 291–302.

Hutchings, John J. "Pediatric AIDS: An overview." *Children Today* 17 (3) (May-June 1988): 4–7.

Katz, Samuel, and Wilfert, Catherine. "Human immunodeficiency virus infection of newborns." *New England Journal of Medicine* 320 (25) (June 22, 1989): 1687–1689.

Klug, Ruth Maring. "Children with AIDS." *American Journal of Nursing* 86 (10) (October 1986): 1126–1132.

Kubler-Ross,. Elisabeth. *AIDS: The Ultimate Challenge.* New York: Macmillan, 1987.

Lewert, George. "Children and AIDS." *Social Casework* 69 (6) (June 1988): 348–354.

Lloyd, David W. "Legal issues for child welfare agencies in policy development regarding HIV infection and AIDS in children." *Children's Legal Rights Journal* 8 (2) (Spring 1987): 8–11.

Lockhart, Lettie, and Wodarski, John. "Facing the unknown: Children and adolescents with AIDS." *Social Work* 34 (3) (May 1989).

Magee, P., and Senizaiz, F. L. "AIDS: A case management approach. The Illinois experience." *Child and Adolescent Social Work Journal* 4 (3) (Fall-Winter 1987): 130–141.

Miller, Jaclyn, and Carlton, Thomas O. "Children and AIDS: A need to rethink child welfare practice." *Social Work* 33 (6) (November-December 1988): 553–555.

Nicholas, Stephen W., et al. "Human immunodeficiency virus infection in childhood, adolescence, and pregnancy: A status report and national research agenda." *Pediatrics* 83 (2) (February 1989): 293–308.

Olson, Sydney. "Pediatric HIV: More than a health problem." *Children Today* 17 (3) (May-June 1988): 8–9.

Osterholm, M. T., and MacDonald, K. L. "Facing the complex issues of pediatric AIDS: A public health perspective." *Journal of the American Medical Association* 258 (1987): 2736.

Quackenbush, Marcia, and Villarreal, Sylvia. *Does AIDS Hurt? Educating Young Children about AIDS.* Santa Cruz, CA: Network Publications, 1988.

Pizzo, Philip, et al. "Effect of continuous intravenous infusion of zidovudine (AZT) in children with symptomatic HIV infection." *New England Journal of Medicine* 319 (14) (October 6, 1988).

Rendon, Mario, Gurdin, Phyllis, Bassi, Jorge, and Weston, Martha. "Foster care for children with AIDS: A psychosocial perspective." *Child Psychiatry and Human Development* 19 (4) (Summer 1989).

Rubinstein, A. "Pediatric AIDS." *Current Problems in Pediatrics* 16 (7) (July 1986): 361–409.

Ryder, Robert, et al. "Perinatal transmission of the human immunodeficiency virus type 1 to infants of seropositive women in Zaire." *New England Journal of Medicine* 320 (25) (June 22, 1989).

Schwarz, S. K., and Rutherford, A. W. "AIDS in infants, children and adolescents." *Journal of Drug Issues* 19 (1) (Winter 1989): 75–92.

Scott, Gwendolyn B., et al. "Mothers of infants with the acquired immunodeficiency syndrome." *Journal of the American Medical Association* 285 (3) (January 18, 1985): 363–366.

Septimus, Anita. "Psycho-social aspects of caring for families of infants infected with human immunodeficiency virus." *Seminars in Perinatology* 13 (1) (February 1989): 49–54.

Taylor-Brown, Susan. "The impact of AIDS on foster care: Examination of a family-centered approach to foster care." Paper. International Foster Care Conference, Ypsilanti, Michigan, August 1989.

Tourse, Phyllis, and Gundersen, Luanne. "Adopting and fostering children with AIDS: Policies in progress." *Children Today* 17 (3) (May-June 1988): 15–19.

Urwin, Charlene. "AIDS in children: A family concern." *Family Relations* 37 (2) (April 1988).

Wiener, Lori. "Helping clients with AIDS: The role of the worker." *Public Welfare* 44 (4) (Fall 1986): 38–41.

Williams, Anne D. "Nursing management of the child with AIDS." *Pediatric Nursing* 15 (3) (May-June 1989): 259–261.

Woodruff, Geneva, and Sterzin, Elaine Durkat. "The transagency approach: A model for serving children with HIV infection and their families." *Children Today* 17 (3) (May-June 1988): 9–14.

B. Adolescents

DiClemente, Ralph, Boyer, Cherrie, and Morales, Edward. "Minorities and AIDS: Knowledge, attitudes, and misconceptions among black and Latino adolescents." *American Journal of Public Health* 78 (1) (January 1988): 55–57.

DiClemente, R. J., Zorn, J., and Temoshok, L. "Adolescents and AIDS: A survey of knowledge, attitudes and beliefs about AIDS in San Francisco." *American Journal of Public Health* 76 (1986): 1443–1445.

Goodman, Elizabeth, and Cohall, Alwyn. "Acquired immunodeficiency syndrome and adolescents: Knowledge, attitudes, beliefs, and behaviors in a New York City adolescent minority population." *Pediatrics* 84 (1) (July 1989): 36–42.

Haffner, D. "The AIDS epidemic: Implications for the sexuality education of our youth." *SIECUS Report* 16 (6) (July-August 1988); *see also* "Safe sex and teens." *SIECUS Report* 17 (1) (September-October 1988).

Hein, Karen. "AIDS in adolescence: Exploring the challenge." *Journal of Adolescent Health Care* 10 (3) (Supplement, May 1989).

Hein, Karen. "Commentary on adolescent acquired immunodeficiency syndrome: The next wave of the human immunodeficiency virus epidemic?" *The Journal of Pediatrics* 114 (1) (January 1989): 144–149.

Jones, Robert, Judkins, Bonnie, and Timbers, Gary. *Adolescents with AIDS in Foster Care: A Case Report.* Morgantown, NC: BIABH Study Center, Appalachian State University, 1988.

Kegeles, Susan, Adler, Nancy, and Irwin, Charles. "Sexually active adolescents and condoms: Changes over one year in knowledge, attitudes and use." *American Journal of Public Health* 78 (4) (April 1988).

Kegeles, S., Adler, N., and Irwin, C. "Adolescents and condoms: Associations of beliefs with intentions to use." *American Journal of Diseases of Childhood* 143 (8) (August 1989): 911.

Madaras, Lynda. *Lynda Madaras Talks to Teens About AIDS.* New York: Newmarket Press, 1989.

Mantell, J. E., and Schinke, S. P. "The crisis of AIDS for adolescents: The need for preventive risk-reduction." In Roberts, A. R. (editor), *Crisis Intervention Handbook.* New York: Springer, 1988.

Overby, Kim, Lo, Bernard, and Litt, Iris. "Knowledge and concerns about acquired immunodeficiency syndrome and their relationship to behavior among adolescents with hemophilia." *Pediatrics* 83 (2) (February 1989).

Quackenbush, Marcia, and Nelson, Mary, with Clark, Kay (editors). *The AIDS Challenge: Prevention Education for Young People.* Santa Cruz, CA: Network Publications, 1988.

Remafedi, Gary. "Preventing the sexual transmission of AIDS during adolescence." *Journal of Adolescent Health Care* 9 (2) (March 1988).

Rickert, Vaughn, Jay, M. Susan, Gottlieb, Anita, and Bridges, Christie. "Adolescents and AIDS: Female's attitudes and behaviors toward condom purchase and use." *Journal of Adolescent Health Care* 10 (1989): 313.

Strunin, L., and Hingson, R. "Acquired immunodeficiency syndrome and adolescents: Knowledge, beliefs, attitudes and behaviors." *Pediatrics* 79 (1987): 825–828.

Wachter, Oralee. *Sex, Drugs and AIDS.* New York: Bantam Books, 1987.

C. Government Publications

AIDS: A Public Health Challenge. Volume 1: Assessing the Problem. Volume 2: Managing and Financing the Problem. Volume 3: Resource Guide. Washington, DC: U.S. Government Printing Office, 1987.

AIDS and Teenagers: Emerging Issues. Hearing before the Select Committee on Children, Youth and Families. One Hundredth Congress. First Session. Hearing held in Washington, DC, June 18, 1987. For sale by the Superintendent of Documents, U.S. Government Printing Office, Washington, DC 20402.

AIDS and Young Children: Emerging Issues. Hearing before the Select Committee on Children, Youth and Families. House of Representatives, One Hundredth Congress. First Session. Hearing held in Berkeley, CA, February 21, 1987. For sale by the Superintendent of Documents, U.S. Government Printing Office, Washington, DC 20402.

Margolis, Stephen, Baughman, Lela, Flynt, J. William, and Kotler, Martin. *AIDS Children and Child Welfare.* Macro Systems, for Assistant Secretary for Planning and Evaluation, U.S. Dept. of Health and Human Services, March 31, 1989.

Report of the Presidential Commission on the Human Immunodeficiency

Virus Epidemic. Washington, DC: Superintendent of Documents, U.S. Government Printing Office, June 1988.

Select Committee on Children, Youth, and Families. *Continuing Jeopardy: Children and AIDS.* A Staff Report of the Select Committee, One Hundredth Congress. Second Session. Washington, DC: U.S. Government Printing Office, 1988.

U.S. Department of Education. *AIDS and the Education of Our Children. A Guide for Parents and Teachers.* Available, free of charge, from: Consumer Information Center, Department ED, Pueblo, Colorado 81009; 1988: 28 pp.

U.S. Department of Health and Human Services, Public Health Service, Health Resources and Service Administration, Bureau of Health Care Delivery and Assistance, Division of Maternal and Child Health, Rockville, MD, in conjunction with The Children's Hospital of Philadelphia. *Report of the Surgeon General's Workshop on Children with HIV Infection and Their Families.* Washington, DC: U.S. Government Printing Office, DHS Publication No. HRS-D-MC 87-1, April 1987.

II. General References

A. Education

Aids Education and Prevention. Official Journal of the International Society for AIDS Education. Articles, book and media reviews. Guilford Publications. Journals Department R, 72 Spring Street, New York, NY 10012; 1-800-365-7006.

Cates, Willard, and Bowen, G. Stephen. "Education for AIDS prevention: Not our only voluntary weapon." *American Journal of Public Health* 79 (7) (July 1989).

Centers for Disease Control. "Guidelines for effective school health education to prevent the spread of AIDS." *MMWR Supplement* 37 (S-2) (January 29, 1988).

Coomer, C. M. "AIDS in schools: Avoiding a crisis." *Social Work in Education* 11 (1) (Fall 1988): 64–67.

Forrest, Jacqueline D., and Silverman, Jane. "What public school teachers teach about preventing pregnancy, AIDS and sexually transmitted diseases." *Family Planning Perspectives* 21 (2) (March-April 1989).

"Guidelines for effective school health education to prevent the spread of AIDS." *New York State Journal of Medicine* 88 (5) (May 1988): 266–272.

Kenney, Asta, Guardado, Sandra, and Brown, Lisanne. "Sex education and AIDS education in the schools: What states and large school districts are doing." *Family Planning Perspectives* 21 (2) (March-April 1989).

Lamb, George A., and Liebling, Linette G. "The role of education in AIDS prevention." *New England Journal of Public Policy* 4 (1) (Winter-Spring 1988): 315–322.

MacFarlane, M. "Equal opportunities: Protecting the rights of AIDS-linked children in the classroom." *American Journal of Law and Medicine* 14 (4) (1989): 377–430.

Raper, Jim, and Alderidge, Jerry. "What every teacher should know about AIDS." *Childhood Education* 64 (3) (February 1988): 146–149.

Ward, Laurien. "Drama: An effective way to educate about AIDS." *Social Casework* 69 (6) (June 1988): 393–396.

B. Grief

Geiss, S., Fuller, R., and Rush, J. "Lovers of AIDS victims: Psychosocial stresses and counseling needs." *Death Studies* 10 (1986).

Grollman, Earl (editor). *Explaining Death to Children.* Boston: Beacon Press, 1967.

Kubler-Ross, Elisabeth. *On Children and Death.* New York: Collier Books/Macmillan, 1983.

Kubler-Ross, Elisabeth. *On Death and Dying.* New York: Macmillan, 1969.

Moynihan, Rosemary, Christ, Grace, and Silver, Les Gallo. "AIDS and terminal illness." *Social Casework* 69 (6) (June 1988): 380–388.

Strang, Rosemary W. "AIDS: Ministering to the dying." *Charities USA* 13 (3) (March 1986): 5–8.

C. HIV Testing and Counseling

Buckingham, Stephan L. "The HIV antibody test: Psychosocial issues." *Social Casework* 68 (7) (September 1987): 387–393.

Cates, Willard, and Handsfield, H. Hunter. "HIV counseling and testing: Does it work?" *American Journal of Public Health* 78 (12) (December 1988).

Galea, Robert, Lewis, Benjamin, and Baker, Lori. "Voluntary testing for antibodies among clients in long-term substance abuse treatment." *Social Work* 33 (3) (May-June 1988): 265–268.

Goldblum, P., and Marks, R. "The HIV testing debate." *FOCUS: A Guide to AIDS Research* 3 (12) (November 1988).

Jaffe, L., and Wortman, R. "Guidelines to the counseling and HTLV-III antibody screening of adolescents." *Journal of Adolescent Health Care* 9 (January 1988): 84–86.

McCusker, Jane, et al. "Effects of HIV antibody test knowledge on subsequent sexual behaviors in a cohort of homosexually active men." *American Journal of Public Health* 78 (4) (April 1988).

Shernoff, Michael. "Pre and post test counseling for individuals taking the HIV antibody test." *SIECUS Report* 16 (1) (September-October 1987).

D. General Articles, Monographs, and Books on AIDS/HIV

AIDS: A Guide for Hispanic Leadership. Washington, DC: The National Coalition of Hispanic Health and Human Service Organizations, 1989.

Allen, James, and Curran, James. "Prevention of AIDS and HIV infection: Needs and priorities for epidemiologic research." *American Journal of Public Health* 78 (4) (April 1988).

Becker, Marshall, and Joseph, Jill. "AIDS and behavioral change to reduce risk: A review." *American Journal of Public Health* 78 (4) (April 1988).

Blachman, M. "Seropositive women: Clinical issues and approaches." *FOCUS: A Guide to AIDS Research* 3 (3) (February 1988). This monthly newsletter is available from AIDS Health Project, University of California, San Francisco, Box 0884, San Francisco, CA 94143-0884.

Bridge, T. Peter, et al. *Psychological, Neuropsychiatric and Substance Abuse Aspects of AIDS.* New York: Raven Press, 1988.

Buckingham, S. L., and Rehms, S. J. "AIDS and women at risk." *Health and Social Work* 12 (1) (1987): 5–11.

Buckingham, Stephen, and Van Gorp, Wilfred G. "AIDS dementia complex: Implications for practice." *Social Casework* 69 (6) (June 1988): 371–375.

Caputo, Larry. "Dual diagnosis: AIDS and addiction." *Social Work* 30 (4) (July-August 1985): 361–364.

Christ, Grace, and Wiener, Lori. "Psychosocial issues in AIDS." In Devita, V., Hellman, S., and Rosenberg, S. (editors), *AIDS: Etiology, Diagnosis, Treatment, and Prevention*. Philadelphia: Lippincott, 1985.

Cutler, John, and Arnold, R. C. "Venereal disease control by health departments in the past: Lessons from the past." *American Journal of Public Health* 78 (4) (April 1988).

DesJarlis, D., and Friedman, S. "Transmission of human immunodeficiency virus among intravenous drug users." In DeVita, V., Hellman, S., and Rosenberg, S. (editors), *AIDS: Etiology, Diagnosis, Treatment and Prevention*. Second Edition. Philadelphia: J. B. Lippincott, 1988.

Dunkel, Joan, and Hatfield, Shellie. "Countertransference issues in working with persons with AIDS." *Social Work* 31 (2) (March-April 1986): 114–117.

Edson, T. (editor). *The AIDS Caregivers Handbook*. New York: St. Martin's Press, 1988.

Faltz, B. *AIDS and Substance Abuse: A Training Manual for Health Care Professionals*. San Francisco: University of California, San Francisco AIDS Health Project, Box 0884, San Francisco, CA 94143-0884, 1987.

Faulstich, Michael. "Psychiatric aspects of AIDS." *American Journal of Psychiatry* 144 (5) (May 1987): 551–556.

Feldblum, Paul, and Fortney, Judith. "Condoms, spermicides, and the transmission of human immunodeficiency virus: A review of the literature." *American Journal of Public Health* 78 (1) (January 1988).

Flaskerud, Jacquelyn, and Rush, Cecilia. "AIDS and traditional health beliefs and practices of black women." *Nursing Research* 38 (4) (July/August 1989): 210–215.

Friedland, Gerald, et al. "Lack of transmission of HTLV III/LAV infection to household contacts with AIDS or AIDS related complex with candidiasis." *New England Journal of Medicine* 314 (6) (February 6, 1986).

Friedland, G., and Klein, R. "Transmission of HIV." *New England Journal of Medicine* 317 (18) (October 1987).

Furstenberg, A. L., and Olson, M. M. "Social work and AIDS." *Social Work in Health Care* 9 (4) (1984): 45–62.

Gong, Victor, and Rudnick, Norman (editors). *AIDS: Facts and Issues.* New Brunswick, NJ: Rutgers University Press, 1986.

Hammonds, E. "Race, sex, AIDS: The construction of 'Other.'" *Radical America* 20 (6) (1987).

Hastings Center: Institute of Society, Ethics, and the Life Sciences. "AIDS: The emerging ethical dilemmas." *Hastings Center Report* (Supplement) (August 1985).

"Healing AIDS." Special Issue. *Holistic Nursing Practice* 3 (4) (August 1989).

Honey, Ellen. "AIDS and the inner city: Critical issues." *Social Casework* 69 (6) (June 1988): 365–370.

Hopkins, Donald R. "AIDS in minority populations in the United States." *Public Health Reports* 102 (6) (November-December 1987): 677–681.

Hsiung, G. D. (guest editor). "Selected topics on acquired immunodeficiency syndrome." *The Yale Journal of Biology and Medicine* 60 (6) (November-December 1987): 505–600.

Imagawa, David, et al. "Human immunodeficiency virus type 1 infection in homosexual men who remain seronegative for prolonged periods." *New England Journal of Medicine* 320 (22) (June 1, 1989): 1458. *See also* "Silent HIV infections": 1487.

Journal of Drug Issues. Special Issue on AIDS. Volume 19 (1) (Winter 1989).

Lang, Jennifer, Spiegel, Judith, and Strigle, Stephen (editors). *Living with AIDS: A Self Care Manual.* AIDS Project Los Angeles, Inc., 7362 Santa Monica Blvd., W. Hollywood, CA 90046, 1986.

Leishman, Katie. "Heterosexuals and AIDS." *The Atlantic Monthly* 259 (2) (February 1987): 39.

Leukefeld, Carl, and Fimbres, Manuel. *Responding to AIDS: Psychosocial Initiatives.* Silver Spring, MD: National Association of Social Workers, 1987.

Lopez, Diego, and Getzel, George S. "Strategies for volunteers caring for persons with AIDS." *Social Casework* 68 (1) (January 1987): 47–53.

Macklin, Eleanor (editor). *AIDS and Families*. New York: Haworth Press, 1989.

Macks, Judy. "Women and AIDS: Countertransference issues." *Social Casework* 69 (6) (June 1988): 340–347.

Marmor, M., et al. "The epidemic of acquired immunodeficiency syndrome (AIDS) and suggestions for its control in drug abusers." *Journal of Substance Abuse Treatment* 1 (4) (1984): 237–247.

Mohr, R., Patten, J., Kaplan, L., and Gilbert, J. "Family therapy and AIDS: Four case studies." *The Family Therapy Networker* 12 (1) (January–February 1988).

Reamer, Frederic G. "AIDS and ethics: The agenda for social workers." *Social Work* 33 (5) (September–October 1988): 460–464.

Rounds, Kathleen. "AIDS in rural areas: Challenges to providing care." *Social Work* 33 (3) (May–June 1988): 257–261.

Rowe, W., Plum, G., and Crossman, C. "Issues and problems confronting the lovers, families and communities associated with a person with AIDS." *Journal of Social Work and Human Sexuality* 6 (2) (1988).

Ryan, Caitlan. "AIDS in the workplace." *Public Welfare* 44 (3) (Summer 1986): 29–33.

Ryan, Caitlan, and Rowe, M. "AIDS: Legal and ethical issues." *Social Casework* 69 (2) (June 1988).

Safyer, Andrew, and Spies-Karotkin, Geraldine. "The biology of AIDS." *Health and Social Work* 13 (4) (Fall 1988).

Schilling, Robert, et al. "Developing strategies for AIDS prevention research with black and Hispanic drug users." *Public Health Reports* 104 (1) (January–February 1989).

Science. Special AIDS Issue. Volume 239. February 5, 1988.

Selik, Richard, Castro, Kenneth, and Pappaioanou, Marguerite. "Racial/ethnic differences in the risk of AIDS in the United States." *American Journal of Public Health* 78 (12) (December 1988).

Shernoff, Michael. "Integrating safer sex counseling into social work practice." *Social Casework* 69 (6) (June 1988).

Stulberg, Ian, and Buckingham, Stephan L. "Parallel issues for AIDS patients, families and others." *Social Casework* 69 (6) (June 1988): 355–359.

Surgeon General's Report on Acquired Immune Deficiency Syndrome. United States Public Health Service, Department of Health and Human Services, October 1986.

Walker, Gillian. "AIDS and family therapy." Parts I and II, *Family Therapy Today* 2 (4) (April 1987) and (6) (June 1987).

Walker, Gillian. "An AIDS journal." *The Family Therapy Networker* (January-February 1988).

APPENDIX E

American Academy of Pediatrics Reprints[1]

Contents

1. American Academy of Pediatrics, Task Force on Pediatric AIDS. "Pediatric Guidelines for Infection Control of Human Immunodeficiency Virus (Acquired Immunodeficiency Virus) in Hospitals, Medical Offices, Schools, and Other Settings." *Pediatrics* 82 (5) (November 1988): 801–807.

2. American Academy of Pediatrics, Task Force on Pediatric AIDS. "Perinatal Human Immunodeficiency Virus Infection." *Pediatrics* 82 (6) (December 1988): 941–944.

3. American Academy of Pediatrics, Task Force on Pediatric AIDS. "Infants and Children with Acquired Immunodeficiency Syndrome: Placement in Adoption and Foster Care." *Pediatrics* 83 (4) (April 1989): 609–612.

---

[1]Reprinted with permission. The recommendations in these statements do not indicate an exclusive course of treatment or procedure to be followed. Variations, taking into account individual circumstances, may be appropriate.

Task Force on Pediatric AIDS

Pediatric Guidelines for Infection Control of Human Immunodeficiency Virus (Acquired Immunodeficiency Virus) in Hospitals, Medical Offices, Schools, and Other Settings*

Acquired immunodeficiency syndrome (AIDS), the most severe manifestation of infection with the human immunodeficiency virus (HIV), has been diagnosed in more than 900 children younger than 13 years of age throughout the United States as of May 1988, 77% of whom were infected in utero or perinatally secondary to maternal infection. Risk factors for maternal infection include intravenous drug abuse or sexual contact with partners who are intravenous drug abusers or bisexual. The remainder of children, including a high proportion of hemophiliacs, have been infected by blood or clotting factor infusion between 1979 and 1985. In addition, adolescents have acquired infection through sexual activity and intravenous drug use, as well as transfusion of contaminated blood or blood factors.

The criteria for diagnosis of AIDS in children differ in some ways from those for adults, and the most recently published diagnostic criteria (*Morbidity and Mortality Weekly Report*, Aug 14, 1987) include the expanded spectrum of disease, such as recurrent bacterial infections and encephalopathy, as well as including children with presumptive diagnosis of AIDS-associated diseases such as lymphoid interstitial pneumonitis. There is no accurate estimate of the numbers of infected asymptomatic children or of infected children with milder symptoms that do not meet the criteria for the diagnosis of AIDS. Although most cases of pediatric HIV infection have been identified in New York City, Newark, Miami, and Los Angeles,

*The recommendations in this statement do not indicate an exclusive course of treatment or procedure to be followed. Variations, taking into account individual circumstances, may be appropriate.

cases are appearing in other locations. Thus, HIV infection in childhood is becoming more widespread, but in many states it is still rare.

Because the cause of AIDS is a virus transmissible from human to human, pediatric health care workers must adjust infection control guidelines to meet this new threat. However, in formulating these guidelines, physicians must constantly bear in mind that HIV is not highly contagious and that transmission ordinarily requires repeated sexual contact or intravenous inoculation.[1,2] In fact, results of prospective studies suggest that the risk of HIV acquisition by accidental needle stick with contaminated needles is less than 1%,[3] and the risk from other types of nonsexual ("casual") exposure appears to be considerably smaller. Despite the tens of thousands of exposures of health care workers to blood and body fluids, only five infections acquired by contamination of skin or mucous membranes have been reported.[4-6] Thus, the guidelines are suggested as reasonable ways to meet the threat of HIV transmission in pediatric health care settings, taking into account both the potential devastating effect of infection and the rarity of its occurrence. Detailed recommendations not specifically directed at the pediatric health field have recently been published by the Centers for Disease Control[7] and describe certain matters not considered here, such as serologic testing, handling of laundry, etc. The Centers for Disease Control recommend universal precautions for blood and body fluids of all patients, whether known to be HIV seropositive or of unknown HIV status. The AAP Task Force does not believe that universal precautions can be recommended for children without taking into account the regional prevalence of infection rate in children and the distinction between the transmission capabilities of blood-contaminated and blood-free body fluid.

BASIC PREMISES

The guidelines that follow are based on the following facts and assumptions:

1. HIV has been isolated from blood (including lymphocytes, macrophages, and plasma), other internal body fluids such as CSF and pleural fluid, human milk, semen, cervical secretions, saliva, and urine. Epidemiologically, only blood, semen, cervical secretions, and (rarely) human milk have been implicated as the means of transmission of the virus from one person to another. HIV has been documented to be transmitted from an infected person to a person who was not infected by three routes:

sexual intercourse (either heterosexual or male homosexual), parenteral inoculation of blood (most often among drug users who share syringes and needles for injection), and congenital or perinatal transmission from a women to her fetus or newborn.[1,2,8]

2. Whereas body fluids, such as tears, saliva, urine, and stool, may contain HIV in low concentration, there is no evidence that transmission has occurred by contamination with these fluids.[9] No studies reported in the literature or cases reported to the Centers for Disease Control suggest transmission of HIV by urine, feces, saliva, tears, or sweat. Similarly, no studies or reports have suggested transmission of HIV in school or day-care settings or during contact sports such as football, boxing, or wrestling.

3. The risk of HIV infection to health care workers, including physicians and nurses, who are taking care of persons who have AIDS or are infected with HIV is extremely low.[10] The number of AIDS cases reported in health care workers is proportional to the number of adults employed in health care settings, and 95% of these persons give a history of a specific risk of infection unrelated to their employment. Six prospective studies have evaluated 2,421 health care workers who have been exposed one or more times to blood or other potentially infectious body fluids of persons with AIDS or HIV infection.[2,3,10-13] Most of these workers were exposed to blood from an infected person, and most had sustained a needle-stick injury. Only four workers are known to have seroconverted to HIV, all following a needle-stick injury, and one worker was found to be seropositive 10 months after exposure (heterosexual transmission to this worker could not be excluded). No health care worker in the prospective studies has seroconverted after mucous membrane or cutaneous exposure or after exposure to any secretions or excretions from an infected patient. A study in dentists has found a similarly low rate of HIV infection.[14] Overall, the risk of HIV infection after direct exposure by needle stick to blood from an infected person is less than 1%. The risk from other types of exposure, including exposure of nonintact skin or mucous membranes, appears to be much lower. Much of the concern about the risk of infection in the health care setting has arisen from nonprospective case reports of infection after exposure of skin or mucous membranes. In addition to the cases reported in the prospective studies, six health care workers and one research laboratory worker (who was cut while working with concentrated virus) from the United States and four from other countries have been reported to have seroconverted after parenteral exposure. Five other health care workers and one research laboratory worker who have not reported other risks for infection have been found to be infected, although

seroconversion proximate to a specific injury or exposure was not documented. Three of these health care workers apparently became infected after contact with blood from an infected patient onto nonintact skin (dermatitis, abrasion, etc).[4]

Two of the health care workers who became infected were providing nursing or home health care without following recommended precautions.[5,15] One was a mother who was assisting with care for her child who had unknowingly been infected with HIV through a blood transmission. The mother had extensive contact with the child's blood, secretions, and excretions during a lengthy hospitalization of the child but did not wear gloves and often did not wash her hands immediately after exposure.

4. Studies of household contacts of patients with AIDS have failed to document infection except for those with known risk factors suggesting that the route of transmission was sexual or perinatal, not "casual contact."[1,16,17] HIV was transmitted from an infected person only by sexual contact or sharing of equipment for injection of drugs. HIV was not transmitted by close household or family contact, even by the sharing of personal items such as razors, toothbrushes, towels, clothes, eating utensils, and drinking glasses or of bedroom, bathroom, and kitchen facilities. Family members helped the infected person bathe, dress, and eat and interacted with hugs, kisses on the cheek, and kisses on the lips. One of the studies included the family members of 35 children (mostly infants) infected through transfusion,[18] and another included 125 infants or children less than 4 years of age who had both clinical and serologic evidence of HIV infection.[19] In the former study, 31 siblings lived with the infected children, and in the latter study 90 children (age range not stated) lived in the families with infected adults and children; none of these children became infected even though they shared items, slept in the same beds, and participated normally in family activities and interactions, including hugging and kissing.

One case report, however, does indicate that transmission within a household setting might occur, although the means of transmission from a young boy (infected at about 18 months of age by transfusion) to his brother who was approximately 4 years old is not known.[20] The report does cite one instance in which the younger brother bit the older, but the skin of the older boy was unbroken and it is not clear that this act resulted in transmission.

Other reports definitely indicate that biting did not transmit HIV from an infected biter to the person bitten.[21,22] In one of the reports,[21] 30 health care workers were bitten and/or scratched by a neurologically impaired adult, the injuries often resulting in puncture wounds of the skin. One report, however, suggests transmission of HIV by a bite from an infected woman to her sister; the bite occurred soon after the infected woman had been hit in the mouth and her mouth was actively bleeding when she bit her sister.[23] In this instance, the transmission more likely occurred from blood than from saliva.

5. Serologic screening for HIV infection of all children who come for medical care is not currently justified for the following reasons: it would not detect all infected infants (some may be antibody-negative owing to failure to mount an antibody response), it would result in many false-positive test results, it would only be retrospective in situations in which urgent medical care had already been given, and it would involve extraordinary costs.

6. Children who are ill but in whom HIV infection has not yet been diagnosed, as well as children who have an asymptomatic infection, may nevertheless carry infectious virus in their blood. Therefore, it is preferable to treat all children in high-prevalence areas as potentially carrying infections communicable by blood or blood-contaminated body fluids. Such a policy would also reduce the transmission of other more common contagious diseases, such as hepatitis B.[24] However, this recommendation should be tempered by local conditions and community decisions about the acceptable level of risk. In many large urban areas, infection rates are already high enough to convince most physicians that these precautions should be taken. Hospitals in other areas should undertake periodic anonymous serosurveys to decide when to undertake the recommendations that follow. The serosurveys could be done on random populations of hospitalized children, on cord blood samples of newborns (which reflect the serologic status of adult women), on specimens from women seeking prenatal care, or on adolescents. These surveys should be conducted in consultation with local health departments or the Centers for Disease Control. Another index that could be used to generate acceptance of precautions is simply the confirmation of indigenous perinatal HIV infection in a particular area. In any case, the decision to consider an area "high prevalence" must be a local decision.

GUIDELINES FOR HOSPITAL INFECTION CONTROL IN HIGH-PREVALENCE AREAS

1. All children who are in the hospital should be treated as if carrying blood-borne infections. Gloves should be worn for contact with blood or blood-containing fluids and for any procedures that involve exposure to blood (Figure). A distinction is made between blood, blood-contaminated

fluids, and tissue fluids (which are considered potentially infectious) and excreted fluids (which are not considered to carry a significant risk). However, if an excretion such as stool contains blood, it must be handled as a high-risk source. Procedures that involve spilling or splattering of blood or blood-contaminated body fluids should be done wearing gloves, gowns, masks, and some form of barrier eye protection. Handwashing after patient contact should be routine, particularly after contact with blood.

Gloves are not required for prevention of HIV transmission while changing diapers in usual circumstances. This recommendation is based on the doubtful importance of urine and stool in HIV transmission and on considerations of practicality. Handwashing after changing diapers is required to reduce the transmission of other pathogens.

HANDWASHING IS NECESSARY AFTER PHYSICAL CONTACT WITH ALL PATIENTS*

Body Fluids and Procedures for Which Gloves are Recommended
  Blood
  Blood-contaminated fluids
  Intubation
  Endoscopy
  Dental procedures
  Wound irrigation
  Phlebotomy
  Finger and/or heel sticks
  Arterial puncture
  Vascular catheter placement
  Tracheostomy suctioning
  Rinsing of used instruments
  Lumbar Puncture
  Amniocentesis
  Puncture of other cavities (eg, pleural, pericardial, peritoneal and synovial)

Body Fluids† and Procedures for Which Only Handwashing is Recommended
  Urine
  Stool
  Vomitus
  Tears
  Nasal secretions
  Oral secretions
  Diaper changing

Figure Infection control requirements for exposure to blood and other body fluids of HIV-infected patients and of all children in areas of high HIV prevalence. *Masks and barrier eye protection should also be used whenever splattering is likely. †Body fluids that are not contaminated with blood.

2. In the delivery room, personnel are exposed to maternal blood and body fluids, and thus to the prevalence of infection in adult women. Newborn infants should be handled with gloves until blood and amniotic fluid have been removed from the skin. Placentas and umbilical cords (at birth) should also be handled with gloves. Personnel assisting in the resuscitation of the newborn should use mechanical suction equipment. In emergencies, when mouth suction of the airway is performed, a trap should always be placed in the line. A separate report regarding "Care of the Potentially HIV-Infected Newborn" will be issued by the Task Force.

3. To avoid the necessity for mouth-to-mouth resuscitation, emergency equipment such as endotracheal tubes and breathing bags should be available wherever likely to be needed.

4. Medical personnel should not recap needles. They should dispose of syringes, needles, and other sharp instruments in puncture-resistant containers. Educational efforts should be intensified.

5. Children known to be HIV positive do not need isolation in single rooms unless they have other infections for which a single room is indicated or unless they require protective isolation. Disposable food trays are not necessary. The use of a playroom by these children should be determined using the criteria described in "Guidelines for Infection Control in Schools in High-Prevalence Areas" and "Guidelines for Infection Control in Day-Care Centers."

GUIDELINES FOR HOSPITAL INFECTION CONTROL IN LOW-PREVALENCE AREAS

1. During patient care, the risk of HIV transmission from exposure to blood either splashing on skin or mucous membranes or by needle stick is low, even when the patient is known to be infected. When the prevalence of HIV infection in the general population of children is low, the probability of a health care worker acquiring HIV infection from a patient is exceedingly low. In most nonurban areas of the United States, the prevalence of HIV in children is less than 1 : 1,000. In those areas, the risk to health care workers is negligible. If the prevalence of HIV infection were 1 : 1,000, and the risk of an accidental needle stick were 1 : 100 patients, then the incidence of a needle stick from an infected patient would be 1 : 100,000. The rate of transmission from the needle stick of an infected patient has been less than 1%. Thus in low-prevalence areas, transmission might occur once in 10,000,000 patients. For a more extensive analysis, see Appendix.

2. Reducing the risk of HIV infection of health care workers to zero is

not possible. When the risk of infection is low, the cost of preventing transmission—even for such simple devices as gloves—is extremely high if measured in dollars per case prevented. (If gloves cost 10 cents per pair, and only one pair is used per patient, it would cost $1 million to prevent a case of AIDS in a low-prevalence area, assuming the gloves were 100% effective in preventing transmission and assuming every case of HIV transmission results in AIDS [Appendix]). In addition to the direct costs, policies that purport to reduce the risk to zero, by treating all children as if they were infected, increase the false belief that the risk of infection is high and lend support to other irrational policies based on those false beliefs. However, we recommend that hospitals in all areas be required to provide gloves to employees who are particularly risk-averse and who wish to use them.

3. Because of these considerations, prevention policies should be based on the prevalence of the virus. In low-prevalence areas, routine precautions such as the use of gloves for venipunctures are not warranted, although individuals who are particularly concerned might choose to wear them. Physicians and hospitals are encouraged to assess the prevalence of infection periodically through anonymous surveys of blood samples obtained for other purposes.

4. Known HIV-infected patients admitted to hospitals in low-prevalence areas should be handled according to the precautions described in "Guidelines for Hospital Infection Control in High-Prevalence Areas."

5. Even in low-prevalence areas, newborn infants should be handled with gloves just after birth, because they are covered with large amounts of maternal blood, and such precautions will also reduce the risk of other blood-borne infections.

GUIDELINES FOR INFECTION CONTROL IN THE EMERGENCY ROOM AND OPERATING ROOM

1. Personnel working in emergency rooms may be subject to repetitious exposure to blood and, although any one exposure carries minimal risk of contagion, risk throughout time will be small but cumulative. Therefore, all personnel working in emergency rooms throughout the United States should wear gloves in situations in which there may be contact with blood or blood-contaminated body fluids (Table). However, because the risk from any single exposure remains extremely small, the emergency care of a child should never be delayed because gloves are not immediately available.

TABLE.

Transmission Rates to Health Care Workers*

Incidence of HIV	No. of Patients With HIV/yr	yr/ Risky Stick	Transmission Likely to Occur Once Every (yr)
1:50	200	2	50
1:1,000	10	10	1,000

*Assumptions: Hospital with 10,000 admissions per year; accidental needle sticks = 1:100 patients = 100 needle sticks per year; transmission rate = 1:100 high-risk needle sticks.

2. If splattering of blood is likely during operative procedures, eg, in orthopedics, barrier eye protection and masks should be worn.

3. During emergency situations in which the risk of exposure to blood or body fluids is increased (eg, trauma, "stat" or "medical code blue"), gloves should be worn during the resuscitation effort. Barrier eye protection and masks should be used for all tracheal intubations when bloody secretions are anticipated.

4. Mouth-to-mouth resuscitation should be avoided when another route and equipment are available, eg, bag respirators and tracheal airways. However, mouth-to-mouth resuscitation is not considered to carry a likely risk of infection and should be used when urgently needed.

5. If personnel clothing is contaminated with blood or blood-contaminated body fluids, it should be changed as soon as practical.

GUIDELINES FOR INFECTION CONTROL IN CLINICS AND PHYSICIANS' OFFICES IN HIGH-PREVALENCE AREAS

1. Handwashing is the most important precaution in this setting, as in others. Exposure to blood or blood-contaminated body fluids (Figure) necessitates the use of gloves. Blood spills should be cleaned using disinfectant. HIV is rapidly inactivated by common germicides, including sodium hypochlorite (household bleach) at a dilution of 1:10 to 1:100.[25]

2. Instruments that become contaminated with blood or body fluids must be subjected to the generally accepted methods for cleaning and sterilization. Instruments that will not withstand heat must be subjected to chemical disinfection.

3. There is no need for separate examining rooms or visiting rooms for

HIV-infected patients, unless the patient is sufficiently immunosuppressed to require reverse isolation or has another infection that is contagious.

4. Needles should be placed uncapped in closed puncture-proof containers, which then should be disposed of as infectious waste.

HEALTH CARE WORKERS WITH HIV INFECTION

No known HIV infections have been transmitted from health care workers to patients, and, indeed, there are few circumstances (except dentistry) in which health care workers are likely to introduce their blood into patients. If the health care worker is wearing gloves, blood from an accidental needle stick typically collects under the glove and the patient is not exposed to a significant inoculum. Thus, HIV-infected health care workers have not presented a hazard to their patients or co-workers as a result of their occupational activities. Therefore, routine screening of health care workers is not indicated, and there is no obligation to inform patients of workers' HIV status. Because pediatricians are generally not involved with invasive procedures, no precautions are necessary for HIV-infected individuals unless they have a weeping dermatitis of the hands or an opportunistic infection with a contagious agent. In the latter circumstances, wearing gloves or discontinuing patient care during the infection are necessary.

GUIDELINES FOR INFECTION CONTROL IN SCHOOLS IN HIGH-PREVALENCE AREAS

1. HIV-infected children who are old enough to attend school can be admitted freely to all activities, to the extent that their own health permits. The child's physician should have access to consultative expertise to assist in decision making.

2. Because all infected children will not necessarily be known to school officials in high-prevalence areas, and because blood is a potential source of contagion, policies and procedures should be developed in advance to handle instances of bleeding. Such policies and procedures should be based upon the understanding that, even within an area of high prevalence, the risk of HIV-infection resulting from a single cutaneous exposure to blood from a school-aged child or adolescent with unknown serologic status is minute. Because of this minimal risk, the only mandatory precautionary action should be washing exposed skin with soap and water.

Lacerations and other bleeding lesions should be managed in a manner that minimizes direct contact of the care giver with blood. Schools in high-prevalence areas should provide access to gloves so that individuals who wish to further reduce a minute risk may opt for their use. Under no circumstance should the urgent care of a bleeding child be delayed because gloves are not immediately available.

GUIDELINES FOR INFECTION CONTROL IN DAY-CARE CENTERS

Studies continue to show lack of transmission from HIV-infected individuals by nonsexual contact, even under conditions of intimacy,[17,26] such as those that occur among children in day care. Recommendations concerning placement of infected children in foster homes will be made in a separate report. Here, we make the following recommendations relative to the admission of infected children to day-care centers, which supercede a prior recommendation from the Committee on Infectious Diseases.[27]

1. HIV-infected children should be admitted to day care if their health, neurologic development, behavior, and immune status are appropriate. The decision as to whether a child with known HIV infection may attend day care or be placed in foster care should be made on an individual case-by-case basis. This decision is best made by qualified persons, including the child's physician, who are able to evaluate (a) whether the child will receive optimal care in the setting under consideration and (b) whether an infected child poses a potential threat to others. Most infected children, particularly those too young to walk, pose no risk to others. HIV-infected children who persistently bite others or who have oozing skin lesions may theoretically transmit the virus, although such has not been conclusively demonstrated (see "Basic Premises"). Medical evaluation should be ongoing, to evaluate changes in the child's health.

2. If the child's personal physician is uncertain as to the efficacy or safety of placement within a school or group setting, consultation should be sought with individuals or groups having particular expertise regarding HIV infection and AIDS. States, municipalities, and professional groups should make available such expert help.

3. Screening of children for the presence of HIV antibody when they seek entrance to day care is not warranted or recommended. First, the risk of HIV transmission in the day-care setting is only hypothetical at present. Second, in populations of young children in which the prevalence of HIV infection is low, screening will likely result in a greater number of false-positive results than correctly identified infected individuals. Those with

false-positive results will experience a great deal of unnecessary anxiety as well as the expense of medical evaluation.

4. Parents of children in the day-care center have no "right" to information regarding HIV status of other children. Information regarding a child who has immunodeficiency, whatever its etiology, should be available to those caretakers who need to know (particularly the child's physician) to protect the child against other infections. This need to know, however, does not require knowledge of HIV status.

5. Where available, day-care centers that are designed to meet the specific needs of children infected with HIV may represent an acceptable alternative placement, particularly to provide a supportive environment for the children, but these centers are not necessary for reasons of infection control. This alternative should not be used to isolate or segregate infected children.

6. Some children may be unknowingly infected with HIV or other infectious agents, such as hepatitis B virus; these agents may be present in blood or body fluids. Thus, responsible individuals in all day-care and foster care settings in high-prevalence areas, and individuals in any day-care center in which there is a known infected child, should adopt precautions for blood spills from all children as described in "Guidelines for Infection Control in Schools in High-Prevalence Areas." All child care personnel and educators should be informed about these procedures. For example, soiled surfaces should be promptly cleaned with disinfectants, such as household bleach (a 1:10 to 1:100 dilution of bleach to water prepared daily). Disposable towels or tissues should be used whenever possible and properly discarded, and mops should be rinsed in the disinfectant. Cleaning personnel should avoid the risk of having their mucous membranes or any open skin lesions exposed to blood or blood-contaminated body fluids (by using disposable gloves, for example).

Task Force on Pediatric AIDS
Stanley A. Plotkin, MD, Chairman
Hugh E. Evans, MD
Norman C. Fost, MD, MPH
Gerald Merenstein, MD
S. Kenneth Schonberg, MD
Gwendolyn B. Scott, MD
Martin W. Sklaire, MD
Esther H. Wender, MD
James R. Allen, MD (Consultant)

APPENDIX

Infection Control Statement

The risk to health care workers of acquiring HIV infection from accidental needle sticks will vary widely. The following analysis should help hospitals assess the risk as well as the costs and benefits of implementing universal precautions on a routine basis.

If the incidence of HIV infection in the population were 1:1,000 and the risk of an accidental needle stick were 1:100 patients, then the incidence of a needle stick from an infected patient would be 1:100,000 patients. Not all needle sticks result in transmission; current estimates are that transmission occurs in less than 1:100 needle sticks from infected patients. Thus, in these areas, transmission might occur once in 10 million patients. In a higher prevalence area, where 1:50 patients had HIV infection, a transmission might occur once for every 500,000 patients (Table).

The benefits of routine universal precautions, assuming they are 100% effective, will be prevention of one case of HIV infection in a health care worker in the interval listed in the fourth column of the Table, as well as possible reduction of anxiety among health care workers. There will be other benefits in preventing transmission of diseases that are more common than HIV infection, such as hepatitis B. The costs will include the direct costs of supplies, as well as the added costs of disposal of such materials, which can be substantial. If, for example, the cost of gloves, gowns, and disposal were 50 cents per patient, the cost to prevent one case of HIV infection in a health care worker would be $50 million in the area in which the one of 1,000 patients is infected, and $250,000 in the higher prevalence area.

Barrier eye protection should also be used whenever splattering is likely. Handwashing is necessary after physical contact with all patients.

REFERENCES

1. Friedland GH, Klein RS: Transmission of the human immunodeficiency virus. *N. Engl J Med* 1987;317:1125–1135
2. Gerberding JL, Bryant-LeBlanc CE,, Nelson K, et al: Risk of transmitting human immunodeficiency virus, cytomegalovirus, and hepatitis B virus to health care workers exposed to patients with AIDS and AIDS-related conditions. *J Infect DIS* 1987;156:1–8
3. Henderson DK, Saah AJ, Szk BJ, et al: Risk of nosocomial infection with human T-cell lymphotropic virus type III/lymphadenopathy-associated virus in a large cohort of intensively exposed health care workers. *Ann Intern Med* 1986;104:644–647

4. Centers for Disease Control: Update: Human immunodeficiency virus infections in health care workers exposed to bloods of infected patients. *MMWR* 1987;36:285–286

5. Centers for Disease Control: Apparent transmission of human T-lymphotropic virus type III/lymphadenopathy-associated virus from a child to a mother providing health care. *MMWR* 1986;35:76–79

6. Weiss SH, Saxinger WC, Rechtman D, et al: HTLV-III infection among health care workers: Association with needle-stick injuries. *JAMA* 1985;254:2089–2093

7. Centers for Disease Control: Update: Recommendations for prevention of HIV transmission in health-care settings. *MMWR* 1987;36(suppl 1):1–18

8. Zeigler JB, Cooper DA, Johnson RO, et al: Postnatal transmission of AIDS-associated retrovirus from mother to infant. *Lancet* 1985;1:896–898

9. Ho DD, Byington RE, Schooley RT, et al: Infrequency of Isolation of HTLV-III virus from saliva in AIDS, letter. *N Engl J Med* 1985;313:1606

10. Centers for Disease Control: Update: Acquired immunodeficiency syndrome and human immunodeficiency virus infection among health care workers. *MMWR* 1988; 37:229–234

11. McEvoy M, Porter K. Mortimer P, et al: Prospective study of clinical, laboratory, and ancillary staff with accidental exposures to blood or body fluids from patients infected with HIV. *Br Med J* 1987;294:1595–1597

12. Health and Welfare Canada: National surveillance program on occupational exposure to HIV among health care workers in Canada. *Can Dis Weekly Rep* 1987;37:163–166

13. Kuhls TL, Viker S, Parris NB, et al: Occupational risk of HIV, HBV and HSV-2 infections in health care personnel caring for AIDS patients. *Am J Public Health* 1987;77:1306–1309

14. Klein RS, Phelan JA, Freeman K, et al: Low occupational risk of human immunodeficiency virus infection among dental professionals. *N Engl J Med* 1988;318:86–90

15. Grint P, McEvoy M: Two associated cases of the acquired immunodeficiency syndrome (AIDS). *PHLS Commun Dis Rep* 1985; 42:4

16. Curran JW, Jaffe HW, Hardy AM, et al: Epidemiology of HIV infection and AIDS in the United States. *Science* 1988;239:610–616

17. Lifson AR: Do alternate modes for transmission of human immunodeficiency virus exist? A review. *JAMA* 1988;259:1353–1356

18. Roger MF, White CR, Sanders R, et al: Can children transmit human T-lymphotropic virus type III/lymphadenopathy-associated virus (HTLV-III/LAV) infection? (Communication 176). Abstracts of the Second International Conference on AIDS, Paris, France, June 23–25, 1986, p 107

19. Fischl MA, Dickinson GM, Scott GB, et al: Evaluation of heterosexual partners, children, and household contacts of adults with AIDS. *JAMA* 1987;257:640–644.

20. Wahn V, Kramer HH, Voit T, et al: Horizontal transmission of HIV infection between two siblings. *Lancet* 1986;2:694

21. Tsolukas C, Hadjis T, Theberge L, et al: Risk of transmission of HTLV-III/LAV from human bites (poster 211). Abstracts of the Second International Conference on AIDS, Paris, France, June 23–25, 1986, p 125

22. Drummond JA: Seronegative 18 months after being bitten by a patient with AIDS. *JAMA* 1986;256:2342–2343

23. Anonymous: Transmission of HIV by human bite. *Lancet* 1987;2:522

24. Seeff LB, Wright EC, Zimmerman HJ, et al: Type B hepatitis after needle-stick ex-

posure: Prevention with hepatitis B immune globulin: Final report of the Veterans Administration Cooperative Study. *Ann Intern Med* 1978;88:285–293

25. Martin LS, McDougal JS, Loskoski SL: Disinfection and inactivation of human T lymphotropic virus type III/lymphadenopathy-associated virus. *J Infect Dis* 1985;152:400–403

26. Lifson AR, Rogers MF, White C, et al: Unrecognized modes of transmission of HIV: Acquired immunodeficiency syndrome in children reported with risk factors. *Pediatr Infect Dis J* 1987;6:292

27. American Academy of Pediatrics, Committee on Infectious Diseases: Health guidelines for the attendance in day-care and foster care settings of children infected with human immunodeficiency virus. *Pediatrics* 1987;79:466–471

Task Force on Pediatric AIDS

Perinatal Human Immunodeficiency Virus Infection*

Infection with human immunodeficiency virus (HIV), the causative agent of acquired immunodeficiency syndrome (AIDS) has become a significant medical problem during the 1980s. Hundreds of infants and thousands of women have been reported to have AIDS. In addition, there are thousands more women infected with HIV, at risk for AIDS, and capable of transmitting HIV to their fetuses/infants if they become pregnant.

DEFINITIONS

Perinatal, the time period including pregnancy through 28 postnatal days; congenital (intrauterine) infection, infection acquired transplacentally; intrapartum infection; infection acquired during the time of delivery; postnatal infection, infection acquired after pregnancy and delivery; HIV

---

*The recommendations in this statement do not indicate an exclusive course of treatment or procedure to be followed. Variations, taking into account individual circumstances, may be appropriate.

infection, asymptomatic or symptomatic infection with HIV; AIDS, meeting the Centers for Disease Control definition for AIDS.

EPIDEMIOLOGIC FEATURES OF AIDS AND HIV

The primary risk factor for AIDS in infants is congenital (and possibly intrapartum) exposure to a mother infected with HIV. Other risks have included transfusion of blood or clotting factor concentrates. However, since the institution of routine testing of blood donors, these risks have become extremely small. Because the majority of women with AIDS (78%) are of childbearing age, it is important that the physician inquire about risk factors in women of childbearing age to provide optimal care and prevention of HIV transmission. The primary risk factors for AIDS in the reported cases in women are IV drug abuse (49%), heterosexual transmission from a person known to be at risk of HIV infection (28%), and transfusion or clotting factor therapy before blood was screened in middle 1985 (11%).[1,2] Although the sex distribution of pediatric AIDS cases is relatively even (54% boys, 46% girls), the racial distribution of pediatric AIDS is uneven: blacks 54%, Hispanics 24%, whites 21%, and others 1%.[3]

RISKS AND MEANS OF CONGENITAL/INTRAPARTUM HIV INFECTION

The seroprevalence rate in an unselected population of childbearing women has been reported to range from 0.7/1,000 in New Mexico[4] to 20/1,000 in an inner New York City hospital.[5] In childbearing women who are IV drug abusers, the seropositive rate is 30%.[4] Hoff et al[6] reported seroprevalence rates in childbearing women in Massachusetts by type of hospital. They found 8/1,000 in the inner city hospitals, 2.6/1,000 in metropolitan hospitals, 2.2/1,000 in urban-suburban hospitals, 0.3/1,000 in suburban hospitals, and 1.2/1,000 in suburban-rural hospitals.[6] The rate for similar populations in New York City is 15.8/1,000 and for upstate New York it is 1.8/1,000.[4]

The risk of congenital or intrapartum transmission of HIV from an infected woman to her fetus or newborn depends on multiple factors that are not yet clearly defined. The best estimates of the risk for congenital or intrapartum transmission from an infected woman range from 30% to 50%, although reports of transmission have ranged from 0% to 65%.[7-11] The relevance of the timing of maternal infection, presence or absence of symptoms of AIDS in the mother, or other variables that influence transmission and infection in the fetus is unknown. Cesarean section has not been proven to be protective. Additional studies are necessary to define more precisely the risk and variables associated with perinatal transmission of HIV.

A few case reports suggest that women who were infected with HIV immediately postpartum (through blood transfusion) transmitted HIV to their infants through breast-feeding.[12,13] Others have found that infants breast-fed as many as 7 months after birth did not become infected with HIV if they were born to women infected prepartum with HIV, suggesting that the relative risk of breast-feeding compared with intrauterine transmission is low.[8] Other types of postpartum transmission from a mother to her newborn (eg, physical affection such as touching and kissing) have not been documented.

DIAGNOSIS OF HIV INFECTION IN INFANTS

Because there is transplacental passage of maternal antibody to HIV in all infants born to seropositive mothers, the diagnosis of HIV infection in newborns is extremely difficult with currently available laboratory methods. Both the enzyme immunoassay (or enzyme-linked immunosorbent assay) and a confirmatory Western blot test are expected to be positive in the serum of both infected and uninfected infants born to a seropositive mother. Passive acquired HIV antibody decreases to undetectable levels in 50% of infants by 10 months, 75% of infants by 12 months, and most infants by 15 months. Unfortunately, some HIV-infected infants fail to elaborate HIV antibody and will, therefore, be HIV antibody negative but can be identified as HIV infected by viral culture and/or antigen detection. Thus, HIV seronegativity does not completely exclude congenital HIV infection.[8,14]

HIV infection is probable in an infant who, on serial specimens assayed by the same technique, has persistent or increasing titers of antibody to HIV or who demonstrates the appearance of new HIV-specific antibody bands on diagnostic tests such as Western blot or radioimmunoprecipitation assay. Additional tests currently under study include assays for HIV-specific IgM, HIV antigen, and viral nucleic acids and viral culture.[15,16] Positive viral culture of infant's blood or tissue is the definitive means of diagnosis but sensitivity is not established in infants. The sensitivity and specificity of the detection of HIV antigen and viral nucleic acids in infants is unknown.

CLINICAL FEATURES OF AIDS IN INFANTS

The incubation period of HIV infection in children may vary depending on the route of transmission. The majority of infants with perinatally acquired disease will appear normal at birth but within the first 24 months of life will have clinical illness. A small number of infected infants have remained asymptomatic for as many as 8 years.

Clinical features associated with HIV infection in infants include failure to thrive, generalized lymphadenopathy, hepatosplenomegaly, parotitis, persistent oral candidiasis, and chronic or recurrent diarrhea. Developmental disabilities and neurologic dysfunction are frequently seen. Bacterial infections with common organisms (*Streptococcus pneumonia* and *Haemophilus influenzae* type b) causing pneumonia, sepsis, meningitis, bone and joint infection, and otitis media are common and frequently recurrent. Lymphoid interstitial pneumonia has been reported in about 40% of infants and children with AIDS. Cardiomyopathy, hepatitis, and renal disease have also been described.

Craniofacial dysmorphic features have been reported in a small number of infants with HIV infection.[17-19] It is uncertain whether this is specifically due to HIV or whether other factors are involved.

Hyper-γ-globulinemia, particularly IgG, is usually present, although a few infected children may have hypo-γ-globulinemia.

Reported overall mortality in children with AIDS is 65% with the majority of deaths occurring during the first 24 months of life.

RISKS TO PERINATAL HEALTH CARE WORKERS (Appendix)

In health care workers, there are no known instances of HIV infection acquired through exposure to infants at delivery. The quantitative risk of acquisition of HIV infection by nonparenteral exposure has not been established, but it is clearly of a low magnitude. Nevertheless, medical history and examination do not reliably identify all mothers infected with HIV, and during delivery and initial care of the infant, health care workers are exposed to large amounts of maternal blood. In view of the utility of gloves in the prevention of other blood-borne diseases, and the low added costs involved, it is prudent for health care workers to use gloves for handling the placenta or the baby before he or she has been washed.[20,21]

RECOMMENDATIONS

1. Because the placenta and infant may be heavily contaminated with maternal blood, gloves should be used for handling the placenta or infant until the blood has been removed from the infant's skin. Hands should be washed immediately after gloves are removed and/or when skin surfaces are contaminated with blood.

2. Personnel assisting in the resuscitation of the newborn should use mechanical (adapted wall) suction equipment. Traps should be used in the line if mouth suction of the airway is performed in an emergency if mechanical suction is not available.

3. Infants of known seropositive mothers may be cared for in the normal nursery and do *not* require isolation in a private room or cubicle. Gloves should be worn for contact with blood or blood-containing fluids and for procedures that involve exposure to blood. Gloves are not required for prevention of HIV transmission while changing diapers in usual circumstances. Of course, hand washing after changing diapers is always required to reduce the transmission of other pathogens.[22]

4. Currently, a definitive determination that an infant < 15 months of age is infected with HIV should be based on either (a) a diagnosis of AIDS based on Centers for Disease Control criteria or (b) a combination of antibody to HIV and a compatible immunologic profile and clinical course or (c) laboratory evidence of HIV in blood or tissues (culture or antigen detection).

5. In the United States and other countries where safe nutrition other than breast-feeding is available, HIV-infected mothers should be advised against breast-feeding their infants to avoid that possible route of HIV infection.

6. Presently, in most areas, prevalence of HIV infection in pregnant women does not warrant the cost of universal screening. However, serologic testing should be offered to pregnant women at increased risk for HIV infection. This may include routine screening of mothers (or newborns) in high seroprevalent areas. Counseling, guidance, and information should be offered to the woman who is seropositive or at high risk regarding the implications of a current or future pregnancy to both herself and the baby.

7. To prevent or better treat HIV infections there is a need to provide:

(a) serologic surveys of anonymous specimens from infants to help define geographic prevalence of maternal HIV infection in areas where prevalence is unknown; (b) development and evaluation of new laboratory tests for the early identification of HIV infection in the newborn and young infant; (c) educational initiatives regarding AIDS, its transmission, and methods to prevent infection, including information concerning sexual and contraceptive behaviors; (d) counseling and easy access to drug treatment programs for individuals who are at increased risk for HIV infection secondary to such IV drug abuse; and (e) development and timely execution of carefully designed experimental protocols for the treatment of infants with HIV infection and its complications.

Task Force on Pediatric AIDS,
1987–1988
Stanley A. Plotkin, MD, Chairman
Hugh E. Evans, MD
Norman C. Fost, MD, MPH
Gerald Merenstein, MD
S. Kenneth Schonberg, MD
Gwendolyn B. Scott, MD
Martin W. Sklaire, MD
Esther H. Wender, MD

Consultant
James R. Allen, MD, MPH

APPENDIX

The risk to health care workers of acquiring HIV infection in the perinatal setting will vary widely. The following analysis should help hospitals assess the risk, as well as the costs and benefits of implementing universal precautions on a routine basis.

Example 1: Low Prevalence Area

If the incidence of HIV infection in the maternal population is 1:1,000, then 1,000 deliveries would be required for a health care worker to be exposed to the HIV virus. Mere contact with such patients does not result in transmission; there must also be either a needlestick, blood coming in contact with mucous membranes, or abraded or cut skin. Not all needlesticks or blood on skin results in transmission: the risk of transmission to persons with needlesticks from infected patients is approximately 1:250.[23] Conclusive data for the risk of cutaneous exposure to perinatal fluids are not available. The risk of transmission for three estimates is as follows.

If transmission rate from blood fluids is:	No. of deliveries needed for transmission to occur	No. of years for transmission if 5,000 deliveries per year
1:100	100,000	20
1:250	250,000	50
1:1,000	1,000,000	200

Example 2: High Prevalence Area

If the incidence of HIV in the maternal population were 1:50, the following analysis would apply.

If transmission rate from blood fluids is:	No. of deliveries needed for transmission to occur	No. of years for transmission if 5,000 deliveries per year
1:100	5,000	1
1:250	12,500	2.5
1:1,000	50,00	10

The *benefits* of routine universal precautions, assuming they are 100% effective, will be prevention of one case of HIV infection in a health care worker in the interval listed in the last column, as well as possible reductoin of anxiety among the workers. There will be other benefits in preventing transmission of diseases that are more common than HIV infection, such as hepatitis B. The *costs* will include the direct costs of supplies and the added costs of disposal of such materials, which can be substantial.

REFERENCES

1. AIDS Weekly Surveillance Report—United States, AIDS Program, Centers for Disease Control, Feb 29, 1987

2. Guinan M E, Hardy A: Epidemiology of AIDS in women in the United States, 1981 through 1986. *JAMA* 1987; 257:2039

3. Hopkins D R: AIDS in minority populations in the United States, *Public Health Rep* 1987; 102:677

4. Centers for Disease Control: HIV infection in the United States. *MMWR* 1987; 36:801

5. Landesman S, Minkoff H, Holman S, et al: Serosurvey of HIV infection in partuients: Implications for human immunodeficiency virus testing programs of pregnant women. *JAMA* 1987; 258:2701

6. Berardi V, Hoff R, Wieblan B, et al: Seroprevalence of HIV among childbearing women: Estimation by testing samples of blood from newborns. *N Engl J Med* 1988; 318:525

7. Semprini A, Vucetich A, Pardi G, et al: HIV infection and AIDS and newborn babies of mothers positive for HIV antibody. *Br Med J* 1987; 294:610

8. Mok J, et al: Infants born to mothers seropositive for HIV. *Lancet* 1987; 1:1164

9. Minkoff H L: Care of the pregnant woman infected with HIV. *JAMA* 1987; 258:2714

10. Scott G B, Mastrucci M, Hutto S, et al: Pediatric HIV infection: Factors influencing case identification and prognosis, abstracted. *Pediatr Res* 1987; 21:334A

11. Stewart G, Tyler J, Cunningham A, et al: Transmission of human T-cell lymphotropic virus type III (HTLV-III) by artificial insemination by donor. *Lancet* 1985; 2:891

12. Ziegler J B, Cooper D A, Pekovish D, et al: Postnatal transmission of AIDS associated retrovirus from mother to infant. *Lancet* 1985; 1:1980

13. Lepage P, et al: Postnatal transmission of HIV from mother to child. *Lancet* 1987; 2:400

14. Borkowsky W, et al: HIV infections in infants negative for anti-HIV by ELISA. *Lancet* 1987; 1:1168

15. Centers for Disease Control: Classification system for HIV infection in children under 13 years of age. *MMWR* 1987; 36:225

16. Centers for Disease Control: Update: Serologic testing for antibody to HIV. *MMWR* 1988; 36:833

17. Marion R, Hutcheon G, Wiznia A, et al: Fetal AIDS syndrome score. *Am J Dis Child* 1987; 141:429

18. Bamji M, Iosub S, Stone R K, et al: More on human immunodeficiency virus embryopathy. *Pediatrics* 1987; 80:512–516

19. Rogers M F, Thomas P A, Starcher E T, et al: Acquired immunodeficiency syndrome in children: Report of the Centers for Disease Control National Surveillance, 1982 to 1985. *Pediatrics* 1987; 79:1008–1014

20. Centers for Disease Control: Recommendations for assisting in the prevention of perinatal transmission of human T-lymphocyte type III lymphadenopathy associated virus and acquired immunodeficiency syndrome. *MMWR* 1985; 34:721

21. Centers for Disease Control: Recommendations for prevention of HIV transmission in healthcare settings. *MMWR* 1987;36(suppl 2):3S

22. American Academy of Pediatrics, AIDS Task Force: Pediatric guidelines infection control of HIV (AIDS Virus) in hospitals, medical offices, schools, and other settings. *Pediatrics* 1988; 82:801–807

23. Henderson D K, Saah A J, Szk B J, et al: Risk of nosocomial infection with human T-cell lymphotrophic virus type III/lymphadenopathy associated virus in a large cohort of intensively exposed health care workers. *Ann Intern Med* 1986; 104:644

Task Force on Pediatric AIDS

Infants and Children With Acquired Immunodeficiency Syndrome: Placement in Adoption and Foster Care*

The transmission of human immunodeficiency virus (HIV) from infected mothers to their infants has been well established. The majority of infants so infected are born to women who have acquired HIV through IV drug use or through sexual contact with IV drug-using partners. Some of these mothers are unable to care for their infants. In addition, many infected mothers become seriously ill or die, leaving children who must be cared for by others. Thus, many infants and children who are infected or are at high risk for infection may require placement in an adoptive or foster care setting. The HIV-infected infant or child places a serious burden on any family. This burden, when anticipated, may make adoption and foster care placement exceedingly difficult. However, such family-based care is clearly in the best interest of the child.

CARE FOR THE CHILD WITH ACQUIRED IMMUNODEFICIENCY SYNDROME (AIDS)

If an infant or child is known to be infected with HIV or is already ill with AIDS, what are some of the implications for the care givers, including adopting or foster care families?

First, the family must bear the physical and emotional burden of caring for a child who will require ongoing medical treatment, will suffer from intermittent bouts of increasingly severe illness, and, in most cases, will ultimately die. A majority of these children can be expected to have

---

*The recommendations in this statement do not indicate an exclusive course of treatment or procedure to be followed. Variations, taking into account individual circumstances, may be appropriate.
PEDIATRICS (ISSN 0031 4005). Copyright © 1989 by the American Academy of Pediatrics.

developmental delay and many may also show behavioral regression, resulting in increased care-giving demands.

A second issue is the fear of spread of the viral infection to family members, friends, and classmates. The evidence to date indicates that this type of spread of HIV infection is virtually nonexistent. In a number of studies involving more than 17,000 family members in contact with AIDS patients, only one documented case of casual, nonsexual household transmission has occurred. In this case, a 4-year-old boy, who lived in the same household as his younger brother who had become infected by transfusion at age 18 months, became infected. A mechanism of transmission has not been established in this case.[1] The types of family contact that have not resulted in the spread of HIV infection include sharing of eating utensils, bathroom facilities, and toothbrushes; and hugging, kissing, and other types of nonsexual physical affection. However, it is theoretically possible that blood from an infected child coming in contact with broken skin surface or mucous membranes of a noninfected person could result in transmission of HIV infection. There is no evidence that transmission has occurred through contact with body fluids other than blood, eg, saliva, urine, or feces. Most experts consider transmission by contact with these fluids to be highly unlikely[1]; therefore, both infected and noninfected children may safely be placed in the same foster care or adoptive home.

A third issue, with powerful emotional implications, is the socal stigma associated with AIDS. The public's fear of contagion plus the association of AIDS with homosexuality, promiscuity, and drug abuse have created the social stigma that extends to the child with AIDS. The child who is known to harbor the virus or who is ill with the disease may expect to experience ridicule, avoidance by others in the community, and restriction from many normal childhood activities. Many parents, therefore, choose to keep their child's condition a secret, even from their child, who, they fear, may divulge the information.

RECOMMENDATIONS

Infected Infant or Child

All infants or children who are identified as HIV infected or in whom AIDS has been diagnosed should receive special support services regardless of who the legal guardian is. If such children are being considered for adoption or foster cared placement, the adoptive or foster care family should be accurately informed of the child's health status prior to placement and these additional support services should be provided.

Education and Counseling. Families should be fully informed of the nature of medical treatments that will be required and the child's probable medical course. They should receive up-to-date information regarding immunizations, management of potential exposure to childhood infections, and the pros and cons of current therapies.

The family should also receive extensive education regarding the risks of transmission of the virus from the child to others. Family members should be reassured that HIV infection is not spread through casual contact and thus there is virtually no risk of transmission. The families should be given specific guidelines for the procedures to be used when caring for the child. Lacerations or other bleeding lesions should be managed in a manner that prevents contact of the care giver's skin or mucous membranes with blood. In most circumstances, the proper use of bandages (or other cloth materials) will be sufficient. Wearing latex gloves is also a useful means for preventing contact. The care giver's hands should be washed promptly after caring for bloody lesions, and spilled blood should be cleaned with a bleach solution (household bleach at a dilution of 1:10). As in the care of any child, hand washing should promptly follow the handling of body fluids such as urine, stool, vomitus, and oral and nasal secretions. In child care settings, general disinfection of body fluids other than blood should be accomplished with a weak solution of bleach (60 mL [¼ cup, 2 oz] of bleach to 3.8 L [1 gal] of water).[2] This mixture constitutes a 1:64 dilution of 5.25% sodium hypochlorite. These precautions are aimed at preventing the spread of viral and bacterial infections and are not specifically required to prevent the transmission of AIDS. Although biting has not been shown to result in HIV transmission, if the infected child bites, appropriate behavior management aimed at ending this behavior, including the provision of closer supervision, should be taught to the parents. Again, this approach is appropriate for all families, not just those who have a child infected with HIV.

Along with these precautions, normal family interaction, especially physical affection, should be encouraged.

Financial Support. The burden of caring for a sick child should not be compounded by the threat of financial hardship. The family should be provided with continued support covering 100% of the medical care expenses of their sick child. At the least, this support entails Medicaid coverage. In addition, the recently enacted Medicare Catastrophic

Coverage Act of 1988 (Public Law 100-360) contains provisions to supplement this support for young children with HIV infection, with coverage for services frequently not included within Medicaid. Moreover, financial support should not be limited to medical costs. Children with HIV infection and their families have interrelated psychosocial, medical, and educational needs. Therefore, additional financial aid in the form of supplemental maintenance payments, as provided through Title IV-E programs (Foster Care and Adoptive Assistance Act) should be used to support the adoptive or foster care placement of these children. Foster care and adoption agencies should also seek additional funding for special services, such as the following, through grants from federal, state, and local sources.

Support for Respite Care. Children with HIV infection can be expected to tax the energies and emotional stamina of their care givers. Yet, periodic relief from this burden in the form of evening or weekend babysitting or day care may be difficult to obtain because of the social stigma associated with the illness. Adoptive or foster care agencies, in collaboration with other community resources, should develop respite care services such as day-care programs or baby-sitting services for these families. In some communities with a high prevalence of pediatric AIDS, special day-care programs have been developed specifically to serve children with this diagnosis. Such programs can provide valuable psychologic support as well as respite care. However, when such special programs are not available, existing day-care services should be open to those HIV-infected or HIV-seropositive children who are well enough to participate in day-care activities and who do not need to be protected from the threat of infection from other children. Families are not obligated to inform day-care staff of the child's HIV status inasmuch as the evidence, to date, indicates that casual transmission of HIV infection is virtually nonexistent.[1]

Psychologic Counseling. Care-giving families should have access to knowledgeable psychologic counseling services without financial obligaton. When several families with children who have HIV infection live in close proximity, family group support services should be developed.

Social and Legal Counseling. Care-giving families of HIV-infected children can be expected to encounter difficulties with community services or institutions that may require expert legal counsel or social service support. Examples of such situations include local regulations regarding school attendance and policies of landlords toward rental housing for families with an AIDS patient. Social service and legal counsel with expertise in issues associated with AIDS should be available to these families without financial obligation.

Infant or Child at Risk, But Not Yet Determined to Have HIV Infection

Foster care or adoption may be anticipated in situations in which the infant or child is currently healthy but may be at risk for later HIV infection due to perinatal transmission.[3] Because some parents may be reluctant or refuse to accept an infant or child in whom there is substantial risk of AIDS developing, foster care placement or adoption may be difficult or impossible unless this risk is partially alleviated by HIV antibody testing. When HIV antibody test results are negative, the infant or child has a low risk for perinatally transmitted HIV infection (although an occasional infant will test antibody negative even though they are infected with the virus). However, positive results on an HIV antibody test are difficult to interpret for infants 15 to 18 months of age because HIV antibody moves freely across the placenta, and its presence in the infant may reflect only the mother's infection. Current estimates of the proportion of infants with positive results on an HIV antibody test who will later manifest HIV infection range from 30% to 50%.[3] The need to clarify risk to improve the possibility of an adoptive or foster care placement, should be tempered by: (1) understanding the complexity and limitations of HIV antibody testing in identifying the HIV status of the very young child and (2) awareness of the ethical issues posed by the fact that a positive result on an HIV antibody test of the infant identifies the biologic mother as having HIV infection.

The widespread testing of all infants and children awaiting adoption or foster placement is not warranted, given the variability of prevalence of AIDS infection in childbearing women.[3] However, in populations that have high seropositive prevalence among women of childbearing age, foster and adoptive parents should have access to information about antibody status. Access to this information may improve the ability of agencies to place into foster or adoptive care such high-risk infants and children who prove to be uninfected.

The Task Force believes that the determinations of what constitutes "high prevalence" cannot be made as a hard and fast rule that governs all jurisdictions. One example of a local factor that might influence this determination is the mobility of the population that will affect the ability of any health care unit to predict the status of patients it serves. Anonymous seroprevalence surveys of the relevant population (women of childbearing age) is the best way to establish the current prevalence of HIV seropositivity in any jurisdiction. It will then be necessary for those health care professionals in that locale with the greatest expertise in HIV infection and epidemiology, to establish necessary practice based on known prevalence and other local factors.[3]

In response to the legitimate need for preplacement HIV testing of the infant or child in areas of high prevalence of HIV infection in childbearing women, procedures should be established by foster care and adoption agencies in collaboration with health care facilities, to accomplish the following.

1. Develop the expertise to provide prospective foster care or adoptive families with comprehensive and up-to-date information regarding all aspects of pediatric HIV infection.

2. Establish a process that would accomplish, with the appropriate consent of the infant's legal guardian, the preplacement HIV testing of infants or children, initiated either: (a) at the request of the prospective adopting or foster care parents through the physician who is responsible for that child's care, or (b) through the request of the infant's physician in response to his or her judgment that the mother is at high risk for HIV infection and that the infant's health supervision and/or placement may be affected by knowing the infant's antibody status.

3. Provide comprehensive and up-to-date interpretation of the meaning of test results, taking into account the age and health status of the child and the reliability of the test.

4. Establish a record-keeping system to contain information regarding the child's test results with access to such information strictly limited to those who need to know, but specifically including the informed adoptive or foster care family and the physician responsible for the infant's medical care.

5. Establish a procedure whereby all infants who have positive results on HIV antibody tests are retested on a regular basis to distinguish between passively transmitted antibody and true HIV infection in the infant.

Task Force on Pediatric AIDS
Stanley A. Plotkin, MD, Chairman
Louis Z. Cooper, MD
Hugh E. Evans, MD
Norman C. Fost, MD, MPH
Gerald Merenstein, MD
S. Kenneth Schonberg, MD
Gwendolyn B. Scott, MD
Martin N. Sklaire, MD

Esther H. Wender, MD
James R. Allen, MD (Consultant)

REFERENCES

1. American Academy of Pediatrics, Task Force on Pediatrics AIDS: Pediatric guidelines for infection control of human immunodeficiency virus (acquired immunodeficiency virus) in hospitals, medical offices, schools, and other settings. *Pediatrics* 1988; 82:801–807

2. American Academy of Pediatrics, Committee on Early Childhood, Adoption, and Dependent Care: *Health in Day Care: A Manual for Health Professionals*. Elk Grove Village, IL, American Academy of Pediatrics, 1987, p 61

3. American Academy of Pediatrics, Task Force on Pediatric AIDS: Perinatal human immunodeficiency virus infection. *Pediatrics* 1988; 82:941–944

Courage to Care

Contributors

Gary R. Anderson, M.S.W. Ph.D.
Associate Professor
Hunter College School of Social Work
City University of New York
New York, New York

Virginia Anderson, M.D.
Clinics Director
New York City Department of Health
Bureau of Child Health
Brooklyn, New York

J. Burt Annin, J.D.
Director, CWLA AIDS Training Institute
Child Welfare League of America
Washington, DC

Patricia Beckler, M.S.W.
Assistant Professor
New Mexico State University
Los Cruces, New Mexico

Mary G. Boland, R.N., M.S.N.
Director, Children's Hospital AIDS Program
Children's Hospital of New Jersey
Newark, New Jersey

Toni Cabat, M.S.W.
Project Coordinator, Women and Infants Project
Albert Einstein College of Medicine
Bronx, New York

Sema Coppersmith, M.S.W.
Director, Project SMILE

413

Children's Home Society of Florida
Miami, Florida

Karl W. Dennis
Executive Director
Kaleidoscope
Chicago, Illinois

Kenneth J. Doka, Ph.D.
Professor of Gerontology
The College of New Rochelle
New Rochelle, New York

Jean Emery, M.S.W.
Director, CWLA AIDS Program
Child Welfare League of America
Washington, DC

Phyllis Gurdin, M.S.W.
Director, Specialized Foster Care Program
Leake and Watts Children's Home
Yonkers, New York

Olga C. Hernandez, B.S.N., M.P.H.
Director of Health Services
Covenant House
New York, New York

Robin James, M.S.W.
Coordinator of Case Management
Gay Men's Health Crisis
New York, New York

Elisabeth Kubler-Ross, M.D.
The Elisabeth Kubler-Ross Center
Head Waters, Virginia

Carolyn Lelyveld, M.S.
Director, Bronx Municipal Hospital Day Care Center
Bronx, New York

A. Damien Martin, Ed.D.
Executive Director
The Hetrick Martin Institute
New York, New York

Kathleen McGowan, M.S.W.
Director of Staff Development
Catholic Charities of Chicago
Chicago, Illinois

James Oleske, M.D., M.P.H.
Professor of Pediatrics
Division of Allergy, Immunology,
* and Infectious Diseases*
The University of Medicine and
* Dentistry of New Jersey*
Newark, New Jersey

Joe Pietrangelo, M.S.W.
Director, Children with AIDS Training Project
Center for Development of Human Services
Buffalo State College
New York, New York

Arye Rubinstein, M.D.
Professor of Pediatrics, Microbiology,
* and Immunology*
Albert Einstein College of Medicine
Bronx, New York

Anita Septimus, M.S.W.
AIDS Social Worker, Department of Social Services
Albert Einstein College of Medicine
Bronx, New York

Sandra M. Stehno, Ph.D.
Assistant to the President
Kaleidoscope
Chicago, Illinois

Elaine Durkot Sterzin, L.C.S.W.
Clinical Supervisor, Project WIN
Brighton, Massachusetts

Steven E. Torkelsen, D.S.W.
Senior Vice President, External Relations
Covenant House
New York, New York

Dionne Warwick
Ambassador of Health
The Warwick Foundation
Washington, DC

Marianne West, M.S.W.
Foster Care Administrator
Kaleidoscope
Chicago, Illinois

Geneva Woodruff, Ph.D.
Project Director, Project WIN
Brighton, Massachusetts

Terry P. Zealand, Ed.D.
Executive Director
AIDS Resource Foundation for Children
Newark, New Jersey